T0229286

Essentials of Sleep Medicine for the Primary Care Provider

Editor

TEOFILO LEE-CHIONG, Jr

SLEEP MEDICINE CLINICS

www.sleep.theclinics.com

Consulting Editor
TEOFILO LEE-CHIONG, Jr

June 2020 • Volume 15 • Number 2

ELSEVIER

1600 John F. Kennedy Boulevard • Suite 1800 • Philadelphia, Pennsylvania, 19103-2899

http://www.theclinics.com

SLEEP MEDICINE CLINICS Volume 15, Number 2
June 2020, ISSN 1556-407X, ISBN-13: 978-0-323-77706-3

Editor: Colleen Dietzler
Developmental Editor: Donald Mumford

Sleep Medicine Clinics (ISSN 1556-407X) is published quarterly by Elsevier Inc., 360 Park Avenue South, New York, NY 10010-1710. Months of issue are March, June, September and December. Business and Editorial Offices: 1600 John F. Kennedy Blvd., Ste. 1800, Philadelphia, PA 19103-2899. Customer Service Office: 3251 Riverport Lane, Maryland Heights, MO 63043. Periodicals postage paid at New York, NY and additional mailing offices. Subscription prices are $218.00 per year (US individuals), $100.00 (US and Canadian students), $518.00 (US institutions), $264.00 (Canadian individuals), $252.00 (international individuals) $135.00 (International students), $587.00 (Canadian and International institutions). Foreign air speed delivery is included in all *Clinics* subscription prices. All prices are subject to change without notice. **POSTMASTER:** Send change of address to *Sleep Medicine Clinics*, Elsevier Health Sciences Division, Subscription Customer Service, 3251 Riverport Lane, Maryland Heights, MO 63043. Customer Service: **Tel: 1-800-654-2452 (U.S. and Canada); 314-447-8871 (outside U.S. and Canada). Fax: 314-447-8029. E-mail: journalscustomerservice-usa@elsevier.com (for print support); journalsonline-support-usa@elsevier.com (for online support).**

Reprints. For copies of 100 or more of articles in this publication, please contact the Commercial Reprints Department, Elsevier Inc., 360 Park Avenue South, New York, NY 10010-1710. Tel.: 212-633-3874; Fax: 212-633-3820; E-mail: reprints@elsevier.com.

Sleep Medicine Clinics is covered in *MEDLINE/PubMed (Index Medicus).*

SLEEP MEDICINE CLINICS

SERIES OF RELATED INTEREST

Clinics in Chest Medicine
Available at: https://www.chestmed.theclinics.com/

THE CLINICS ARE AVAILABLE ONLINE!
Access your subscription at:
www.theclinics.com

Contributors

CONSULTING EDITOR

TEOFILO LEE-CHIONG, Jr, MD
Professor of Medicine, National Jewish Health;
Professor of Medicine, University of Colorado,
Denver, Colorado, USA; Chief Medical Liaison,
Philips Respironics, Pennsylvania, USA

EDITOR

TEOFILO LEE-CHIONG, Jr, MD
Professor of Medicine, National Jewish Health;
Professor of Medicine, University of Colorado,
Denver, Colorado, USA; Chief Medical Liaison,
Philips Respironics, Pennsylvania, USA

AUTHORS

IMRAN M. AHMED, MD
Sleep-Wake Disorders Center, Department of
Neurology, Montefiore Medical Center, Albert
Einstein College of Medicine, Bronx, New York,
USA

GALIA V. ANGUELOVA, MD, MSc
Center for Sleep and Wake Disorders,
Haaglanden Medical Center, The Hague, The
Netherlands

RICHARD BARNETT BERRY, MD
Professor of Medicine, Medical Director of the
UF Health Sleep Disorders Center, University
of Florida Sleep Medicine Fellowship Director,
Department of Sleep Medicine, UF Health
Sleep Center, University of Florida, Gainesville,
Florida, USA

HELEN J. BURGESS, PhD
Biological Rhythms Research Laboratory,
Department of Behavioral Sciences, Rush
University Medical Center, Chicago, Illinois,
USA

JACOB F. COLLEN, MD
Assistant Professor of Medicine, Program
Director, Sleep Medicine Fellowship,
Department of Pulmonary, Critical Care, and
Sleep Medicine, Walter Reed National Military
Medical Center, Bethesda, Maryland,
USA

MARIE NGUYEN DIBRA, MD
Clinical Assistant Professor, Division of
Pulmonary, Critical Care, and Sleep Medicine,
Department of Sleep Medicine, UF Health
Sleep Center, University of Florida, Gainesville,
Florida, USA

SYLVIE DUJARDIN, MD
Sleep Medicine Center Kempenhaeghe,
Heeze, The Netherlands

MATTHEW R. EBBEN, PhD
Associate Professor, Department of
Neurology, Center for Sleep Medicine, Weill
Cornell Medical College of Cornell University,
New York, New York, USA

JACK D. EDINGER, PhD
Professor, Department of Medicine, National
Jewish Health, Denver, Colorado, USA

JONATHAN S. EMENS, MD
Departments of Psychiatry and Medicine,
Oregon Health & Science University, VA

Portland Health Care System, Portland, Oregon, USA

NEIL FREEDMAN, MD
Division Head, Pulmonary, Critical Care, Allergy and Immunology, Department of Medicine, NorthShore University HealthSystem, Evanston, Illinois, USA

MICHAEL A. GRANDNER, PhD, MTR, CBSM
Director, Sleep and Health Research Program, Department of Psychiatry; Assistant Professor, Departments of Medicine and Psychology, College of Medicine; Director, Behavioral Sleep Medicine Clinic, Banner-University Medical Center, Member, Sarver Heart Center, University of Arizona, Tucson, Arizona

JONATHAN P. HINTZE, MD
Clinical Assistant Professor, Division of Pediatric Sleep Medicine, University of South Carolina School of Medicine Greenville, Greenville Health System, Greenville, South Carolina, USA

ANNEMARIE IDA LUIK, PhD
Assistant Professor, Department of Epidemiology, Erasmus MC University Medical Center, Rotterdam, the Netherlands

MEIR H. KRYGER, MD, FRCP(C)
Professor, Pulmonary, Critical Care, and Sleep Medicine, Department of Internal Medicine, Yale School of Medicine, New Haven, Connecticut; VA Connecticut Healthcare System, West Haven, Connecticut

ARTHUR G.Y. KURVERS, MD
Center for Sleep and Wake Disorders, Haaglanden Medical Center, The Hague, The Netherlands

JAAP LANCEE, PhD
Assistant Professor, Department of Clinical Psychology, University of Amsterdam, PsyQ Amsterdam, Amsterdam, the Netherlands

TAN KAH LEONG ALVIN, MBChB, MRCS
Adjunct Assistant Professor, Principal Staff Registrar, Department of Otorhinolaryngology, Head and Neck Surgery, Changi General Hospital, Singapore, Singapore

CHRISTOPHER J. LETTIERI, MD
Professor of Medicine, Department of Pulmonary, Critical Care, and Sleep Medicine, Walter Reed National Military Medical Center, Bethesda, Maryland, USA

RAFFAELE MANNI, MD
Unit of Sleep Medicine and Epilepsy, C. Mondino National Neurological Institute, Pavia, Italy

BRIENNE MINER, MD, MHS
Geriatric and Sleep Medicine Fellow, Department of Internal Medicine, Yale School of Medicine, New Haven, Connecticut

RENEE MONDERER, MD
Sleep-Wake Disorders Center, Department of Neurology, Montefiore Medical Center, Albert Einstein College of Medicine, Bronx, New York, USA

BRIAN JAMES MURRAY, MD, FRCPC, D,ABSM
Associate Professor, Neurology and Sleep Medicine, Sunnybrook Health Sciences Centre, University of Toronto, Toronto, Ontario, Canada

JING HAO NG, BDS (Singapore), MDS Orthodontics (Singapore), MOrth RCS (Edinburgh, UK)
Associate Consultant, Department of Orthodontics, National Dental Centre, Singapore, Singapore

SEIJI NISHINO, MD, PhD
Director, Sleep and Circadian Neurobiology Laboratory, Professor, Department of Psychiatry and Behavioral Sciences, Stanford University School of Medicine, Stanford University, Palo Alto, California, USA

LINO NOBILI, MD, PhD
Department of Neuroscience, Centre of Sleep Medicine, Centre for Epilepsy Surgery, Niguarda Hospital, Milan, Italy; Department of Neuroscience (DINOGMI), University of Genoa, Genoa, Italy

DIRK PEVERNAGIE, MD, PhD
Sleep Medicine Center Kempenhaeghe, Heeze, The Netherlands; Departments of Internal Medicine and Paediatrics, Faculty of

Medicine and Health Sciences, Ghent University, Ghent, Belgium

ANGELIQUE PIJPERS, MD, PhD
Sleep Medicine Center Kempenhaeghe, Heeze, The Netherlands

HSU PON POH, MBBS, MD
Head, Adjunct Professor, Department of Otorhinolaryngology, Head and Neck Surgery, Changi General Hospital, Singapore, Singapore

PAOLA PROSERPIO, MD
Department of Neuroscience, Centre of Sleep Medicine, Centre for Epilepsy Surgery, Niguarda Hospital, Milan, Italy

ROSELYNE M. RIJSMAN, MD, PhD
Center for Sleep and Wake Disorders, Haaglanden Medical Center, The Hague, The Netherlands

THOMAS G. SCHELL, DMD, DABDSM
Owner, Dr. Thomas G Schell and Dr. Patrick C Noble PLLC, Lebanon, New Hampshire, USA; Adjunctive Administrative Assistant Professor, Department of Surgery, Dartmouth Geisel School of Medicine, Hanover, New Hampshire, USA

WONG HANG SIANG, MBBS, MRCP
Consultant, Department of Respiratory and Critical Care Medicine, Changi General Hospital, Singapore, Singapore

ANNEMIEKE VAN STRATEN, PhD
Professor, Department of Clinical Psychology, EMGO Institute for Health and Care Research, VU University, Amsterdam, the Netherlands

SHINICHI TAKENOSHITA, MD, MPH
Visiting Assistant Professor, Sleep and Circadian Neurobiology Laboratory, Department of Psychiatry and Behavioral Sciences, Stanford University School of Medicine, Stanford University, Palo Alto, California, USA

MICHELE TERZAGHI, MD
Unit of Sleep Medicine and Epilepsy, C. Mondino National Neurological Institute, Pavia, Italy

MICHAEL THORPY, MD
Sleep-Wake Disorders Center, Department of Neurology, Montefiore Medical Center, Albert Einstein College of Medicine, Bronx, New York, USA

MONIQUE H.M. VLAK, MD, PhD
Center for Sleep and Wake Disorders, Haaglanden Medical Center, The Hague, The Netherlands

MARY H. WAGNER, MD
Associate Professor of Pediatric Pulmonology, University of Florida Sleep Medicine Fellowship Co-Director, Department of Sleep Medicine, Director of the Pediatric Sleep Laboratory, UF Health Sleep Disorders Center, UF Health Sleep Center, Gainesville, Florida, USA

EMERSON M. WICKWIRE, PhD
Assistant Professor and Director, Insomnia Program, Department of Psychiatry, Sleep Disorders Center, Division of Pulmonary and Critical Care Medicine, Department of Medicine, University of Maryland School of Medicine, Baltimore, Maryland, USA

SCOTT G. WILLIAMS, MD
Associate Professor of Medicine, Chief of Sleep Medicine, Department of Pulmonary, Critical Care, and Sleep Medicine, Walter Reed National Military Medical Center, Bethesda, Maryland, USA

MOK YINGJUAN, MBBS, MRCP
Adjunct Assistant Professor, Consultant, Department of Respiratory and Critical Care Medicine, Changi General Hospital, Singapore, Singapore

MIMI YOW, BDS (Singapore), FDS RCS (Edinburgh), MSc (London) (Orthodontics), FAMS (Craniofacial Orthodontics)
Head, Cleft and Craniofacial Deformity Programme, Senior Consultant, Clinical Associate Professor, Department of Orthodontics, National Dental Centre, Singapore, Singapore

TANJA VAN DER ZWEERDE, MSc
PhD-candidate, Department of Clinical Psychology, EMGO Institute for Health and Care Research, VU University, Amsterdam, the Netherlands

Contents

history, a review of medications, as well as a social and family history. Physical examination should include a general medical examination with careful attention to the upper airway and the neurologic examination. Appropriate objective testing with a polysomnogram and a multiple sleep latency test if needed will help confirm the diagnosis and direct the appropriate treatment plan.

CPAP or APAP therapy because of pressure intolerance. Several additional factors should be considered when choosing the type of PAP device for a given patient, including associated symptoms and comorbid medical problems, cost, access to online data management and patient portals, and the portability for the device for patients who travel frequently.

or impossible to correct and can affect the patient in serious ways. As this field evolves, new information is discovered, and new products are introduced at a rather rapid pace, continuing education and prudent practice are critical to ethical care in the practice of dental sleep medicine.

Positional therapy appears to be an attractive strategy for many patients with positional obstructive sleep apnea (OSA). However, under the American Academy of Sleep Medicine OSA guidelines, positional therapy is considered as only an alternative therapy, because previous research has demonstrated poor treatment tolerance and adherence. Recent technological advances have renewed interest in positional therapy, with the invention of new sophisticated vibratory positional therapy devices. These devices have shown great promise with efficacy, markedly improved patient tolerance, and long-term adherence. We review the literature on positional therapy and explore the most current evidence on the new positional therapy devices.

This article provides an updated practical guide for the treatment of primary restless legs syndrome (RLS). Articles that appeared after the American Academy of Neurology guideline search were reviewed according to the same evidence rating schedule. We found limited evidence for nonpharmacologic treatment options. In moderate to severe primary RLS, pharmacologic options may be considered, including iron supplementation, an $\alpha2\delta$ ligand, a dopamine agonist, a combination of an $\alpha2\delta$ ligand and a dopamine agonist, or oxycodone/naloxone. This article includes treatment options in case of augmentation.

Patient education and behavioral management represent the first treatment approaches to the patient with parasomnia, especially in case of disorders of arousal (DOA). A pharmacologic treatment of DOA may be useful when episodes are frequent and persist despite resolution of predisposing factors, are associated with a high risk of injury, or cause significant impairment, such as excessive sleepiness. Approved drugs for DOA are still lacking. The most commonly used medications are benzodiazepines and antidepressants. The pharmacologic treatment of rapid eye movement sleep behavior disorder is symptomatic, and the most commonly used drugs are clonazepam and melatonin.

This article focuses on melatonin and other melatonin receptor agonists, and specifically their circadian phase shifting and sleep-enhancing properties. The circadian system and circadian rhythm sleep-wake disorders are briefly reviewed, followed by a summary of the circadian phase shifting, sleep-enhancing properties, and possible safety concerns associated with melatonin and other melatonin receptor agonists. The recommended use of melatonin, including dose and timing, in the latest American Academy of Sleep Medicine Clinical Practice Guidelines for the treatment of intrinsic circadian rhythm disorders is also reviewed. Lastly, the practical aspects of treatment and consideration of clinical treatment outcomes are discussed.

Sleep in the Aging Population

Brienne Miner and Meir H. Kryger

There are normal changes to sleep architecture throughout the lifespan. There is not, however, a decreased need for sleep and sleep disturbance is not an inherent part of the aging process. Sleep disturbance is common in older adults because aging is associated with an increasing prevalence of multimorbidity, polypharmacy, psychosocial factors affecting sleep, and certain primary sleep disorders. It is also associated with morbidity and mortality. Because many older adults have several factors from different domains affecting their sleep, these complaints are best approached as a multifactorial geriatric health condition, necessitating a multifaceted treatment approach.

Sleep, Health, and Society

Michael A. Grandner

Biological needs for sleep are met by engaging in behaviors that are largely influenced by the environment, social norms and demands, and societal influences and pressures. Insufficient sleep duration and sleep disorders such as insomnia and sleep apnea are highly prevalent in the US population. This article outlines some of these downstream factors, including cardiovascular and metabolic disease risk, neurocognitive dysfunction, and mortality, as well as societal factors such as age, sex, race/ethnicity, and socioeconomics. This review also discusses societal factors related to sleep, such as globalization, health disparities, public policy, public safety, and changing patterns of use of technology.

Preface
Why Sleep Medicine Is Essential

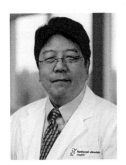

Teofilo Lee-Chiong, Jr, MD
Editor

While science continues to better understand the reasons why we sleep, such as physiologic drive and neurocognitive health, it is equally essential to recognize the mechanisms why we *don't* sleep. Three general reasons are responsible for this lack of sleep. We *can't* sleep due to sleep apnea, insomnia, or restless legs syndrome. We *won't* sleep as a result of social media and school or work schedules. Finally, we *shouldn't* sleep because of shift work or occupation as a commercial driver or pilot. Addressing these diverse factors requires a comprehensive approach that incorporates an understanding of anatomy and physiology, behavioral sciences and psychology, and public health and societal transformation.

We are increasingly more aware of how sleep affects our health. What is less certain is whether this knowledge leads to actions that optimize our sleep. Are we integrating better sleep habits into our general lifestyle? Are consumer-targeted wearables and mobile activity-monitoring technologies helping us achieve our desired sleep-work-life balance? Not infrequently, our efforts to adopt better sleep behaviors are thwarted by demands on our time by family, peers, school, or work. Having both personal and societal determinants, sleep optimization can only be attained if the community supports each individual's need for sleep, respects choices regarding sleep behaviors, and allocates enough time for adequate sleep for everyone. Corporations must develop strategies that foster sleep health, incorporating proper sleep behaviors among its employees and discouraging unnecessary after-work activities. Society at large also plays a major role in regulating work schedules of workers in more high-risk occupations, including pilots, public transportation crews, and hospital staff.

There is great global disparity in the availability of sleep health care, with many nations having well-established sleep medicine systems, yet others struggling to address the needs of their vulnerable populations with limited resources. For instance, it is estimated that nearly 425 million adults have moderate to severe obstructive sleep apnea globally today, and it is widely held that the majority remain either undiagnosed or untreated. Although we have accurate diagnostic tools and effective therapies for many sleep-related disorders, sleep testing and treatments are still unavailable for many, and adequate numbers of sleep health professionals are lacking in parts of the world. Primary care resources are essential but are, at present, underutilized. Incorporating sleep medicine into primary care can enhance efficiency and quality of care, increase access, and improve health outcomes.

All of us are eyewitnesses to, as well as participants of, an ongoing social transformation of sleep. Among the most primordial of physiologic

sleep.theclinics.com

Sleep Med Clin 15 (2020) xv–xvi
https://doi.org/10.1016/j.jsmc.2020.04.001
1556-407X/20/© 2020 Published by Elsevier Inc.

drives, sleep, today, is being reshaped by life-style, technology, pharmacology, and policy. This rapidly evolving part of human behavior and communal life has a wide-ranging impact on personal health, relationships, performance, and public safety. For many, adequacy of sleep is deemed both necessary yet unattainable, and solutions for sleep disorders are considered effective but remain inaccessible or unafford-able. As we continue to imagine what our sleep *should* or *could* be, it is essential we remember that sleeping is not an evolutionary error of physiology or simply a momentary pause in a highly scheduled calendar; rather, it exists side by side with waking life, and neither endures without the other.

Teofilo Lee-Chiong, Jr, MD
National Jewish Health
Denver, CO 80206, USA

University of Colorado
School of Medicine
Aurora, CO 80045, USA

E-mail address:
Lee-ChiongT@njc.org

Internet-Delivered Cognitive Behavioral Therapy for Insomnia
Tailoring Cognitive Behavioral Therapy for Insomnia for Patients with Chronic Insomnia

Tanja van der Zweerde, MSc[a],*, Jaap Lancee, PhD[b,c],
Annemarie Ida Luik, PhD[d], Annemieke van Straten, PhD[a]

KEYWORDS

- Chronic insomnia • Insomnia • Internet • Cognitive behavioral therapy (CBT)
- CBT for Insomnia (CBTI) • Online psychological treatment • Tailoring treatment

KEY POINTS

- Insomnia is an important public health issue with high prevalence, disease burden, and economic costs. Insomnia is preferably treated with cognitive behavioral therapy (CBTI).
- Both face-to-face and Internet-delivered CBT for Insomnia (I-CBTI) are evidence-based effective treatments.
- I-CBTI has yet to reach its full potential in both scope and scale. More developments toward improved effectiveness could further improve I-CBTI.
- I-CBTI can be successfully offered to a wide and varied range of insomnia sufferers and is suggested to be effective irrespective of demographic variation or baseline severity.
- Research should focus on working mechanisms and moderators of effects, aimed at implementation of tailored Internet treatments to successfully treat more people.

PRECISION MEDICINE FOR INSOMNIA DISORDER

Insomnia is a common mental disorder, characterized by complaints of dissatisfaction with sleep quantity, sleep quality, or both. Persons with insomnia suffer from these symptoms 3 or more nights per week, for at least 3 months, which results in significant distress or impaired daytime functioning (*Diagnostic and Statistical Manual of Mental Disorders, 5th Edition: DSM-5*[1]; for full criteria see **Table 1**). Approximately one-third of the population suffers from occasional insomnia symptoms, whereas approximately 7% to 10%

This article originally appeared in September, 2019 issue of *Sleep Medicine Clinics* (Volume 14, Issue 3).
Disclosure Statement: The online cognitive behavioral therapy for insomnia program, i-Sleep, was developed at the VU University Amsterdam by Annemieke van Straten and further developed in collaboration with Jaap Lancee (University of Amsterdam) and T. van der Zweerde (VU University). The authors have no commercial interest in this program. Annemarie Luik has previously worked in a position funded by Big Health Inc. (Sleepio); she currently has no commercial or financial interest in Big Health Inc.
[a] Department of Clinical Psychology, EMGO Institute for Health and Care Research, VU University, Van der Boechorststraat 7, Amsterdam 1081 BT, the Netherlands; [b] Department of Clinical Psychology, University of Amsterdam, Nieuwe Achtergracht 129, Amsterdam 1018 WS, the Netherlands; [c] PsyQ Amsterdam, Amsterdam, the Netherlands; [d] Department of Epidemiology, Erasmus MC University Medical Center, Dr. Molewaterplein 40, Rotterdam 3015 GD, the Netherlands
* Corresponding author.
E-mail address: t.vander.zweerde@vu.nl

Table 1			
DSM-5 and ICSD-3 diagnosis of insomnia disorder			
Classification System	**Duration**	**Frequency**	**Sleep Complaints**
DSM-5	≥3 mo	≥3 nights per week	Difficulty initiating sleep, maintaining sleep, and/or early morning awakening with inability to return to sleep despite adequate opportunity for sleep.
			Resulting in significant impairment of daytime functioning and/or significant distress.
			Not better explained by another sleep-wake disorder, physiologic effects of substances or coexistent conditions.
ICSD-3	≥3 mo	≥3 nights per week	Difficulty initiating sleep, maintaining sleep, waking up earlier than desired, resistance to going to bed at appropriate time, and/or difficulty sleeping without intervention.
			Fatigue/malaise, impaired attention/concentration/memory, impaired performance (social, familial, occupational, or academic), mood disturbance/irritability, daytime sleepiness, behavioral problems (eg, hyperactivity, impulsivity, or aggression), reduced motivation/energy/initiative, proneness to judgment errors or to physical accidents, and/or concerns about or dissatisfaction with sleep.
			Reported sleep-wake complaints cannot be explained purely by inadequate opportunity or circumstance for sleep: enough time has been allotted for sleep and the environment is safe, dark, quiet, and comfortable.
			Sleep-wake difficulty is not better explained by another sleep disorder (intoxication and acute withdrawal are ruled out).

Abbreviations: DSM-5, diagnostic and statistical manual of mental disorders, 5th Edition: DSM-5; ICSD-3, international classification of sleep disorders. Third Edition.

fit clinical criteria for an insomnia diagnosis.[2,3] People typically suffer from insomnia for multiple years[3] before diagnosis. Insomnia also increases the risk for other mental and physical health problems, and persons with insomnia often develop comorbid mental health problems, such as depression or anxiety.[4–6] The economic burden of insomnia is considerable: poor sleepers cost society up to 10 times as much as good sleepers.[7,8] The high prevalence, costs, burden, and risk of insomnia warrant efficacious treatment. Precision medicine offers the potential to realize the best use of limited time and resources in (mental) health care. Internet-delivered therapy can facilitate a precision medicine approach, as components, intensity, order, reminders, and guidance can be tailored to suit the specific needs of the patient, but at the same time needs fewer resources than face-to-face solutions for precision medicine.

COGNITIVE BEHAVIORAL THERAPY FOR INSOMNIA

Currently, many people seeking help for insomnia are prescribed a pharmacologic treatment, mostly benzodiazepines or benzodiazepine receptor agonists (the so-called "Z-drugs": zolpidem, zopiclone, zaleplon[9]). As short-term treatment, pharmacotherapies are effective in relieving insomnia[10–12]; however, pharmacotherapy has negative side effects, such as headaches, drowsiness and dizziness, can alter sleep microstructure, and potentially leads to dependency and addiction when used long-term.[11–13] When a person quits medication, the person can also suffer from rebound effects.[14] Furthermore, the evidence for longer-term effects of pharmacotherapies is limited.[15–17] Despite these concerns, in the United States, use of prescription sleep aids has increased in recent years.[10] Other psychoactive medications such as antidepressants or antipsychotics are also used to treat insomnia, even though their effectiveness has not adequately been demonstrated in clinical trials.[18]

Fortunately, evidence-based alternatives to pharmacotherapy for persons with insomnia are available. Since the 1990s, a collection of different treatment components (educational, behavioral, and cognitive) has been offered as a combined treatment: cognitive behavioral therapy for insomnia (CBTI). An overview of the different components of CBTI is listed in **Table 2**.[21]

Multiple reviews have concluded that CBTI is effective and has effects that last longer than those of pharmacologic treatments for insomnia. As a result, CBTI has a substantial evidence base for the treatment of insomnia.[16,22–29] Large posttreatment effects are reported on insomnia severity (Hedges '$g = 0.98$), self-rated sleep efficiency

Table 2
Core cognitive behavioral therapy for insomnia components

Component	Content
Psycho-education	Information about the process and function of normal and disturbed sleep.
Sleep hygiene and lifestyle advice	Information about a healthy lifestyle that can promote sleep (eg, low caffeine and alcohol intake), about behaviors and habits that hinder sleep, about adjustments that can be made to improve their sleep (eg, a suitable bedroom and bedtime routine). Fixed hours are set for bed and rising times aiming to stabilize the circadian rhythm.
Stimulus control	Person's associations between bed and sleep are reaffirmed by advice to get out of bed when awake >15 min, and only go back to bed when sleepy. The bed is to be used for sleep and sexual activity only.
Sleep restriction therapy	Person's time in bed is restricted to the average time a patient slept the past week (typically with a minimum of 5 hours). This heightens the homeostatic sleep drive (ie, patients are more tired), making them fall asleep easier and strengthens the bed-sleep association. When this results in less fragmented sleep, the sleep window is elongated slowly (see Refs.[19,20]).
Relaxation techniques	Different relaxation and breathing exercises are used to teach patients to unwind and take more breaks during the day, for example, progressive muscle relaxation or meditation exercises.
Cognitive restructuring	Persons identify and challenge misconceptions (such as "I have to sleep 8 h a night") and worries that keep them awake. These might be related to sleep or to other non–sleep-related issues. Unhelpful thoughts are unpacked and challenged using cognitive techniques, such as gathering evidence for and against a certain belief or statement, and gathering evidence for a more helpful alternative.

(g = 0.71) and sleep quality (g = 0.65[29]). A recent meta-analysis[30] demonstrated that CBTI has positive long-term effects that last up to a year, showing an effect of clinically significant magnitude. Because of these favorable effects, international guidelines recommend CBTI as a first-line treatment rather than prescribing medication, or combining the 2 modalities if necessary.[31,32]

Online Cognitive Behavioral Therapy for Insomnia

Although CBTI is recommended therapy for insomnia, many patients with insomnia do not receive CBTI. Several important reasons for this discrepancy can be identified. First, estimates are that only 50% of persons with insomnia actively seek help.[33] Second, given the high prevalence of insomnia[2] and the relatively small number of trained CBTI therapists, there is a discrepancy between the demand for treatment and available resources. Moreover, health care budgets are not sufficient to provide face-to-face CBT to everyone, even if therapists were available.

Third, general practitioners (GPs), often the first point of contact for persons with insomnia who seek treatment, rarely refer to psychological treatments for insomnia.[34]

As a potential solution to some of these issues CBTI could be offered in an online format (I-CBTI). Because I-CBTI requires less therapist input than face-to-face therapy, the same number of therapists can treat many more people. Furthermore, I-CBTI might be less stigmatizing and more easily accessible to patients. Going to a health care professional, such as a GP, is required in most cases to obtain access to online treatment, but patients may nonetheless regard this as a smaller and more easily accomplished step than being referred to mental health care facilities for help.

CBTI in an online format is similar to CBTI delivered face-to-face, containing mostly the same elements in the same order. Typically, I-CBTI is offered through secured Web sites that include informative texts, videos, graphs, and illustrations. Participants provide information to the program via (interactive) questionnaires and a sleep diary.

Many variations of I-CBTI exist, including variations that (1) use a mix of face-to-face sessions and I-CBTI, (2) use support and feedback from a health care professional, and (3) use fully automated support and feedback, either personalized or not. In most treatments, the number of sessions and their order is fixed, but some programs have opt-in elements in which participants can select components that they feel are relevant for them,[35] or provide a mix of fixed and optional components.[36]

EFFICACY OF INTERNET-DELIVERED COGNITIVE BEHAVIORAL THERAPY FOR INSOMNIA

In 2004, Ström and colleagues[37] published the first randomized controlled study investigating Internet-based treatment for insomnia. Since then, many more studies and digital programs for insomnia have been developed. To our knowledge, 13 different I-CBTI programs have been studied in a randomized controlled trial (Refs.[35–49]; **Table 3**), of which most programs were developed for adults except 1 program for adolescents.[49] Although the number of online treatments for insomnia is expected to continue to grow rapidly, only a small percentage has been evidence-based so far, leaving many more programs without any evidence base accompanied by unknown efficacy and risks, potentially even causing harm.

GUIDANCE IN ONLINE COGNITIVE BEHAVIORAL THERAPY FOR INSOMNIA PROGRAMS

Most programs offer at least some form of therapeutic guidance, either automated or by a therapist, that is, human feedback. Common elements are feedback on sleep diaries that a person keeps, as well as motivational messages to help participants adhere to the program, and providing additional instructions and explanations when necessary. Participants usually receive online feedback and motivational support for every session they complete. Providing human feedback takes an estimated 15 to 30 minutes per online participant per session and can be provided by psychologists, other health care professionals, or by clinical psychology students.[36,52,54,57] Automated feedback also is used.[35,39,48] Extensive programming ensures that participants receive tailored messages suited to their situation and sleep patterns.

Research on online treatments for other psychological disorders reports that support promotes adherence and increases effects[58]; however, only 2 studies have investigated these effects in online insomnia treatment. Both report that support, even if it is very limited, improves effectiveness.[59,60] More research is needed to identify the optimal form and dosage of support. If I-CBTI is to offer a true alternative to pharmacotherapy and be implemented on a large scale, personal (online) support or guidance could present a challenge. Current and future developments not yet applied to I-CBTI could be used to enhance automated support and guidance, for example, by using avatars and/or artificial intelligence.

EFFECTS OF INTERNET-DELIVERED COGNITIVE BEHAVIORAL THERAPY FOR INSOMNIA
Effects on Insomnia of Internet-Delivered Cognitive Behavioral Therapy for Insomnia

Overall, I-CBTI is effective and effect sizes seem in the same range as those of face-to-face treatments,[61] in line with research in, for example, Internet treatment for depression.[62] As such, it is suggested to be a viable treatment option. Since the meta-analysis by Zachariae and colleagues,[61] many trials have been published investigating an existing I-CBTI program (eg, Refs.[35–46,48,50–54,56,57,59,63–67]), and new programs have been introduced (eg, Refs.[45,47]). These studies reliably show positive effects (see **Table 3**).

The few direct comparisons that have been made between online and face-to-face CBTI have reported mixed results. Lancee and colleagues[52] found that face-to-face therapy substantially outperformed its online alternative. Blom and colleagues[36] compared I-CBTI with group therapy and did not report differences in effects. More research directly comparing face-to-face CBTI with I-CBTI is needed to compare effects of different treatment modalities and their moderators.

Effects of Internet-Delivered Cognitive Behavioral Therapy for Insomnia on Other (Mental) Health Symptoms and Daily Functioning

Insomnia is often comorbid with psychological complaints. Insomnia plays a role in the onset of anxiety disorders, bipolar disorders, and suicidality, but is most notably related to depression.[68] Patients suffering from a major depressive episode have an 80% chance of also reporting insomnia symptoms.[2] In addition, a person suffering from insomnia is at greater risk for depression.[69] Residual insomnia complaints after successful depression treatment also predict depression relapse.[70]

Table 3
Different Internet-delivered cognitive behavioral therapy for insomnia (all components) programs studied

Study	Program	Population	Scheduled Sessions	Support	Delivery	Indications of Effect Size[a]
Ström et al,[37] 2004	—	Adults	Order fixed, structured program at patients own[b] pace (5 sessions/wk)	Automated	Text-based	BAASS = 0.81.[37]
Suzuki et al,[35] 2008	—	Adults	Patients pick any 3 or more (4 sessions/2 wk)	Automated	Interactive Web platform	0.09–0.33 for SOL, TST, and SE.[35]
Vincent & Lewycky,[38] 2009	—	Adults	Fixed, structured program at patients own pace (5 sessions/6 wk)	None	Interactive Web platform	Range 0.14–0.75 for sleep diary variables.[38]
Espie et al,[39] 2012	Sleepio	Adults	Fixed, structured program at patients own pace (6 sessions/6 wk)	Automated, personalized	Interactive, virtual therapist	SCI = 0.89[50]; SCI = 1.11.[51]
Lancee et al,[40] 2012	—	Adults	Fixed, structured program at patients own pace (6 sessions)	None	Text-based	ISI = 1.00[52]; 1.05[43]; SLEEP50 Insomnia = 1.44[40]
Ho et al,[41] 2014	—	Adults	Fixed, structured program at patients own pace (6 sessions/6 wk)	Weekly phone support vs no support	Interactive Web platform	ISI = 0.53[41]
Van Straten et al,[42] 2014	I-Sleep	Adults	Fixed, structured program at patients own pace (text-based: 6[42], interactive: 5,[53] over 5–8 wk).	Weekly personal online therapist support	Text-based[42], updated to interactive Web platform[53]	PSQI = 1.06[42]; ISI 2.36[53]
Blom et al,[36] 2015	—	Adults	Some elements fixed, some optional (8 sessions over 8 wk).	Weekly personal online therapist support	Text-based	ISI = 0.85[54], 1.8[36]

(continued on next page)

Table 3
(continued)

Study	Program	Population	Scheduled Sessions	Support	Delivery	Indications of Effect Size[a]
Thiart et al,[44] 2016	Get.On Recovery	Adults	Fixed, structured program at patients own pace (6 sessions)	Weekly personal online therapist support	Interactive Web platform	ISI = 1.45[55]
Bernstein et al,[45] 2017	GO! To sleep	Adults	Fixed, structured program at patients own pace (6 sessions/ 6 wk)	None	Interactive Web platform	n/a
Horsch et al,[47] 2017	Sleepcare	Adults	Fixed, structured program at patients own pace (6–7 wk)	Automated, personalized	Fully automated interactive app	ISI = 0.66[47]
Hagatun et al,[46] 2017; Ritterband et al,[48] 2017	SHUT-I	Adults	Fixed, structured program at patients own pace (6 sessions/ 6 wk)	Automated, personalized	Interactive Web platform	ISI = 1.14[56]
de Bruin et al,[49] 2015	—	Adolescents	Fixed weekly online sessions (6 sessions/ 6 wk)	Weekly personal feedback from a coach or therapist	Text-based	HSDQ insomnia scale = 1.26[49]

Abbreviations: BAASS, beliefs and attitudes about sleep scale; C-E, cost-effectiveness; ES, effect size; HSDQ, Holland sleep disorder questionnaire; ISI, insomnia severity index; n/a, not available; P HQ-9, patient health questionnaire-9; PSQI, Pittsburgh sleep quality index; SCI, sleep condition indicator; SE, sleep efficiency; SOL, sleep onset latency; TST, total sleep time; —, no specific title for this program.

[a] Between-group (cognitive behavioral therapy for insomnia vs placebo, wait list, or no treatment) Cohen's *d* reported from publications when available; reported effect sizes are between-group unless otherwise indicated; this is a selection of studies and not an exhaustive overview. For programs with more than 3 randomized controlled trials (RCTs) available, the effect sizes of the most recent 3 RCTs were reported. Reporting on insomnia severity measure when available; sleep diary otherwise; and different measure if neither are available.

[b] Patient-paced programs commonly have a 1 week per session minimum.

Similar to face-to-face CBTI,[71,72] I-CBTI also has been shown to have antidepressant effects.[73] Most participants studied in these meta-analyses,[72,73] however, were not recruited for depression specifically, and severely depressed persons were not included in these studies. Three recent I-CBTI studies specifically assessing I-CBTI as a treatment for depressive symptoms and insomnia showed promising results. Blom and colleagues[57] found I-CBTI to be more effective than online depression treatment on insomnia and equally effective on depressive symptoms. Christensen and colleagues[64] and van der Zweerde and colleagues[53] demonstrated that I-CBTI reduced both depressive symptoms and insomnia symptoms in people suffering from both.[53,64]

Depressive symptoms are not the only psychiatric complaints influenced by I-CBTI. A large study by Freeman and colleagues[51] on 3755 students showed that I-CBTI also leads to positive changes in psychotic symptoms. Improving insomnia has been suggested to have beneficial effects on other aspects of (mental) health and quality of life as well.[50] This is particularly important because daytime complaints and impaired daily functioning are often the reason to seek treatment.[74] There is also evidence of I-CBTI improving work performance and cognitive complaints.[50,65,66]

FACTORS INFLUENCING INTERNET-DELIVERED COGNITIVE BEHAVIORAL THERAPY FOR INSOMNIA EFFECTS

Even though CBTI treatments are effective overall, the treatment does not work for everyone, up to an estimated 30% of persons with insomnia do not respond to treatment.[75] Why this is the case and which factors (eg, genetic, environmental, biological, lifestyle) play a role here is largely unknown. More research is needed to enable precision medicine approaches taking into account specific patient characteristics that influence the changes of treatment success.

Clear mediators and moderators of I-CBTI effects have yet to be determined. Some influential variables have been suggested by earlier research on CBTI (**Table 4**). It is yet unclear whether these factors differ between CBTI and I-CBTI, but it seems likely that comparable processes play a role in both treatment modalities.

Cognitive and Behavioral Factors

The importance of cognitive processes in insomnia treatment has been well documented over the past 20 years (eg, Refs.[92–94]). Cognitive processes, such as worrying and dysfunctional beliefs, have been studied as mediators of the effects of CBTI treatment, with varying results.[43,56,76–80] Overall, although not all studies study the same specific outcomes and cognitive processes, cognitive factors do seem to play a role. Two important factors worth mentioning are insomnia-related worrying and dysfunctional beliefs.[81,95] Harvey[81] suggests patients with insomnia perceive worrying to be beneficial to them (which may in itself be seen as a dysfunctional belief). At the same time, worrying also heightens arousal, making sleeping difficult. Dysfunctional beliefs (eg, "Without a good night's rest I will not be able to function at work tomorrow") are a topic of worry, and can also aggravate the perceived consequences of poor sleep.

Behavioral factors such as habits incompatible with sleep, varying bedtimes, and spending too much time in bed are commonly seen among bad sleepers and influence effects of treatment. Harvey and colleagues[78] recently concluded that the effects of these behavioral factors depend on the type of treatment (behavioral treatment [BT], cognitive therapy [CT], or a combination) a person undergoes.[78] They observed that behavioral processes mediated the results for BT but not for CT. Notably, the cognitive mediators studied (worry, unhelpful beliefs about sleep, and monitoring behavior for sleep-related threat) were significant mediators of the effect of BT as well as CT. When patients report a high level of disturbance in both behavioral and cognitive sleep-related processes, they achieved better treatment results when they received the combined CBT.[78]

Delivery-Mode–Specific Factors

Online delivery may not be suited for everyone suffering from insomnia. Blom and colleagues[86] looked at patient-reported factors that facilitate and hinder uptake of I-CBTI. They found that having more than one psychological problem next to insomnia makes it more difficult to adhere to an I-CBTI program and may warrant different delivery modes or more intensive (human) support. A review on Internet therapy aimed at behavior changes emphasized that the intensity of a program should be high and that reminders, preferably text-messages, are important tools to enhance adherence.[88]

Sleep as a Perpetuating Factor in Other Psychiatric Problems

Disturbed sleep is seen in 60% of psychiatric patients,[96] and is often a perpetuating factor, for example, in depression.[70] Treating insomnia also

Table 4
Factors that have been suggested to play a role in precision medicine for insomnia

Factors	Characteristic	Supported on Sequence	Level of Research Support
Mediators	Type of problem (cognitive or behavioral)	BT for primarily behavioral problems, CT for primarily cognitive problems, combined CBT when both are present.	• Empirical results on cognitive process vary,[43,56,76–80] their influence remains unclear. • Empirical evidence does show insomnia-related worrying and dysfunctional beliefs about sleep mediate treatment effects.[81] • Behavioral processes mediated results for BT, but not for CT in RCT.[78]
Predictors of treatment effects			
Demographic[a] Age		Higher chance of treatment success with younger age.	• Meta-analytic evidence based on data from 49 studies.[82] • However: no evidence from older populations, age range in 90% of studies is quite small.[82]
Educational level		Higher chance of treatment success with higher educational level.	• Observational study of intervention group only (Vincent et al, 2001) showed education moderated effects.[83] • Not found to moderate effects in meta-analysis.[82]
Clinical	Higher (>6 h) initial total sleep time[b]	Risk of dropout.	• Empirical evidence higher TST predicts dropout from dropped-out participants in RCT.[84]
	Lower initial total sleep time (<6 hr)	Lower chance of treatment success.	• Empirical evidence from RCT results.[85]
	Lower initial insomnia severity	Lower change of treatment success, may predict dropout.	• Empirical evidence from dropped-out participants in RCT.[84]
	Higher initial sleep efficiency[b]	Lower chance of treatment success.	• Suggested in 2014 conference abstract, results not published to our knowledge.[83]
	Other sleep disorders	Lower chance of treatment success.	• Observational study of intervention group only (Vincent et al, 2001) showed sleep comorbidity moderated effects.[83]

(continued on next page)

Table 4
(continued)

Factors	Characteristic	Supported on Sequence	Level of Research Support
	Other psychiatric or medical disorders	Chance of lower adherence.	• Empirical RCT evidence shows psychiatric comorbidities warrant more intensive delivery modes/more intensive (human) support/scheduled program reminders. • Meta-analytic evidence of effect sizes equal to effect sizes in non-comorbid samples.[73] • Psychiatric comorbidities do not seem to decrease treatment effects and comorbidities may benefit from CBTI as well.[53,57,64,86–88] • Meta-analytic evidence shows the positive response to CBTI on insomnia symptoms does not appear to be moderated by the type of comorbid condition (psychiatric/medical).[89]
	Insomnia subtype	Different treatment (elements) may be indicated depending on for example, level of distress.	Insomnia subtypes identified by Blanken and colleagues,[90] further research and clinical application needed.

Abbreviations: BT, behavioral therapy; CBTI, cognitive behavioral therapy for insomnia; CT, cognitive therapy; RCT, randomized controlled trial; TST, total sleep time.

[a] Research suggests only 2.2% of variance in CBTI treatment effects on sleep efficiency (SE) was due to demographics (conference abstract by Espie and colleagues,[83] 2014).

[b] Paradoxical insomnia could also play a role when TST and/or SE are high but patients experience an insomnia problem nonetheless.[91]

improves depression (eg, Refs.[53,64]); however, it is unclear how and why: more research into the mechanisms by which treating insomnia improves mood is needed. Often, mediation analysis is used to study such mechanisms (eg, Ref.[79]). To do this successfully, the mediator should be measured during and after intervention but before the effects occur and the sample size should be substantial.[97] I-CBTI has made it possible to do large trials adequately powered to assess mediation. These studies suggest that improvement of insomnia symptoms is preceding the improvements in depression (eg, Refs.[50,51]). Recently, network approaches have been developed to investigate changes in specific symptoms, instead of full questionnaires only. This new tool called Network Intervention Analysis (NIA[98]) can be used to study trial data using specific symptoms. This approach demonstrated that depression symptoms clear up *after* specific insomnia symptoms.[98] NIA could be used on other datasets in the field of I-CBTI to provide more insight into working mechanisms and hence into optimizing treatment response in patients with insomnia.

PERSONALIZING INTERNET-DELIVERED COGNITIVE BEHAVIORAL THERAPY FOR INSOMNIA

In psychotherapy, an important question is: what works for whom? As discussed previously, more knowledge on the working mechanisms of I-CBTI will likely lead to better treatments, but efficacy of the treatment also could depend on person-specific factors. It has been suggested that online CBT effects on anxiety and depression are moderated by age (older people reporting fewer beneficial effects) but not by other "person, problem, program, or provider characteristics."[82] For insomnia treatment, research by Cheng and colleagues[67] showed that I-CBTI effectively reduces symptoms across a wide range of demographic characteristics. Their large study was the first to identify different potential factors influencing the scope of treatment benefit, such as age, gender, socioeconomic status, and baseline severity, but also comorbidities in mental and physical health. They did not find any demographic variables to be associated with treatment efficacy and concluded that I-CBTI can be successfully offered to a wide and varied range of persons with insomnia complaints.[67] Luik and colleagues[83] suggested in their review that being younger and more highly educated improves one's chances of success.[99,100] They also reported on clinical predictors of treatment success. The limited available research suggests that comorbid sleep disorders other than insomnia, a higher initial sleep efficiency, lower baseline severity of insomnia, and longer total sleep time at the start of treatment may put a person at risk of improving little or not at all from I-CBTI.[83]

I-CBTI does not work for everyone suffering from insomnia.[75] The insomnia subtypes introduced by Blanken and colleagues[90] might offer a promising approach for tailoring treatment. Their 5 subtypes are as follows: (1) highly distressed; (2) moderately distressed, intact response to pleasurable emotions; (3) moderately distressed, weak response to pleasurable emotions; (4) low distress, low reactivity to environment and life events; and (5) low distress and high reactivity to environment and life events.[90] These stable subtypes have been shown to differ in biologically based traits and life history and treatment response.[90] Future research should focus on whether different insomnia treatments have different effects on the subtypes; that is, their clinical relevance. Specific subtypes may be present that will or will not respond well to I-CBTI. For example, a person whose subtype is particularly characterized by high presleep arousal might benefit more from mindfulness or acceptance-based techniques than from cognitive therapies.

COST-EFFECTIVENESS

Insomnia is a problem accompanied by substantial health care and societal costs, the latter for example, due to productivity loss and absence from work.[7] Treatment of insomnia could therefore potentially lead to large cost savings. Unfortunately, the cost-effectiveness of I-CBTI (or CBTI in general), has not been studied often. At least 3 studies have examined the cost-effectiveness of CBTI. These studies seem to suggest that the treatment is indeed cost-effective when offered in a face-to-face format,[101] to employees in online format,[44] and to adolescents online or in group format.[102] A pragmatic randomized controlled trial is currently under way studying whether I-CBTI can be offered cost-effectively in the general practice.[103]

IMPLEMENTATION

I-CBTI has several advantages that could facilitate implementation. It can be administered without scheduling appointments, and no travel time is required. This makes it suitable for those living remotely or with reduced mobility, limited time or busy schedules, and for those experiencing stigma preventing them from seeking face-to-face help. In addition, I-CBTI reduces waiting lists because much less resource is needed. However, online therapy also has some disadvantages that could impede implementation. A person has to invest a significant amount of time, which might require more self-discipline without face-to-face contact. In addition, people may have particular concerns about data privacy when data are shared online.[104] This makes it critical that programs adhere to respective regulations concerning data security. Also, not all persons suffering from insomnia may want online therapy: some insist on seeing a therapist, but equally some will prefer online treatment. Another concern might be related to personal safety. It may be preferable to keep a health care professional involved when a patient with insomnia is taking any online treatment. Automated systems can have algorithms to deal with certain safety issues. For example, when a program detects certain problems in the patient's answers (eg, suicide risk), patients could be automatically advised to contact their GP or health care professional, or a professional could be alerted to contact the patient automatically.

After determining effectiveness, working mechanisms, and costs associated with the treatment, the next big question is how best to implement on-line insomnia treatments. Whether or not a treatment is offered with or without support is an important factor in the implementation process. Accessible online treatments that are offered without human feedback are very scalable. Currently, a number of online programs can be freely purchased, but most programs are provided via research programs, health insurance programs, or at a (primary or secondary) care facility. Ideally, the guidelines recommending CBT for insomnia[31,32] should facilitate easy access to reimbursed treatment for diagnosed patients seeking help. Siversten and Nordgreen[105] have advised implementation of a varied range of modalities in which CBTI is offered, ranging from self-help material to online treatment to face-to-face conversations. Face-to-face therapy should then, due to scarcity of therapists, be provided only to those patients not helped (enough) through any of the other methods; that is, using a stepped-care approach.[105]

SUMMARY

There is ample evidence that I-CBTI is an effective treatment for those suffering from insomnia. This enables tailoring precision medicine to individual needs and characteristics. I-CBTI has the potential to play an important role in precision medicine because of its flexibility, accessibility, low costs, and multiple tailoring options. More research is needed looking into the moderators, mediators, and working mechanisms underlying the effects of I-CBTI on insomnia and other psychopathology to reach this potential. Then, we can offer efficacious treatment to those currently not benefiting from I-CBTI treatment, for reasons yet unknown. This would provide a strong incentive to implement I-CBTI on a larger scale, reaching more people, offering a true and perhaps preferable alternative to pharmacotherapy.

RESEARCH AGENDA

We suggest the following gaps in current research should be addressed:

1. Establishing patient characteristics influencing treatment success to facilitate a precision medicine approach.
2. Further specifying (sub)types of patients with insomnia and identifying optimal ways to offer subtype-specific treatment in a stepped-care and cost-effective manner.
3. Determining the working mechanisms of I-CBTI to be able to specifically target these in treatment.

REFERENCES

1. APA committee. Diagnostic and statistical manual of mental disorders, 5th edition: DSM-5. Washington, DC: American Psychiatric Association; 2013.
2. Ohayon MM. Epidemiology of insomnia: what we know and what we still need to learn. Sleep Med Rev 2002;6:97–111.
3. Morin CM, Bélanger L, LeBlanc M, et al. The natural history of insomnia: a population-based 3-year longitudinal study. Arch Intern Med 2009;169:447–53.
4. Baglioni C, Riemann D. Is chronic insomnia a precursor to major depression? Epidemiological and biological findings. Curr Psychiatry Rep 2012;14:511–8.
5. Suh S, Kim H, Yang HC, et al. Longitudinal course of depression scores with and without insomnia in non-depressed individuals: a 6-year follow-up longitudinal study in a Korean cohort. Sleep 2013;36:369–76.
6. Olfson M, Wall M, Liu SM, et al. Insomnia and impaired quality of life in the United States. J Clin Psychiatry 2018;79.
7. Daley M, Morin CM, LeBlanc M, et al. The economic burden of insomnia: direct and indirect costs for individuals with insomnia syndrome, insomnia symptoms, and good sleepers. Sleep 2009;32:55–64.
8. Kessler RC, Berglund PA, Coulouvrat C, et al. Insomnia and the performance of US workers: results from the America insomnia survey. Sleep 2011;34:1161–71.
9. Hoebert JM, Souverein PC, Mantel-Teeuwisse AK, et al. Reimbursement restriction and moderate decrease in benzodiazepine use in general practice. Ann Fam Med 2012;10:42–9.
10. Bertisch SM, Herzig SJ, Winkelman JW, et al. National use of prescription medications for insomnia: NHANES 1999-2010. Sleep 2014;37:343–9.
11. Glass J, Lanctôt KL, Herrmann N, et al. Sedative hypnotics in older people with insomnia: meta-analysis of risks and benefits. BMJ 2005;331:1169.
12. Buscemi N, Vandermeer B, Friesen C, et al. The efficacy and safety of drug treatments for chronic insomnia in adults: a meta-analysis of RCTs. J Gen Intern Med 2007;22:1335.
13. Manconi M, Ferri R, Miano S, et al. Sleep architecture in insomniacs with severe benzodiazepine abuse. Clin Neurophysiol 2017;128:875–81.
14. Hintze JP, Edinger JD. Hypnotic discontinuation in chronic insomnia. Sleep Med Clin 2018;13:263–70.
15. Holbrook AM, Crowther R, Lotter A, et al. Meta-analysis of benzodiazepine use in the treatment of insomnia. Can Med Assoc J 2000;162:225–33.
16. Smith MT, Perlis ML, Park A, et al. Comparative meta-analysis of pharmacotherapy and behavior

therapy for persistent insomnia. Am J Psychiatry 2002;159:5–11.

17. Riemann D, Perlis ML. The treatments of chronic insomnia: a review of benzodiazepine receptor agonists and psychological and behavioral therapies. Sleep Med Clin 2009;13:205–14.

18. Everitt H, Baldwin D, Stuart B, et al. Antidepressants for insomnia in adults. New Jersey: Cochrane Library; 2018.

19. Kyle SD, Miller CB, Rogers Z, et al. Sleep restriction therapy for insomnia is associated with reduced objective total sleep time, increased daytime somnolence, and objectively impaired vigilance: implications for the clinical management of insomnia disorder. Sleep 2014;37:229–37.

20. American Academy of Sleep Medicine. International classification of sleep disorders. Diagnostic and coding manual 2005;2:51–5.

21. Morin CM, Espie CA. Insomnia: a clinical guide to assessment and treatment. New York: Springer Science & Business; 2007.

22. Murtagh DR, Greenwood KM. Identifying effective psychological treatments for insomnia: a meta-analysis. J Consult Clin Psychol 1995;63:79.

23. Edinger JD, Wohlgemuth WK. The significance and management of persistent primary insomnia: the past, present and future of behavioral insomnia therapies. Sleep Med Rev 1999;3:101–8.

24. Harvey AG, Tang NK. Cognitive behaviour therapy for primary insomnia: can we rest yet? Sleep Med Rev 2003;7:237–62.

25. Montgomery P, Dennis J. A systematic review of non-pharmacological therapies for sleep problems in later life. Sleep Med Rev 2004;8:47–62.

26. Morin CM, Bootzin RR, Buysse DJ, et al. Psychological and behavioral treatment of insomnia: update of the recent evidence (1998–2004). Sleep 2006;29:1398–414.

27. Siebern AT, Suh S, Nowakowski S. Non-pharmacological treatment of insomnia. Neurotherapeutics 2012;9:717–27.

28. Trauer JM, Qian MY, Doyle JS, et al. Cognitive behavioral therapy for chronic insomnia: a systematic review and meta-analysis. Ann Intern Med 2015;163:191–204.

29. Van Straten A, van der Zweerde T, Kleiboer A, et al. Cognitive and behavioral therapies in the treatment of insomnia: a meta-analysis. Sleep Med Rev 2018;38:3–16.

30. Van der Zweerde T, Bisdounis L, Kyle SD, et al. Cognitive behavioral therapy for insomnia: a meta-analysis of long-term effects in controlled studies. Under review.

31. Riemann D, Baglioni C, Bassetti C, et al. European guideline for the diagnosis and treatment of insomnia. J Sleep Res 2017;26:675–700.

32. Qaseem A, Kansagara D, Forciea MA, et al. Management of chronic insomnia disorder in adults: a clinical practice guideline from the American College of Physicians. Ann Intern Med 2016;165:125–33.

33. Morin CM, LeBlanc M, Daley M, et al. Epidemiology of insomnia: prevalence, self-help treatments, consultations, and determinants of help-seeking behaviors. Sleep Med 2006;7:123–30.

34. Everitt H, McDermott L, Leydon G, et al. GPs' management strategies for patients with insomnia: a survey and qualitative interview study. Br J Gen Pract 2014;64:112–9.

35. Suzuki E, Tsuchiya M, Hirokawa K, et al. Evaluation of an Internet-based self-help program for better quality of sleep among Japanese workers: a randomized controlled trial. J Occup Health 2008;50:387–99.

36. Blom K, Tillgren HT, Wiklund T, et al. Internet- vs. group-delivered cognitive behavior therapy for insomnia: a randomized controlled non-inferiority trial. Behav Res Ther 2015;70:47–55.

37. Ström L, Pettersson R, Andersson G. Internet-based treatment for insomnia: a controlled evaluation. J Consult Clin Psychol 2004;72:113.

38. Vincent N, Lewycky S. Logging on for better sleep: RCT of the effectiveness of online treatment for insomnia. Sleep 2009;32:807–15.

39. Espie CA, Kyle SD, Williams C, et al. A randomized, placebo-controlled trial of online cognitive behavioral therapy for chronic insomnia disorder delivered via an automated media-rich web application. Sleep 2012;35:769–81.

40. Lancee J, van den Bout J, van Straten A, et al. Internet-delivered or mailed self-help treatment for insomnia? A randomized waiting-list controlled trial. Behav Res Ther 2012;50:22–9.

41. Ho FYY, Chung KF, Yeung WF, et al. Weekly brief phone support in self-help cognitive behavioral therapy for insomnia disorder: relevance to adherence and efficacy. Behav Res Ther 2014;63:147–56.

42. Van Straten A, Emmelkamp J, De Wit J, et al. Guided Internet-delivered cognitive behavioural treatment for insomnia: a randomized trial. Psychol Med 2014;44:1521–32.

43. Lancee J, Eisma MC, van Straten A, et al. Sleep-related safety behaviors and dysfunctional beliefs mediate the efficacy of online CBT for insomnia: a randomized controlled trial. Cogn Behav Ther 2015;44:406–22.

44. Thiart H, Ebert DD, Lehr D, et al. Internet-based cognitive behavioral therapy for insomnia: a health economic evaluation. Sleep 2016;39:1769.

45. Bernstein AM, Allexandre D, Bena J, et al. "Go! to sleep": a web-based therapy for insomnia. Telemed J E Health 2017;23:590–9.

46. Hagatun S, Vedaa Ø, Nordgreen T, et al. The short-term efficacy of an unguided Internet-based cognitive-behavioral therapy for insomnia: a randomized controlled trial with a six-month nonrandomized follow-up. Behav Sleep Med 2019;17(2):137–55.

47. Horsch CH, Lancee J, Griffioen-Both F, et al. Mobile phone-delivered cognitive behavioral therapy for insomnia: a randomized waitlist controlled trial. J Med Internet Res 2017;9. https://doi.org/10.2196/jmir.6524.

48. Ritterband LM, Thorndike FP, Ingersoll KS, et al. Effect of a web-based cognitive behavior therapy for insomnia intervention with 1-year follow-up: a randomized clinical trial. JAMA Psychiatry 2017;74:68–75.

49. de Bruin EJ, Bögels SM, Oort FJ, et al. Efficacy of cognitive behavioral therapy for insomnia in adolescents: a randomized controlled trial with Internet therapy, group therapy and a waiting list condition. Sleep 2015;38:1913–26.

50. Espie CA, Emsley R, Kyle SD, et al. Effect of digital cognitive behavioral therapy for insomnia on health, psychological well-being, and sleep-related quality of life: a randomized clinical trial. JAMA Psychiatry 2018. https://doi.org/10.1001/jamapsychiatry.2018.2745.

51. Freeman D, Sheaves B, Goodwin GM, et al. The effects of improving sleep on mental health (OASIS): a randomised controlled trial with mediation analysis. Lancet Psychiatry 2017;4:749–58.

52. Lancee J, van Straten A, Morina N, et al. Guided online or face-to-face cognitive behavioral treatment for insomnia: a randomized wait-list controlled trial. Sleep 2016;39:183–91.

53. Van der Zweerde T, Van Straten A, Effting M, et al. Does online insomnia treatment reduce depressive symptoms? A randomized controlled trial in individuals with both insomnia and depressive symptoms. Psychol Med 2019;49(3):501–9.

54. Kaldo V, Jernelöv S, Blom K, et al. Guided Internet cognitive behavioral therapy for insomnia compared to a control treatment–a randomized trial. Behav Res Ther 2015;71:90–100.

55. Thiart H, Lehr D, Ebert DD, et al. Log in and breathe out: Internet-based recovery training for sleepless employees with work-related strain–results of a randomized controlled trial. Scand J Work Environ Health 2015;41:164–74.

56. Chow PI, Ingersoll KS, Thorndike FP, et al. Cognitive mechanisms of sleep outcomes in a randomized clinical trial of Internet-based cognitive behavioral therapy for insomnia. Sleep Med 2018;47:77–85.

57. Blom K, Jernelöv S, Kraepelien M, et al. Internet treatment addressing either insomnia or depression, for patients with both diagnoses: a randomized trial. Sleep 2015;38:267–77.

58. Spek V, Cuijpers PI, Nyklíček I, et al. Internet-based cognitive behaviour therapy for symptoms of depression and anxiety: a meta-analysis. Psychol Med 2007;33:319–28.

59. Lancee J, van den Bout J, Sorbi MJ, et al. Motivational support provided via email improves the effectiveness of Internet-delivered self-help treatment for insomnia: a randomized trial. Behav Res Ther 2013;51:797–805.

60. Jernelöv S, Lekander M, Blom K, et al. Efficacy of a behavioral self-help treatment with or without therapist guidance for co-morbid and primary insomnia—a randomized controlled trial. BMC Psychiatry 2012;12:5.

61. Zachariae R, Lyby MS, Ritterband LM, et al. Efficacy of Internet-delivered cognitive-behavioral therapy for insomnia–a systematic review and meta-analysis of randomized controlled trials. Sleep Med Rev 2016;30:1–10.

62. Andersson G, Cuijpers P. Internet-based and other computerized psychological treatments for adult depression: a meta-analysis. Cogn Behav Ther 2009;38:196–205.

63. Ritterband LM, Thorndike FP, Gonder-Frederick LA, et al. Efficacy of an Internet-based behavioral intervention for adults with insomnia. Arch Gen Psychiatry 2009;66:692–8.

64. Christensen H, Batterham PJ, Gosling JA, et al. Effectiveness of an online insomnia program (SHUTi) for prevention of depressive episodes (the GoodNight Study): a randomised controlled trial. Lancet Psychiatry 2016;3:333–41.

65. Bostock S, Luik AI, Espie CA. Sleep and productivity benefits of digital cognitive behavioral therapy for insomnia: a randomized controlled trial conducted in the workplace environment. J Occup Environ Med 2016;58:683–9.

66. Barnes CM, Miller JA, Bostock S. Helping employees sleep well: effects of cognitive behavioral therapy for insomnia on work outcomes. J Appl Psychol 2017;102:104.

67. Cheng P, Luik AI, Fellman-Couture C, et al. Efficacy of digital CBT for insomnia to reduce depression across demographic groups: a randomized trial. Psychol Med 2019;49:491–500.

68. Pigeon WR, Bishop TM, Krueger KM. Insomnia as a precipitating factor in new onset mental illness: a systematic review of recent findings. Curr Psychiatry Rep 2017;19:44.

69. Li MJ, Kechter A, Olmstead RE, et al. Sleep and mood in older adults: coinciding changes in insomnia and depression symptoms. Int Psychogeriatr 2018;30:431–5.

70. Carney CE, Segal ZV, Edinger JD, et al. A comparison of rates of residual insomnia symptoms following pharmacotherapy or cognitive-

behavioral therapy for major depressive disorder. J Clin Psychiatry 2007;68:254–60.

71. Ballesio A, Aquino MRJV, Feige B, et al. The effectiveness of behavioural and cognitive behavioural therapies for insomnia on depressive and fatigue symptoms: a systematic review and network meta-analysis. Sleep Med Rev 2017;37:114–29.

72. Gebara MA, Siripong N, DiNapoli EA, et al. Effect of insomnia treatments on depression: a systematic review and meta-analysis. Depress Anxiety 2018; 35:717–31.

73. Ye YY, Zhang YF, Chen J, et al. Internet-based cognitive behavioral therapy for insomnia (ICBT-i) improves comorbid anxiety and depression—a meta-analysis of randomized controlled trials. PLoS One 2015;10:e0142258.

74. Kyle SD, Crawford MR, Morgan K, et al. The Glasgow Sleep Impact Index (GSII): a novel patient-centered measure for assessing sleep-related quality of life impairment in insomnia disorder. Sleep Med 2013;14:493–501.

75. Morin CM, Benca R. Chronic insomnia. Lancet 2012;379:1129–41.

76. Okajima I, Nakajima S, Ochi M, et al. Reducing dysfunctional beliefs about sleep does not significantly improve insomnia in cognitive behavioral therapy. PLoS One 2014;9:e102565.

77. Espie CA, Kyle SD, Miller CB, et al. Attribution, cognition and psychopathology in persistent insomnia disorder: outcome and mediation analysis from a randomized placebo-controlled trial of online cognitive behavioural therapy. Sleep Med 2014;15:913–7.

78. Harvey AG, Dong L, Bélanger L, et al. Mediators and treatment matching in behavior therapy, cognitive therapy and cognitive behavior therapy for chronic insomnia. J Consult Clin Psychol 2017;85: 975.

79. Norell-Clarke A, Tillfors M, Jansson-Fröjmark M, et al. How does cognitive behavioral therapy for insomnia work? An investigation of cognitive processes and time in bed as outcomes and mediators in a sample with insomnia and depressive symptomatology. Int J Cogn Ther 2017;10:304–29.

80. Lancee J, Effting M, Van der Zweerde T, et al. Cognitive processes mediate the effects of insomnia treatment: evidence from a randomized wait-list controlled trial. Sleep Med 2019;54:86–93.

81. Harvey AG. A cognitive model of insomnia. Behav Res Ther 2002;40:869–93.

82. Grist R, Cavanagh K. Computerised cognitive behavioural therapy for common mental health disorders, what works, for whom under what circumstances? A systematic review and meta-analysis. J Contemp Psychother 2013;43:243–51.

83. Espie CA, Bostock S, Kyle SD, et al. Who benefits from online CBT for insomnia? Factors associated with change in sleep efficiency in a large online treatment cohort. Sleep 2014;37:A205.

84. Yeung WF, Chung KF, Ho FYY, et al. Predictors of dropout from Internet-based self-help cognitive behavioral therapy for insomnia. Behav Res Ther 2015;73:19–24.

85. Bathgate CJ, Edinger J, Krystal AD. Insomnia patients with objective short sleep duration have a blunted response to cognitive behavioral therapy for insomnia. Sleep 2017;40.

86. Blom K, Jernelöv S, Lindefors N, et al. Facilitating and hindering factors in Internet-delivered treatment for insomnia and depression. Internet Interv 2016;4:51–60.

87. Dong L, Soehner AM, Bélanger L, et al. Treatment agreement, adherence, and outcome in cognitive behavioral treatments for insomnia. J Consult Clin Psychol 2018;86:294.

88. Webb TL, Joseph J, Yardley L, et al. Using the Internet to promote health behavior change: a systematic review and meta-analysis of the impact of theoretical basis, use of behavior change techniques, and mode of delivery on efficacy. J Med Internet Res 2010;12.

89. Wu JQ, Appleman ER, Salazar RD, et al. Cognitive behavioral therapy for insomnia comorbid with psychiatric and medical conditions: a meta-analysis. JAMA Intern Med 2015;175:1461–72.

90. Blanken TF, Benjamins JS, Borsboom D, et al. Robust insomnia disorder subtypes revealed by non-sleep-related traits and life history. Lancet Psychiatry 2019;6(2):151–63.

91. Castelnovo A, Ferri R, Punjabi NM, et al. The paradox of paradoxical insomnia: a theoretical review towards a unifying evidence-based definition. Sleep Med Rev 2018;44:70–82.

92. Perlis ML, Giles DE, Mendelson WB, et al. Psychophysiological insomnia: the behavioural model and a neurocognitive perspective. J Sleep Res 1997;6: 179–88.

93. Riemann D, Spiegelhalder K, Feige B, et al. The hyperarousal model of insomnia: a review of the concept and its evidence. Sleep Med Rev 2010; 14:19–31.

94. Schwartz DR, Carney CE. Mediators of cognitive-behavioral therapy for insomnia: a review of randomized controlled trials and secondary analysis studies. Clin Psychol Rev 2012;32:664–75.

95. Sunnhed R, Jansson-Fröjmark M. Are changes in worry associated with treatment response in cognitive behavioral therapy for insomnia? Cogn Behav Ther 2014;43:1–11.

96. Okuji Y, Matsuura M, Kawasaki N, et al. Prevalence of insomnia in various psychiatric diagnostic categories. Psychiatry Clin Neurosci 2002;56:239–40.

97. Kazdin AE. Understanding how and why psychotherapy leads to change. Psychother Res 2009; 19:418–28.

98. Blanken TF, Van der Zweerde T, Van Straten A, et al. Introducing Network Intervention Analysis to investigate sequential, symptom-specific treatment effects: a demonstration in co-occurring insomnia and depression. Psychother Psychosom 2019; 88(1):52–4.

99. Vincent N, Walsh K, Lewycky S. Determinants of success for computerized cognitive behavior therapy: examination of an insomnia program. Behav Sleep Med 2013;11:328–42.

100. Espie CA, Bostock S, Kyle SD, et al. Who benefits from online CBT for insomnia? Factors associated with change in sleep efficiency in a large online treatment cohort. Sleep 2014;37:A205.

101. Watanabe N, Furukawa TA, Shimodera S, et al. Cost-effectiveness of cognitive behavioral therapy for insomnia comorbid with depression: analysis of a randomized controlled trial. Psychiatry Clin Neurosci 2015;69:335–43.

102. De Bruin EJ, van Steensel FJ, Meijer AM. Cost-effectiveness of group and Internet cognitive behavioral therapy for insomnia in adolescents: results from a randomized controlled trial. Sleep 2016;39:1571–81.

103. Van der Zweerde T, Lancee J, Slottje P, et al. Cost-effectiveness of i-Sleep, a guided online CBT intervention, for patients with insomnia in general practice: protocol of a pragmatic randomized controlled trial. BMC Psychiatry 2016;85.

104. Coulson NS, Smedley R, Bostock S, et al. The pros and cons of getting engaged in an online social community embedded within digital cognitive behavioral therapy for insomnia: survey among users. J Med Internet Res 2016;18. https://doi.org/10.2196/jmir.5654.

105. Siversten B, Vedaa Ø, Nordgreen T. The future of insomnia treatment—the challenge of implementation. Sleep 2013;36:303–4.

Prescription Drugs Used in Insomnia

Sylvie Dujardin, MD[a], Angelique Pijpers, MD, PhD[a], Dirk Pevernagie, MD, PhD[a,b,]*

KEYWORDS

- Chronic insomnia • Prescription drugs • Pharmacotherapy • Sleep-effect

KEY POINTS

- Several prescription drugs are available that at least temporarily improve sleep duration and continuity, objectively and subjectively, with acceptable side effects.
- Prescription drugs used for insomnia promote sleep by a limited number of different mechanisms: enhancing GABAergic neurotransmission, antagonizing receptors for the wake-promoting monoamines, or binding the melatonin receptors. Orexin receptor antagonists comprise a new class of hypnotic drugs.
- The ideal sleeping pill still does not exist.
- When available, cognitive behavioral therapy for insomnia remains the first-line therapy for chronic insomnia.

INTRODUCTION

Various studies have shown the efficacy of cognitive behavioral therapy for insomnia (CBT-I) and were recently confirmed by meta-analysis.[1] The American Academy of Sleep Medicine (AASM) clinical practice guideline and the European guideline for the treatment of insomnia state that this nonpharmacologic therapeutic approach is the treatment of choice for chronic insomnia in adults, regardless of age.[2,3] By acting on different sleep mechanisms, CBT-I helps to tilt the delicate neurobiologic balance from wakefulness to sleep.

Prescription of pharmacologic treatment is to be considered when CBT-I is not available or not effective. In the acute phase of CBT-I, adding pharmacotherapy may have a slightly better effect compared with CBT-I alone, provided the medication is discontinued in the maintenance phase of CBT-I.[4] However, pharmacotherapy is not indicated for chronic use and efforts at discontinuation should be made when this is the case.[3]

Moreover, discontinuation may improve rather than worsen the effects of CBT-I.[5]

Many studies have been conducted to evaluate the pharmacologic treatment of chronic insomnia. Unfortunately, large randomized controlled trials (RCTs) with representative patient populations are lacking. Studies are often weak from a methodologic point of view and, in addition, difficult to compare because of differences in patient samples, diagnostic and inclusion criteria, and outcome criteria. Finally, many studies are sponsored by the industry, which could lead to publication bias.

It is important to keep in mind that in the treatment of insomnia, whether pharmacologic or behavioral, a substantial placebo effect may confound clinical results. In a meta-analysis, the placebo effect was contended to account for almost two-thirds of the drug effect.[6] A recent meta-analysis comparing placebo with no treatment groups confirms the placebo effect in the subjective but not objective sleep measures.[7]

This article originally appeared in June, 2018 issue of *Sleep Medicine Clinics* (Volume 13, Issue 2).
The authors have no disclosures to report.
a Sleep Medicine Center Kempenhaeghe, PO Box 61, Heeze 5590 AB, The Netherlands; b Department of Internal Medicine and Paediatrics, Faculty of Medicine and Health Sciences, Ghent University, Corneel Heymanslaan 10, 9000 Ghent, Belgium
* Corresponding author. Sleep Medicine Center Kempenhaeghe, PO Box 61, Heeze 5590 AB, The Netherlands.
E-mail address: pevernagied@kempenhaeghe.nl

sleep.theclinics.com

This article provides an overview of pharmacologic and biologic features of different hypnotic drugs, with a reference to medical practice in adults with chronic insomnia without comorbidities. The focus is on prescription drugs and discussed are benzodiazepines (BZDs), non-BZD BZD receptor agonists (NBBzRAs), melatonin receptor agonists, orexin receptor antagonists, antidepressants, and antipsychotics. Over-the-counter preparations, including antihistamines, are outside the scope of this article. The main characteristics of the reviewed drugs are summarized in **Table 1**.

The reviewed compounds all have an impact on the neurobiologic processes of sleep and may even change its normal macrostructure and microstructure. Because hypnotic drugs act via different pathways within the central nervous system, they have dissimilar neuropharmacologic profiles. Remarkably, these differential properties have not been translated into evidence that would facilitate clinical decision making based on the pharmacologic signature of the drug.[8]

Practical advice for optimization of drug treatment is outside the scope of this article. For further study, we refer the reader to other references.[9]

BENZODIAZEPINES
Neuropharmacology

BZD receptor agonists constitute the most important class of drugs prescribed for insomnia and encompass BZDs and NBBzRAs. Both groups intensify γ-aminobutyric acid (GABA)$_A$-mediated neurotransmission and are therefore GABA$_A$ agonists.

GABA is the most important and abundant inhibitory neurotransmitter in the nervous system. Stimulating GABAergic action promotes sleep, but the exact locations in the brain are not yet fully disclosed.[10] At very high dose, GABA$_A$ agonists suppress c-Fos expression in the entire central nervous system, including the sleep-wake control centers.[11] At lower dose, GABA$_A$ agonists increase c-Fos expression in ventrolateral preoptic area (VLPO) neurons, albeit less than in natural sleep. The VLPO (and the median preoptic nucleus) contain sleep-active GABAergic neurons that send anatomic projections to the arousal systems, in which GABA release has been shown to increase during sleep.[12] Besides, systemic injection of GABA$_A$ receptor agonists consistently suppressed the expression of c-Fos in the tuberomammillary nucleus (TMN).[11] The VLPO and the TMN mutually inhibit each other.[12] Thus GABA$_A$ agonists might stimulate sleep through reinforcing the relief of the inhibition of the VLPO

by the TMN.[11] Microinjections of triazolam into the perifornical hypothalamus containing hypocretin neurons significantly increased sleep.[13] BZDs might thus also act via inhibition of the hypocretin wake-promoting system.

Pharmacologic Properties

BZDs act as positive allosteric modulators of GABA$_A$ receptors: they increase the effect of GABA binding. GABA$_A$ receptors are located post-synaptically and consist of a pentameric complex forming a chloride channel. When the GABA is released in the synaptic cleft, the chloride channel opens. With BZD, the GABA$_A$ receptor increases the frequency of opening of its chloride-channel. By this mechanism, the cellular membrane of the post-synaptic neuron becomes hyperpolarized, thus inhibiting the activation of the neuron.[14]

The GABA$_A$ receptor carrying the α_1 subunit is believed to be the mediator of the sedative and amnesic effects of BZDs. The anxiolytic, myorelaxant, motor-impairing, and ethanol-potentiating effects are attributed to GABA$_A$ receptor, carrying other α subunits (α subunits 2, 3, 5).[15] Currently available BZDs are nonselective for GABA$_A$ receptors with different α subunits.[14]

Clinical Effects

BZDs have a positive effect on objective and subjective sleep parameters of people with insomnia. Recently, a meta-analysis was performed on two BZDs: triazolam and temazepam.[2] Two studies including a total of 72 patients addressed subjective sleep latencies (SL) and total sleep time (TST).[16,17] In the second study of 34 patients, objective SL and TST also were assessed.[17] Temazepam, 15 mg, decreased subjective SL by 20 minutes and objective SL by 37 minutes versus placebo. It increased subjective TST by 64 minutes and objective TST by 99 minutes versus placebo. The evidence for efficiency of triazolam is scarce. In a study of only subjective data with triazolam, 0.25 mg, improvements of subjective SL and TST (respectively −9 minutes and −25 minutes versus placebo) were not clinically relevant.[18]

Tolerance to hypnotic effect is a frequent manifestation in chronic use of BZDs. It has been shown that after 24 weeks of chronic BZD intake, the subjective sleep quality drops to a level below baseline. This was observed in BZDs with short and long half-life (lorazepam and nitrazepam, respectively).[19] Rebound insomnia is the most frequent symptom following acute withdrawal of BZDs, occurring in up to 71% of subjects.[20] Next to tolerance, dependence is of concern. The prevalence of misuse and dependency of BZDs and

Table 1
Prescription drugs used for insomnia: main characteristics

Drug (Class)	Predominant Mode of Action for Sedative Effect	T_{max} (h)	$T_{1/2}$ (h)	Recommended Use	Dose[a] (mg)	FDA Approved/ CSA IV
BZD						
Triazolam	Nonselective $GABA_A$ agonism	1–2	2–6	Sleep onset insomnia	0.125–0.25	+/+
Temazepam	Nonselective $GABA_A$ agonism	1–2	8–15	Sleep onset and sleep maintenance insomnia	7.5–30	+/+
Quazepam	Nonselective $GABA_A$ agonism	2–3	48–120	Not recommended		+/+
Estazolam	Nonselective $GABA_A$ agonism	1.5–2	8–24	Not recommended		+/+
Flurazepam	Nonselective $GABA_A$ agonism	1.5–4.5	48–120	Not recommended		+/+
NBBzRA						
Zopiclone	$GABA_A$ - $\alpha_{1,2,3}$ agonism	1.5–2	5	Sleep onset and sleep maintenance insomnia	3.75–7.5	+/+
Eszopiclone	$GABA_A$ - $\alpha_{1,2,3}$ agonism[b]	1–1.5	6	Sleep onset and sleep maintenance insomnia	1–3	+/+
Zolpidem	$GABA_A$ - α_1 agonism	1–2	2.6	Sleep onset and sleep maintenance insomnia	1.75–10 6.25–12.5 ER	+/+
Zaleplon	$GABA_A$ - α_1 agonism	~ 1	0.7–1.4	Sleep onset insomnia	5–20	+/+
Orexin receptor antagonists						
Suvorexant	OxR1 and OxR2 antagonism	2–3.5	12	Sleep onset and sleep maintenance insomnia	5–20	+/+
Melatonin and melatonin receptor agonists						
Ramelteon	Melatonin receptor agonism	0.75–1	1–2.5	Sleep onset insomnia	8	+/–
Melatonin	Melatonin receptor agonism	~0.75	~0.75	Not recommended		NA
Circadin®	Melatonin receptor agonism	0.75–3	3.5–4	Sleep onset and sleep maintenance insomnia, age >55 y	2	–/–[c]
Antidepressants						
Doxepin	H1 antagonism	2–8	20	Sleep maintenance insomnia	3–6	+/–
Amitriptyline	H1, alpha1, M1 antagonism	2–8	30	Not recommended		–/–
Trazodone	5HT2A, alpha1 antagonism	1–2	9	Not recommended		–/–
Mirtazapine	H1, 5HT2A/2C antagonism	1–3	25	Not recommended		–/–
Antipsychotics						

(continued on next page)

Table 1
(continued)

Drug (Class)	Predominant Mode of Action for Sedative Effect	T_{max} (h)	$T_{1/2}$ (h)	Recommended Use	Dose[a] (mg)	FDA Approved/ CSA IV
Quetiapine	H1 but also alpha1, M1, 5HT, D2 antagonism	1–2	6	Not recommended		–/–
Olanzapine	H1 but also 5HT, M1, D2, alpha1 antagonism	4–6	20–54	Not recommended		–/–

Abbreviations: Alpha1, alpha-1 adrenergic receptor; CSA IV, Controlled Substance Act schedule IV controlled substances; D2, dopamine receptor D2; ER, extended release; FDA approved, U.S. Food and Drug Administration approved for the treatment of insomnia; GABA, γ-aminobutyric acid; $GABA_A$ - $\alpha_{1,2,3}$, $GABA_A$ receptor alpha subunits 1,2,3; H1, histamine receptor type 1; 5HT, 5-hydroxytryptamine (serotonin); M1, Muscarinic acetylcholine receptor 1; NA, not applicable; OxR1-2, orexin receptors type 1 and 2.

[a] The lowest effective dose should be used to minimize side effects.
[b] Precise mechanism unknown.
[c] European Medicines Agency approval.
Data from Refs.[26,31,74,77,97–99]

related Z-drugs has been estimated to be 5% in a German population. Approximately 20% of BZD users have a problematic intake. Overall, 50% of BZD users list insomnia as the reason for taking the drug.[20]

Important to highlight is that older adults are especially vulnerable, because BZDs increase the risk of cognitive impairment, delirium, falls, fractures, and motor vehicle accidents. Therefore, BZDs of any type should be avoided for the treatment of insomnia, according to the American Geriatrics Society Beers Criteria for Potentially Inappropriate Medication Use in Older Adults.[21] Sleep apnea is a contraindication for BZDs, although the available evidence indicates the effects on respiration are moderate.[22]

BZDs have an effect on the sleep macroarchitecture. Studies on healthy volunteers and those with insomnia have consistently shown that BZDs reduce the percentage of slow wave sleep.[23] Percentage of stage 2 sleep increases, and spectral power of the spindle frequency range (11–14 Hz) is enhanced.[24,25] The effect on rapid eye movement (REM) sleep is variable and less pronounced. In some individuals, a reduction of the amount of REM sleep has been reported.[26]

It seems paradoxic that BZDs improve subjective sleep quality while they decrease slow wave sleep. This paradox can possibly be explained by observations on the microstructure of sleep. In a recent study, the sleep of six chronic BZD abusers versus healthy control subjects was compared. The abusers had significantly more awakenings but fewer fast frequency arousals and lower indexes of non-REM (NREM) instability as measured by Cyclic Alternating Pattern rate. It has been hypothesized that chronic BZD use may affect the function of the thalamic filter. In normal subjects, incoming stimuli are able to produce arousals without awakenings. Potentially, the thalamic filter of chronic BZD users is less adaptive: the response to stimuli is either no reaction (no arousal) or a full awakening.[27]

Medical Prescription

Five BZDs are approved by the Food and Drug Administration (FDA) as prescription insomnia drugs: (1) quazepam, (2) estazolam, (3) flurazepam, (4) triazolam, and (5) temazepam. In Europe, approval varies across countries.

American guidelines support the prescription of triazolam, 0.25 mg, for sleep onset, and temazepam, 15 mg, for sleep onset and sleep maintenance insomnia versus no treatment in adults.[2] Because of lack of data appropriate for statistical analysis, the AASM could not give clinical practice recommendations for the other three FDA-approved drugs (quazepam, estazolam, flurazepam). Their long elimination half-life (>15 hours) is not favorable for use in insomnia.

In European guidelines, the use of BZDs is recommended for short-term treatment (less than 4 weeks), if CBT-I is not effective or not available. Shorter half-life drugs are favored and intermittent dosing is strongly recommended. Long-term treatment of insomnia with BZDs is not recommended because of lack of evidence, side effects, and risks of tolerance and dependence.[3] Prescription should be limited to cases where the impairment is clinically significant and the benefits are expected to outweigh the potential harms. When starting a prescription treatment, the clinician is encouraged to discuss the temporary nature of the prescription with the patient.[28]

NONBENZODIAZEPINE RECEPTOR AGONISTS
Neuropharmacology

NBBzRAs are thought to have a somewhat higher affinity for the GABA$_A$ α1 and α2 receptor subtypes or bind to the complex in a different way than BZDs. Therefore, NBBzRAs are considered to have a more favorable benefit-risk profile (fewer side effects, lower abuse potential) compared with BZDs.[29] The GABA$_A$ α_1 receptor subunit is associated with the most hypnotic effects. These receptors are primarily found on the lamina IV of the sensorimotor cortical regions, substantia nigra pars reticulata, olfactory bulb, ventral thalamic complex, the molecular layer of the cerebellum, pons, inferior colliculus, and globus pallidus.[30] This class of NBBzRAs, also referred to as "Z-drugs," comprise three compounds: (1) zopiclone and eszopiclone, (2) zolpidem, and (3) zaleplon.

Pharmacologic Properties

NBBzRAs are positive allosteric modulators at GABA$_A$ receptors, but they have a chemical structure that is unrelated to other hypnotics, including BZDs. They are all rapidly absorbed after oral administration. NBBzRAs, like BZDs, are primarily metabolized in the liver by the cytochrome P-450 (CYP) 3A4 enzyme.

Zopiclone and its active stereoisomer eszopiclone belong to the group of cyclopyrrolones. They bind to the GABA$_A$ $\alpha_{1, 2, 3}$ subunits. Eszopiclone has a time to maximal concentration (Tmax) of approximately 1 to 1.5 hours, with a half-life time of approximately 6 hours. Zopiclone has a Tmax of 1.5 to 2 hours and a half-life time of approximately 5 hours.

Zolpidem is an imidazopyridine and in therapeutic dosage binds selectively to the GABA$_A$ α_1 subunit. Tmax is 1 to 2 hours, with an additional 30 minutes for the extended-release formula. It has a short half-life time of approximately 2.6 hours.[31,32]

Zaleplon is a pyrazolopyrimidine. In therapeutic dosage, it binds selectively to the GABA$_A$ α_1 subunit. T max is 0.7 to 1.4 hours. It has an ultrashort half-life time of 1 hour and has therapeutic effects usually within 5 to 15 minutes after ingestion.[31,32]

Clinical Effects

Clinical effects of NBBzRAs in treatment of chronic insomnia, including discontinuation effects, are comparable with BZDs.[33,34] Side effects are partial comparable with BZDs.[35] Most commonly reported side effects are amnesia, dizziness, sedation, and headache.[36] An unpleasant, altered, or metallic taste is a typical side effect of (es)zopiclone.[37,38] Somnambulism has been reported with the use of zolpidem and zaleplon.[39,40] Like BZDs, Z-drugs have a potentially higher risk of falls, fractures, and injuries in elderly.[41] Data on whether or not Z-drugs are associated with an increased risk of motor vehicle accidents are controversial.[42,43]

Studies evaluating objective and subjective improvements of sleep parameters of insomniacs using NBBzRAs usually report favorable outcomes. However, many of those studies have methodologic flaws, making it difficult to draw definite conclusions.[2,36]

Of the cyclopyrrolones, the clinical effects of eszopiclone are more extensively studied than those of zopiclone. However, only six studies fit the criteria for systematic review in the AASM clinical practice guideline. In summary, a mean reduction in SL of 14 minutes was seen, TST improved up to 57 minutes, sleep quality was better, and there was less WASO. Studies with 2 mg eszopiclone yielded better statistical significant results than the 3 mg dose.[2]

Zolpidem, 10 mg, showed a mean reduction of SL of 5 to 12 minutes and improvement of TST by 29 minutes. In addition, improvements were seen in WASO, but not in sleep efficiency or number of awakenings.[2]

For zaleplon, only two studies met the inclusion criteria for review, of which one only reported subjective outcomes. Objective polysomnography data showed a significant reduction of SL of approximately 10 minutes. There were no significant differences in TST or sleep quality compared with placebo.[2]

Medical Prescription

The therapeutic dose of zopiclone ranges from 3.75 to 7.5 mg and of eszopiclone from 1 to 3 mg. The therapeutic dose of zolpidem mainly depends on the route of administration (oral tablets, spray, sublingual) varying from 1.75 to 10 mg or 6.25 to 12.5 mg extended-release tablets.[29]

Zaleplon is dosed at 5 to 20 mg. It is advised not to be taken within 4 hours of rise-time, because of the risk of residual sedation and memory impairment.[36] Because of its short half-life time, zaleplon is only suited for sleep-onset insomnia. The others are used for sleep onset and sleep maintenance insomnia. Eszopiclone is the only hypnotic sedative drug that is approved by the FDA for long-term use for the relief of insomnia.[37]

Availability and indication preferences for NBBzRAs vary worldwide. In the United States, NBBzRAs are considered as class IV drugs. As with BZDs and suvorexant, prescription of NBBzRAs should be considered only if nonpharmacologic treatments for insomnia are not available or ineffective. Similarly, prescription should be restricted to a short period of time and intermittent use is recommended when prescription is extended over a longer period of time. Like BDZ, caution should be taken when prescribing NBBzRAs to elderly and careful consideration in case of other drugs metabolized by CYP34A or simultaneous use of central nervous depressants.

OREXIN RECEPTOR ANTAGONISTS
Neuropharmacology

Orexin-producing neurons are located in specific parts of the hypothalamus. These neurons project to most parts of the brain and are active during wake. Orexins stabilize wake through a strong excitatory action on wake-promoting neurons. Orexin knockout mice have many more transitions among wake, NREM, and REM states than do wild-type mice, supporting this model. Similar patterns of sleep-wake disruption are present in human narcolepsy. In addition to promoting wakefulness, orexin plays a role in goal-directed, motivated behaviors.[44,45]

Pharmacologic Properties

There are two types of orexin receptors (OxR1 and OxR2), which are post-synaptic G-protein-coupled receptors. They are expressed in various parts of the brain: OxR1s are highly expressed in the locus coeruleus and OxR2s in the histaminergic TMN.[46,47] There are also two types of orexin neurotransmitters: type A and B (also known as hypocretin 1 and 2). Orexin neurotransmitter type A can bind to OxR1 and OxR2, whereas orexin neurotransmitter type B selectively binds to OxR2. The exact pathways by which dual orexin (hypocretin) receptor antagonists (DORAs) promote sleep, without causing narcoleptic features, are unknown. Presumably antagonism of OxR2s decreases histaminergic activity in the hypothalamus, and in addition antagonism of OxR1 decreases arousal from motivational states, therefore promoting sleep.

Suvorexant has a Tmax of approximately 2 to 3.5 hours, depending on the ingestion of food. It binds to plasma proteins and has a half-life time of approximately 12 hours. Its kinetics are not age-dependent, but gender and weight do play a role. Suvorexant is predominantly metabolized by CYP3A4 enzyme and some involvement of CYP2C19. Approximately 66% is eliminated in feces and 23% in urine.[48]

Clinical Effects

Orexin receptor antagonists are a novel drug class used to treat insomnia. So far, only suvorexant, a DORA, is registered in the United States, Japan, and Australia for the treatment of insomnia. Clinical data available for suvorexant are derived from a limited number of pivotal trials that could be subject to publication bias.[49–51]

In summary, clinical significant improvement was most noticeable in improvement of wake after sleep onset by 16 to 28 minutes, compared with placebo. This might favor suvorexant for sleep maintenance insomnia. However, the total number of awakenings was not statistically altered. TST increased by 10 minutes, compared with placebo, but this was not clinically significant. At higher doses (20 mg), it might improve sleep onset latency, with an average reduction of 22.3 minutes. Sleep efficiency at 20 mg increased on average with 10.4%. Available data were objectively controlled by polysomnography. Subjectively, TST improved but did not reach clinical significance.[49,51]

Reported side effects include somnolence, fatigue, abnormal dreams, and dry mouth, but these were not significantly different from placebo.[49–52] Polysomnographic data of patients with insomnia show a reduced REM latency and an increased REM sleep duration compared with placebo. There is a limited increase of the delta power band and a limited decrease in the γ and β power bands. The largest differences were seen in the first night and diminished over months 1 and 3. The clinical significance of these observations remains unclear.[53]

It should be noted that most of the presented data had an imprecision bias, mainly because of large confidence intervals. Furthermore, studies were sponsored by industry.

Medical Prescription

Suvorexant is FDA-approved for the treatment of insomnia characterized by sleep onset and/or sleep maintenance difficulties. The AASM clinical practice guideline recommends suvorexant only for the treatment of sleep maintenance insomnia.[2] The recommended starting dose is 10 mg, taken approximately 30 minutes before bed time, with sleep opportunity of at least 7 hours. The drug is available in 5, 10, 15, and 20 mg tablets, with 20 mg being the maximum advised daily dose. Dose reduction should be considered in obesity. When patients use moderate CYP3A4 inhibitors, the recommended starting dose is 5 mg, and the highest dose should not exceed 10 mg.[52]

The use of suvorexant is not advised in patients using strong CYP3A4 inhibitors, those with severe hepatic impairment, or with a diagnosis of narcolepsy. There are no available data on use during pregnancy or lactation, which should therefore be avoided. It is not recommended to use suvorexant simultaneously with other central nervous system depressants, including alcohol. Available data suggest that suvorexant has no major respiratory depressant effects.[54–56] However, it is unclear if this is still the case in high-risk patients (severe sleep apnea, severe chronic obstructive pulmonary disease, concomitant use of muscle relaxants). To date, there are only a few postmarketing case reports on side effects.[57,58]

MELATONIN AND MELATONIN RECEPTOR AGONISTS
Neuropharmacology

Endogenous melatonin is secreted by the pineal gland. Melatonin secretion typically starts in late afternoon, reaches a peak in the first half of the night, and disappears on awakening. As such, melatonin secretion is a hormonal signal of the central nervous system that provides different end-organs with information on the nyctohemeral phase of the circadian cycle. The physiologic function of melatonin in humans has not been fully disclosed. It is hypothesized that melatonin entrains peripheral oscillators, but in vivo confirmation of this hypothesis is difficult, given the redundancy within the circadian system.[59]

Neurons of the suprachiasmaticus nucleus carry melatonin receptors, indicating that melatonin can act on the central master clock itself. In in vitro studies, exogenous melatonin had two distinct effects on neurons of the suprachiasmaticus nucleus: an acute inhibitory effect on neuronal firing and a phase-shifting effect.[59] The acute inhibitory effect may mediate the sleep-promoting properties of melatonin, whereas the phase-shifting properties may induce a delay or advance of the sleep phase, depending on the time of administration with respect to the actual circadian phase.[60,61]

Pharmacologic Properties

Natural melatonin and ramelteon are ligands with great affinity for MT1 and MT2 receptors.[61] They are present in various parts of the brain, but also in other tissues, including cardiac and peripheral vessels, retina, kidneys, and other organs.[62]

The pharmacokinetics of melatonin are characterized by a low and variable bioavailability (on average, 15%). Immediate-release melatonin has Tmax and elimination half-life close to 45 minutes.[63,64] The Tmax of prolonged-release melatonin is affected by food intake, and ranges from 45 minutes to 3 hours in the fed state. Its elimination half-life is 3.5 to 4 hours.

The pharmacokinetics of ramelteon are characterized by rapid absorption, with Tmax and elimination half-life, respectively, approximately 1 and 1.5 hours.[65]

Clinical Effects

Experience from patients in whom pinealectomy was performed for medical reasons has shown that melatonin is not an essential factor for inducing and maintaining sleep. Many of these patients do not experience changes in subjective sleep quality or polysomnographic sleep variables following resection of the pineal gland.[66]

The natural melatonin synthesis may be reduced by drugs (eg, BZDs, nonsteroidal anti-inflammatory drugs, calcium channel blockers, and β-blockers).[67] Oral administration of melatonin or ramelteon may reduce subjective SL and increase perceived sleep quality, although effects on sleep maintenance and duration are equivocal.[68]

In a dosage up to 10 mg given at 11:30 PM, short-acting melatonin induced no significant effect on sleep architecture in healthy subjects.[69] Neither were major changes in sleep architecture observed following exogenous administration of 2 mg melatonin with prolonged-release formulation.[70] In a clinical trial, ramelteon increased the percentage of time spent in N2 by approximately 2% points, at the expense of the percentage of time spent in slow wave sleep, but this is unlikely to be clinically significant.[71]

Melatonin and its agonists are considered safe drugs. Overall, side effects are not different from placebo.[2] One potential serious adverse effect with ramelteon, 8 mg, was a single case of reversible leukopenia out of 227 subjects with insomnia treated with the drug. Six-month nightly administration of prolonged-release 2 mg dose in a population of 65 to 80 year olds, and of ramelteon, 8 mg, in adults, did not produce tolerance, rebound insomnia, or withdrawal effects.[71,72] Biologic effects of melatonin outside sleep have been reviewed elsewhere.[61,73]

Medical Prescription

Ramelteon is FDA-approved for the treatment of insomnia characterized by difficulty with sleep onset.[74] Prolonged-release melatonin (Circadin®) is European Medicines Agency–approved for the short-term treatment of primary insomnia characterized by poor quality of sleep, in patients aged 55 or older. In addition, short-acting melatonin is available over-the-counter in many countries. Although evidence is limited, melatonin or ramelteon may be indicated to treat sleep-onset insomnia, because it slightly shortens the SL of patients with insomnia more than placebo.[2]

SEDATING ANTIDEPRESSANTS
Neuropharmacology

Sedating antidepressants promote sleep by antagonizing the effect of wake-promoting monoamines, including histamine, acetylcholine, noradrenaline, and serotonin. Evidence of the sleep-promoting effect of antagonizing histamine (H_1), muscarinic acetylcholine, noradrenaline receptors (α_1-adrenergic) and serotonin ($5HT_2$) receptors has been reviewed in a previous issue of *Sleep Medicine Clinics*.[75]

The neurons producing these monoamines are located in the ascending arousal system in the upper brainstem, its extension into the caudal hypothalamus, and in the basal forebrain. In wake (but not in REM sleep), histamine is released by neurons of the TMN and adjacent posterior hypothalamus, noradrenaline by neurons of the locus coeruleus, and serotonin by neurons of the dorsal and median raphe nuclei. Dopamine neurons located in the ventral periaqueductal gray matter are also part of this arousal system.[12]

Cholinergic neurons in the laterodorsal tegmental and pedunculopontine tegmental nuclei and the basal forebrain are active in wakefulness and REM sleep. Neurons forming the laterodorsal tegmental and pedunculopontine tegmental nuclei constitute an important modulator of the thalamic relay. In general, arousal systems project on multiple regions of the cerebrum, including the hypothalamus, thalamus, limbic system, and neocortex.[12]

Pharmacologic Properties

Doxepin and amitriptyline are sedative tricyclic antidepressants (TCAs) that also affect sleep. At doses recommended for treatment of depression, they are potent boosters of serotonergic and noradrenergic neurotransmission by blocking serotonin (5HT) and noradrenaline reuptake. They have more effect on the 5HT than on the noradrenaline reuptake, in contrast with TCAs that have stimulating effects.[76] Furthermore, doxepin and amitriptyline block histamine H_1 receptors, which accounts for their sedative and weight gain effects. They inhibit α_1-adrenergic receptors,

causing hypotension, and muscarinic M_1 receptors, causing anticholinergic side effects.[29]

At low doses, doxepin and amitriptyline exert their sedating effect through potent H_1-antagonism. At 3 to 6 mg, doxepin almost acts as an H_1 selective antagonist. Low-dose amitriptyline is less selective and exhibits stronger anti-M_1 cholinergic as part of the sedating effect.[29]

Trazodone is chemically unrelated to tricyclic or other known antidepressant agents. Its antidepressant effect is probably caused by inhibition of serotonin uptake and $5HT_{2A/2C}$ antagonism. At lower (hypnotic) doses, $5HT_2$, α_1, and weak H_1 antagonism promotes sleep.[29,48]

Mirtazapine has a tetracyclic chemical structure. α_2-Antagonism results in disinhibition of 5HT and noradrenaline release. Therefore, mirtazapine is classified as a noradrenergic and specific serotonergic antidepressant. $5HT_{2A/2C}$ antagonism and potent H_1 antihistaminic action promote sleep.[48] The combined $5HT_{2C}$ and H_1 antagonism also promotes weight gain.[29] Contrarily to the TCAs, mirtazapine and trazodone have minimal to no effect on M_1 receptors.[48]

The pharmacokinetics of these drugs are diverse. Tmax is longer for doxepin and amitriptyline (2–8 hours) than for trazodone and mirtazapine (1–2 and 1–3 hours, respectively). Doxepin, amitriptyline, and mirtazapine all have elimination half-lives close to 24 hours. Trazodone has a significantly shorter elimination half-life of approximatively 8 to 9 hours.[77] Although the pharmacokinetic profile of trazodone is more apt for use in insomnia than the other antidepressant agents, residual sedation after awakening in the morning is a frequent complaint. Because of variability in clearance, trazodone may accumulate in some individuals over time.[48]

Clinical Effects

Doxepin has been shown to increase objective TST by 26 and 32 minutes (with the 3 and 6 mg dosage, respectively) mainly because of reductions in WASO.[2] Subjective increases in TST are comparable and maintained for up to 4 weeks.[78] Reductions in objective SL are less than clinical threshold with doxepin 3 mg and 6 mg. At these dosages, adverse effects are minimal.[2] Trials in the elderly population have shown no more adverse effects than placebo during up to 4 weeks of treatment with up to 6 mg and 12 weeks with 3 mg.[78–80]

Although a positive effect of amitriptyline has been shown on the sleep of depressed patients, there are no RCTs in the treatment of insomnia without comorbidities.[81]

Placebo-controlled studies of trazodone are also scarce in insomnia. In a study of patient-reported outcomes, trazodone, 50 mg, reduced subjective SL, TST, and WASO, but below threshold for clinical significance.[82] A polysomnography study of trazodone, 150 mg, administered to middle-aged self-reported poor sleepers failed to show a significant improvement in objective TST versus placebo, but confirms the subjective improvement in sleep quality.[83] Consistent with this observation, trazodone, 50 mg, administered to those with primary insomnia significantly improved the subjective ability to sleep. The change in polysomnographic variables was only significant for the number of night-time awakenings (20 awakenings after 7 days of placebo vs 13 after trazodone, 50 mg) and the amount of N1 sleep. Objective sleep efficiency was unchanged.[84]

There are no studies of mirtazapine in insomnia without comorbidities. In a study of depressed patients, TST improved and WASO decreased accordingly when compared with sleep parameters before mirtazapine administration, but there was no placebo control.[85] Acute administration of 30 mg mirtazapine to healthy volunteers did not improve TST versus placebo but improved other measures of sleep continuity.[86] Whether these findings are relevant for the sleep of those with insomnia is unproven.

Many antidepressants delay REM sleep and decrease its duration. This effect seems modest for low-dose doxepin, because it has been shown in some, but not all studies.[79,87] A study on amitriptyline, 75 mg, showed that the REM sleep period dropped to 19 minutes, versus 83 minutes with the use of placebo.[88] No significant REM sleep duration changes were shown for mirtazapine in healthy subjects or trazodone, 50 mg, in subjects with insomnia.[84,86]

In a minority of patients, antidepressants increase restless legs syndrome symptoms and/or periodic limb movements of sleep. This effect might be higher with mirtazapine and amitriptyline than with doxepin (at dose up to 50 mg) or trazodone, 100 mg.[89]

Medical Prescription

Doxepin, amitriptyline, trazodone, and mirtazapine are approved in the United States and many other countries as antidepressants. At much lower dose than needed for their antidepressant effect, they are prescribed for the treatment of insomnia. Only low-dose doxepin (3 to 6 mg) is FDA approved for that indication; any other use is off label.

In the American guidelines, the use of doxepin, 3 to 6 mg, is supported for sleep maintenance, but not for initiation of sleep. The use of amitriptyline, trazodone, or mirtazapine is not recommended.[2] The European guidelines report on sedating antidepressants as a group. These drugs are judged effective in the short-term treatment of insomnia, provided contraindications are carefully taken into account. Long-term treatment is not recommended.[3]

In older subjects, amitriptyline and doxepin greater than 6 mg are to be avoided, and mirtazapine is to be used with caution. Trazodone and doxepin up to 6 mg are not listed in the American Geriatrics Society Beers Criteria for Potentially Inappropriate Medication Use in Older Adults, and thus seem safer.[21] However, trazodone, 50 mg, slightly but significantly reduced next day memory, equilibrium, and muscle endurance versus placebo in subjects with primary insomnia younger than 65 years.[84]

ANTIPSYCHOTICS
Neuropharmacology

Antipsychotic drugs exert their sedative effects by antagonizing the activity of wake-stimulating neurotransmitters, similarly to the antidepressants.[75]

Pharmacologic Properties

All antipsychotic medications interact with dopamine D_2 receptors (most of them are D_2 blockers), and possess numerous other pharmacologic properties, among which various degrees of H_1 histamine, M_1 cholinergic, and α_1-adrenergic receptor antagonism. This triple action can be highly sedating.[29] The second-generation antipsychotics differ from the first generation, because they also possess $5HT_2$ antagonism. Therefore, they are expected to be better sleep promotors.[75]

Quetiapine is the most commonly used antipsychotic for insomnia.[90] Quetiapine is effective as an antipsychotic at doses of 300 to 800 mg. In much lower doses (25 to 50 mg), its hypnotic effect is preserved, because of its high affinity for H_1 receptors.[29]

Clinical Effects

The effects of antipsychotic medications on sleep have mostly been investigated in psychiatric patients. These studies are not relevant to insomnia without psychiatric comorbidity, and the doses given are often much higher than the ones needed for the sedating effect. Although quetiapine is used off label in insomnia, evidence is definitely lacking.[90] A small RCT including healthy people showed improvements in subjective and polysomnographic sleep with quetiapine, 25 mg and 100 mg.[91] In insomnia without psychiatric comorbidity, only one RCT has been published so far. In this study, seven patients took quetiapine, 25 mg daily, during 2 weeks versus six placebo control subjects. Compared with placebo, improvement of subjective TST and SL with quetiapine was not statistically significant.[92] Because of the small size of the study, no firm conclusion could be drawn. Although in these studies quetiapine, 25 to 75 mg, was well tolerated, a concern remains about serious adverse effects on the longer term, encompassing abuse, suicidal ideation, and metabolic adverse effects, even at low doses.[93,94] A significant increase in periodic leg movements during sleep was observed with quetiapine, 100 mg.[91]

No RCT exists on other antipsychotics prescribed for insomnia without psychiatric comorbidity.[94] Monti and colleagues[95] recently reviewed the effects of the second-generation antipsychotics in healthy subjects. The results were either nonsignificant or showed an improvement in measures of SL, WASO, and TST. Most consistent evidence of a positive effect on the sleep parameters of healthy subjects exists for olanzapine, 5 to 10 mg. Of note, the elimination half-life of olanzapine is more than 24 hours, whereas that of quetiapine is less than 8 hours.

Medical Prescription

Because of lack of evidence and potential harm even at low doses, antipsychotics are not approved or recommended for the treatment of insomnia without comorbidities.[3]

SUMMARY

Several prescription drugs are available that, at least temporarily, improve sleep duration and continuity objectively and subjectively, with acceptable side effects. Although new medication classes (eg, DORAs) are becoming available, the ideal sleeping pill still does not exist.

Will such a drug ever overthrow CBT-I as the first-line therapy for chronic insomnia? CBT-I targets many sleep mechanisms. Sleep restriction affects homeostatic sleep pressure, keeping strict bed and rise times, targets circadian timing and relaxation training reduces cognitive arousal. It is unlikely that a single drug will be able to modulate all these mechanisms simultaneously.

However, pharmacologic treatment will remain important for patients in whom CBT-I is not effective or not available. But even then, the use of medication should always be part of a broader treatment plan in which dysfunctional sleep habits are challenged, substance use is optimized, and comorbid conditions are addressed.

In insomnia, the subjective aspects of the sleep complaint are paramount in the diagnostic criteria. Epidemiologic studies increasingly point to a link between insomnia and somatic morbidity and mortality, but until now, only in the subgroup of objectively poor sleepers.[96–99] Although pharmacologic treatment might offer some benefits to this subgroup of insomnia patients, to date, there is no evidence that hypnotics can ameliorate their health risks. It is hoped that further unraveling of the neurobiology and genetics of sleep regulation and the pathophysiology of insomnia will help the development of drugs that not only improve subjective sleep complaints, but also objective health outcomes.

REFERENCES

1. van Straten A, van der Zweerde T, Kleiboer A, et al. Cognitive and behavioral therapies in the treatment of insomnia: a meta-analysis. Sleep Med Rev 2018; 38:3–16.
2. Sateia MJ, Buysse DJ, Krystal AD, et al. Clinical practice guideline for the pharmacologic treatment of chronic insomnia in adults: an American Academy of Sleep Medicine clinical practice guideline. J Clin Sleep Med 2017;13(2):307–49.
3. Riemann D, Baglioni C, Bassetti C, et al. European guideline for the diagnosis and treatment of insomnia. J Sleep Res 2017;26(6):675–700.
4. Morin CM, Vallieres A, Guay B, et al. Cognitive behavioral therapy, singly and combined with medication, for persistent insomnia: a randomized controlled trial. JAMA 2009;301(19):2005–15.
5. Zavesicka L, Brunovsky M, Matousek M, et al. Discontinuation of hypnotics during cognitive behavioural therapy for insomnia. BMC Psychiatry 2008;8:80.
6. Winkler A, Rief W. Effect of placebo conditions on polysomnographic parameters in primary insomnia: a meta-analysis. Sleep 2015;38(6):925–31.
7. Yeung V, Sharpe L, Glozier N, et al. A systematic review and meta-analysis of placebo versus no treatment for insomnia symptoms. Sleep Med Rev 2018;38:17–27.
8. Krystal AD. A compendium of placebo-controlled trials of the risks/benefits of pharmacological treatments for insomnia: the empirical basis for U.S. clinical practice. Sleep Med Rev 2009;13(4):265–74.
9. Minkel J, Krystal AD. Optimizing the pharmacologic treatment of insomnia: current status and future horizons. Sleep Med Clin 2013;8(3):333–50.
10. Wafford KA, Ebert B. Emerging anti-insomnia drugs: tackling sleeplessness and the quality of wake time. Nat Rev Drug Discov 2008;7(6):530–40.

11. Lu J, Greco MA. Sleep circuitry and the hypnotic mechanism of GABAA drugs. J Clin Sleep Med 2006;2(2):S19–26.

12. Saper CB, Scammell TE, Lu J. Hypothalamic regulation of sleep and circadian rhythms. Nature 2005; 437(7063):1257–63.

13. Mendelson W, Laposky A. Effects of triazolam microinjections into the peri-fornicular region on sleep in rats. Sleep Hypnosis 2003;5(3):154–62.

14. Nestler EJ, Hyman S, Holtzmann DM, et al. Molecular neuropharmacology: a foundation for clinical neuroscience. 3rd edition. New York: McGraw-Hill Medical; 2015.

15. Rudolph U, Crestani F, Benke D, et al. Benzodiazepine actions mediated by specific gamma-aminobutyric acid(A) receptor subtypes. Nature 1999;401(6755):796–800.

16. Glass JR, Sproule BA, Herrmann N, et al. Effects of 2-week treatment with temazepam and diphenhydramine in elderly insomniacs: a randomized, placebo-controlled trial. J Clin Psychopharmacol 2008;28(2):182–8.

17. Wu R, Bao J, Zhang C, et al. Comparison of sleep condition and sleep-related psychological activity after cognitive-behavior and pharmacological therapy for chronic insomnia. Psychother Psychosom 2006;75(4):220–8.

18. Roehrs T, Bonahoom A, Pedrosi B, et al. Treatment regimen and hypnotic self-administration. Psychopharmacology (Berl) 2001;155(1):11–7.

19. Oswald I, French C, Adam K, et al. Benzodiazepine hypnotics remain effective for 24 weeks. Br Med J (Clin Res Ed) 1982;284(6319):860–3.

20. Janhsen K, Roser P, Hoffmann K. The problems of long-term treatment with benzodiazepines and related substances. Dtsch Arztebl Int 2015;112(1–2):1–7.

21. Campanelli C. American Geriatrics Society updated beers criteria for potentially inappropriate medication use in older adults: the American Geriatrics Society 2012 beers criteria update expert panel. J Am Geriatr Soc 2012;60(4):616–31.

22. Luyster FS, Buysse DJ, Strollo PJ Jr. Comorbid insomnia and obstructive sleep apnea: challenges for clinical practice and research. J Clin Sleep Med 2010;6(2):196–204.

23. Roehrs T, Roth T. Drug-related sleep stage changes: functional significance and clinical relevance. Sleep Med Clin 2010;5(4):559–70.

24. Bastien CH, LeBlanc M, Carrier J, et al. Sleep EEG power spectra, insomnia, and chronic use of benzodiazepines. Sleep 2003;26(3):313–7.

25. Borbely AA, Mattmann P, Loepfe M, et al. Effect of benzodiazepine hypnotics on all-night sleep EEG spectra. Hum Neurobiol 1985;4(3):189–94.

26. Kilduff T, Mendelson WB. Hypnotic medications: mechanisms of action and pharmacologic effects. In: Kryger M, Roth T, editors. Principles and practice of sleep medicine. 6th edition. Philadelphia: Elsevier; 2017. p. 425–31.

27. Mazza M, Losurdo A, Testani E, et al. Polysomnographic findings in a cohort of chronic insomnia patients with benzodiazepine abuse. J Clin Sleep Med 2014;10(1):35–42.

28. Royant-Parola S, Brion A, Poirot I. Prise en charge de l'insomnie: guide pratique. Issy-les-Moulineaux (France): Elsevier Masson SAS; 2017.

29. Stahl SM. Stahl's essential psychopharmacology: neuroscientific basis and practical applications. Cambridge (England): Cambridge University Press; 2013.

30. Holm KJ, Goa KL. Zolpidem: an update of its pharmacology, therapeutic efficacy and tolerability in the treatment of insomnia. Drugs 2000;59(4): 865–89.

31. Wishart DS, Feunang YD, Guo AC, et al. DrugBank 5.0: a major update to the DrugBank database for 2018. Nucleic Acids Res 2018;46(D1):D1074–82.

32. Drover DR. Comparative pharmacokinetics and pharmacodynamics of short-acting hypnosedatives: zaleplon, zolpidem and zopiclone. Clin Pharmacokinet 2004;43(4):227–38.

33. Erman MK, Zammit G, Rubens R, et al. A polysomnographic placebo-controlled evaluation of the efficacy and safety of eszopiclone relative to placebo and zolpidem in the treatment of primary insomnia. J Clin Sleep Med 2008;4(3):229–34.

34. Walsh JK, Vogel GW, Scharf M, et al. A five week, polysomnographic assessment of zaleplon 10 mg for the treatment of primary insomnia. Sleep Med 2000;1(1):41–9.

35. Gunja N. In the Zzz zone: the effects of Z-drugs on human performance and driving. J Med Toxicol 2013;9(2):163–71.

36. Becker PM, Somiah M. Non-benzodiazepine receptor agonists for insomnia. Sleep Med Clin 2015; 10(1):57–76.

37. Krystal AD, Walsh JK, Laska E, et al. Sustained efficacy of eszopiclone over 6 months of nightly treatment: results of a randomized, double-blind, placebo-controlled study in adults with chronic insomnia. Sleep 2003;26(7):793–9.

38. Wadworth AN, McTavish D. Zopiclone. A review of its pharmacological properties and therapeutic efficacy as an hypnotic. Drugs Aging 1993;3(5): 441–59.

39. Toner LC, Tsambiras BM, Catalano G, et al. Central nervous system side effects associated with zolpidem treatment. Clin Neuropharmacol 2000;23(1): 54–8.

40. Chen YW, Tseng PT, Wu CK, et al. Zaleplon-induced anemsic somnambulism with eating behaviors under once dose. Acta Neurol Taiwan 2014;23(4): 143–5.

41. Treves N, Perlman A, Kolenberg Geron L, et al. Z-drugs and risk for falls and fractures in older adults: a systematic review and meta-analysis. Age Ageing 2018;47(2):201–8.

42. Orriols L, Philip P, Moore N, et al. Benzodiazepine-like hypnotics and the associated risk of road traffic accidents. Clin Pharmacol Ther 2011;89(4): 595–601.

43. Chang CM, Wu EC, Chen CY, et al. Psychotropic drugs and risk of motor vehicle accidents: a population-based case-control study. Br J Clin Pharmacol 2013;75(4):1125–33.

44. Mahler SV, Moorman DE, Smith RJ, et al. Motivational activation: a unifying hypothesis of orexin/hypocretin function. Nat Neurosci 2014;17(10): 1298–303.

45. Bonnavion P, de Lecea L. Hypocretins in the control of sleep and wakefulness. Curr Neurol Neurosci Rep 2010;10(3):174–9.

46. Sakurai T, Amemiya A, Ishii M, et al. Orexins and orexin receptors: a family of hypothalamic neuropeptides and G protein-coupled receptors that regulate feeding behavior. Cell 1998;92(4):573–85.

47. de Lecea L, Kilduff TS, Peyron C, et al. The hypocretins: hypothalamus-specific peptides with neuroexcitatory activity. Proc Natl Acad Sci U S A 1998; 95(1):322–7.

48. Law V, Knox C, Djoumbou Y, et al. DrugBank 4.0: shedding new light on drug metabolism. Nucleic Acids Res 2014;42(Database issue):D1091–7.

49. Herring WJ, Connor KM, Ivgy-May N, et al. Suvorexant in patients with insomnia: results from two 3-month randomized controlled clinical trials. Biol Psychiatry 2016;79(2):136–48.

50. Herring WJ, Snyder E, Budd K, et al. Orexin receptor antagonism for treatment of insomnia: a randomized clinical trial of suvorexant. Neurology 2012;79(23): 2265–74.

51. Michelson D, Snyder E, Paradis E, et al. Safety and efficacy of suvorexant during 1-year treatment of insomnia with subsequent abrupt treatment discontinuation: a phase 3 randomised, double-blind, placebo-controlled trial. Lancet Neurol 2014;13(5): 461–71.

52. Herring WJ, Connor KM, Snyder E, et al. Suvorexant in patients with insomnia: pooled analyses of three-month data from phase-3 randomized controlled clinical trials. J Clin Sleep Med 2016; 12(9):1215–25.

53. Snyder E, Ma J, Svetnik V, et al. Effects of suvorexant on sleep architecture and power spectral profile in patients with insomnia: analysis of pooled phase 3 data. Sleep Med 2016;19:93–100.

54. Sun H, Palcza J, Card D, et al. Effects of suvorexant, an orexin receptor antagonist, on respiration during sleep in patients with obstructive sleep apnea. J Clin Sleep Med 2016;12(1):9–17.

55. Sun H, Palcza J, Rosenberg R, et al. Effects of suvorexant, an orexin receptor antagonist, on breathing during sleep in patients with chronic obstructive pulmonary disease. Respir Med 2015; 109(3):416–26.

56. Uemura N, McCrea J, Sun H, et al. Effects of the orexin receptor antagonist suvorexant on respiration during sleep in healthy subjects. J Clin Pharmacol 2015;55(10):1093–100.

57. Tabata H, Kuriyama A, Yamao F, et al. Suvorexant-induced dream enactment behavior in parkinson disease: a case report. J Clin Sleep Med 2017; 13(5):759–60.

58. Petrous J, Furmaga K. Adverse reaction with suvorexant for insomnia: acute worsening of depression with emergence of suicidal thoughts. BMJ Case Rep 2017.

59. Pevet P. Melatonin receptors as therapeutic targets in the suprachiasmatic nucleus. Expert Opin Ther Targets 2016;20(10):1209–18.

60. Liu C, Weaver DR, Jin X, et al. Molecular dissection of two distinct actions of melatonin on the suprachiasmatic circadian clock. Neuron 1997;19(1): 91–102.

61. Liu J, Clough SJ, Hutchinson AJ, et al. MT1 and MT2 melatonin receptors: a therapeutic perspective. Annu Rev Pharmacol Toxicol 2016;56:361–83.

62. Pandi-Perumal SR, Trakht I, Srinivasan V, et al. Physiological effects of melatonin: role of melatonin receptors and signal transduction pathways. Prog Neurobiol 2008;85(3):335–53.

63. Andersen LP, Werner MU, Rosenkilde MM, et al. Pharmacokinetics of oral and intravenous melatonin in healthy volunteers. BMC Pharmacol Toxicol 2016; 17:8.

64. Harpsoe NG, Andersen LP, Gogenur I, et al. Clinical pharmacokinetics of melatonin: a systematic review. Eur J Clin Pharmacol 2015;71(8):901–9.

65. Sateia MJ, Kirby-Long P, Taylor JL. Efficacy and clinical safety of ramelteon: an evidence-based review. Sleep Med Rev 2008;12(4):319–22.

66. Slawik H, Stoffel M, Riedl L, et al. Prospective study on salivary evening melatonin and sleep before and after pinealectomy in humans. J Biol Rhythms 2016; 31(1):82–93.

67. Auld F, Maschauer EL, Morrison I, et al. Evidence for the efficacy of melatonin in the treatment of primary adult sleep disorders. Sleep Med Rev 2017;34:10–22.

68. Ferracioli-Oda E, Qawasmi A, Bloch MH. Meta-analysis: melatonin for the treatment of primary sleep disorders. PLoS One 2013;8(5):e63773.

69. Stone BM, Turner C, Mills SL, et al. Hypnotic activity of melatonin. Sleep 2000;23(5):663–9.

70. Arbon EL, Knurowska M, Dijk DJ. Randomised clinical trial of the effects of prolonged-release melatonin, temazepam and zolpidem on slow-wave

activity during sleep in healthy people. J Psychopharmacol 2015;29(7):764–76.

71. Mayer G, Wang-Weigand S, Roth-Schechter B, et al. Efficacy and safety of 6-month nightly ramelteon administration in adults with chronic primary insomnia. Sleep 2009;32(3):351–60.

72. Wade AG, Ford I, Crawford G, et al. Nightly treatment of primary insomnia with prolonged release melatonin for 6 months: a randomized placebo controlled trial on age and endogenous melatonin as predictors of efficacy and safety. BMC Med 2010;8:51.

73. Tordjman S, Chokron S, Delorme R, et al. Melatonin: pharmacology, functions and therapeutic benefits. Curr Neuropharmacol 2017;15(3):434–43.

74. Available at: https://www.fda.gov/Drugs/DrugSafety. Accessed January 22, 2018.

75. Krystal AD. Antidepressant and antipsychotic drugs. Sleep Med Clin 2010;5(4):571–89.

76. DeMartinis NA, Winokur A. Effects of psychiatric medications on sleep and sleep disorders. CNS Neurol Disord Drug Targets 2007;6(1):17–29.

77. Buysse DJ, Tyagi S. Clinical pharmacology of other drugs used as hypnotics. In: Kryger M, Roth T, editors. Principles and practice of sleep medicine. 6th edition. Philadelphia: Elsevier; 2017. p. 432–45.

78. Lankford A, Rogowski R, Essink B, et al. Efficacy and safety of doxepin 6 mg in a four-week outpatient trial of elderly adults with chronic primary insomnia. Sleep Med 2012;13(2):133–8.

79. Scharf M, Rogowski R, Hull S, et al. Efficacy and safety of doxepin 1 mg, 3 mg, and 6 mg in elderly patients with primary insomnia: a randomized, double-blind, placebo-controlled crossover study. J Clin Psychiatry 2008;69(10):1557–64.

80. Krystal AD, Durrence HH, Scharf M, et al. Efficacy and safety of doxepin 1 mg and 3 mg in a 12-week sleep laboratory and outpatient trial of elderly subjects with chronic primary insomnia. Sleep 2010;33(11):1553–61.

81. Liu Y, Xu X, Dong M, et al. Treatment of insomnia with tricyclic antidepressants: a meta-analysis of polysomnographic randomized controlled trials. Sleep Med 2017;34:126–33.

82. Walsh JK, Erman M, Erwin CW, et al. Subjective hypnotic efficacy of trazodone and zolpidem in DSMIII-R primary insomnia. Hum Psychopharmacol 1998; 13(3):191–8.

83. Montgomery I, Oswald I, Morgan K, et al. Trazodone enhances sleep in subjective quality but not in objective duration. Br J Clin Pharmacol 1983;16(2): 139–44.

84. Roth AJ, McCall WV, Liguori A. Cognitive, psychomotor and polysomnographic effects of trazodone in primary insomniacs. J Sleep Res 2011;20(4): 552–8.

85. Schmid DA, Wichniak A, Uhr M, et al. Changes of sleep architecture, spectral composition of sleep EEG, the nocturnal secretion of cortisol, ACTH, GH, prolactin, melatonin, ghrelin, and leptin, and the DEX-CRH test in depressed patients during treatment with mirtazapine. Neuropsychopharmacology 2006;31(4):832–44.

86. Aslan S, Isik E, Cosar B. The effects of mirtazapine on sleep: a placebo controlled, double-blind study in young healthy volunteers. Sleep 2002; 25(6):677–9.

87. Krystal AD, Lankford A, Durrence HH, et al. Efficacy and safety of doxepin 3 and 6 mg in a 35-day sleep laboratory trial in adults with chronic primary insomnia. Sleep 2011;34(10):1433–42.

88. Goerke M, Cohrs S, Rodenbeck A, et al. Differential effect of an anticholinergic antidepressant on sleep-dependent memory consolidation. Sleep 2014; 37(5):977–85.

89. Kolla BP, Mansukhani MP, Bostwick JM. The influence of antidepressants on restless legs syndrome and periodic limb movements: a systematic review. Sleep Med Rev 2018;38:131–40.

90. Walsh JK. Drugs used to treat insomnia in 2002: regulatory-based rather than evidence-based medicine. Sleep 2004;27(8):1441–2.

91. Cohrs S, Rodenbeck A, Guan Z, et al. Sleep-promoting properties of quetiapine in healthy subjects. Psychopharmacology (Berl) 2004;174(3):421–9.

92. Tassniyom K, Paholpak S, Tassniyom S, et al. Quetiapine for primary insomnia: a double blind, randomized controlled trial. J Med Assoc Thai 2010; 93(6):729–34.

93. Coe HV, Hong IS. Safety of low doses of quetiapine when used for insomnia. Ann Pharmacother 2012; 46(5):718–22.

94. Thompson W, Quay TAW, Rojas-Fernandez C, et al. Atypical antipsychotics for insomnia: a systematic review. Sleep Med 2016;22:13–7.

95. Monti JM, Torterolo P, Pandi Perumal SR. The effects of second generation antipsychotic drugs on sleep variables in healthy subjects and patients with schizophrenia. Sleep Med Rev 2017;33:51–7.

96. Vgontzas AN, Fernandez-Mendoza J, Liao D, et al. Insomnia with objective short sleep duration: the most biologically severe phenotype of the disorder. Sleep Med Rev 2013;17(4):241–54.

97. Stahl SM. Temazepam. In: Stahl SM, editor. Stahl's Essential Pharmacology: The prescriber's guide. 6th ed. Cambridge (UK): Cambridge University Press; 2017. p. 703–6.

98. Yasui-Furukori N, Takahata T, Kondo T, et al. Time effects of food intake on the pharmacokinetics and pharmacodynamics of quazepam. Br J Clin Pharmacol 2003;55(4):382–8.

99. Available at: https://www.drugs.com. Accessed February 19, 2018.

Hypnotic Discontinuation in Chronic Insomnia

Jonathan P. Hintze, MD[a],*, Jack D. Edinger, PhD[b]

KEYWORDS

- Deprescribing • Discontinuation • Hypnotic • Benzodiazepines • Insomnia • Sleep disorder

KEY POINTS

- Patients with chronic insomnia are commonly prescribed hypnotic medications but discontinuation of these medications is difficult to achieve.
- A gradual taper is preferred over abrupt cessation to avoid rebound insomnia and withdrawal symptoms.
- Written information provided to the patient about medication discontinuation may be helpful.
- Cognitive behavioral therapy or behavioral therapies alone can improve hypnotic discontinuation outcomes.
- There is limited evidence for adjunct medications to assist in hypnotic cessation for insomnia.

INTRODUCTION

Insomnia disorder is common in adults and children. The estimated prevalence ranges from 9% to 15% in the general population, with higher prevalence in certain subpopulations.[1–6] Hypnotic medications are those that tend to produce sleep and are frequently used to treat insomnia.[7] Commonly used hypnotics in adults include benzodiazepines (BZDs), BZD receptor agonists (BzRAs), antihistamines, antidepressants, melatonin receptor agonists, orexin receptor antagonists, and antipsychotics. Although there are currently no medications for pediatric insomnia approved by the US Food and Drug Administration, commonly used medications include antihistamines, alpha agonists, antidepressants, BZDs, BzRAs, and antipsychotics.[8,9] The long-term health consequences of using hypnotics are not well described, and current guidelines recommend medication tapering and discontinuation

when possible.[10] However, hypnotic discontinuation is difficult and often unsuccessful.[11] This article discusses strategies to discontinue hypnotics and evidence supporting their use.

HYPNOTIC TAPER STRATEGIES
Abrupt Hypnotic Cessation

Rapid drug cessation is an option for many medications. However, rebound insomnia and withdrawal symptoms may accompany abrupt hypnotic discontinuation. Rebound insomnia is generally defined as insomnia that is worse relative to baseline. This was first described with the discontinuation of triazolam[12] and has since been reported with several other BZDs[13,14]; sedating antidepressants, including amitriptyline[15] and trazodone[16]; and BzRAs, though with conflicting reports.[14,17–19] Additionally, withdrawal symptoms, largely defined as the emergence of previously absent symptoms, are frequently

This article originally appeared in June, 2018 issue of *Sleep Medicine Clinics* (Volume 13, Issue 2).

Disclosure Statement: J.P. Hintze has no potential conflicts of interest or funding sources. J.D. Edinger conflicts of interest or funding: grant support from Merck, Philips, Respironics, Inc.

[a] Division of Pediatric Sleep Medicine, University of South Carolina School of Medicine-Greenville, Greenville Health System, 200 Patewood Drive, Suite A330, Greenville, SC 29615, USA; [b] Department of Medicine, National Jewish Health, 1400 Jackson Street, Denver, CO 80206, USA

* Corresponding author.

E-mail address: jhintze@ghs.org

sleep.theclinics.com

reported with abrupt discontinuation of BZDs.[20] Consequently, tapering hypnotics is generally preferred to abrupt cessation.

Tapering Hypnotics

Reported tapering strategies vary widely, with no consensus on the optimal tapering protocol. A frequently described approach is a dose reduction of 25% every 1 to 2 weeks until discontinued completely.[21–25] Complete discontinuation rates ranged from 24% to 61% in these studies but there is variability in the frequency of office visits and the follow-up period in these reports. Withdrawal symptoms were commonly reported. A slightly slower wean was used by Lopez-Peig and colleagues.[26] Subjects all took BZDs, and were instructed to reduce their dose by 25% every 2 to 4 weeks. At the end of the taper period, 80.4% had successfully discontinued their BZD, and 64% remained BZD-free at 12 months. Another study weaned subjects from various BZDs by 10% to 25% every 2 to 3 weeks, with an approximately 40% hypnotic abstinence rate maintained at 36 months, without significant sleep dissatisfaction compared with a control group.[27] Drake[28] weaned subjects from temazepam by cutting doses roughly in half every 2 weeks, from 10 mg to 5 mg to 2 mg. Of the subjects, 59% successfully completed the taper, with 52% remaining hypnotic-free at follow-up 12 to 35 weeks later. Lemoine and colleagues[29] reported a similar taper with 2 BzRAs, zopiclone and zolpidem. In that study, subjects were weaned from zolpidem 10 mg to 5 mg for a week, followed by a placebo. Similarly, subjects were weaned from zopiclone 7.5 mg to 3.75 mg for a week, followed by a placebo. This regimen was associated with significantly higher withdrawal symptoms than the control group that was not weaned. In contrast, Raju and Meagher[30] used a more flexible taper protocol, in which subjects were able to control the rate of withdrawal. Given control over the weaning pace, some subjects rapidly discontinued hypnotic use (19 of 68), whereas others preferred a prolonged, yet complete, taper (13 of 68). The remainder did not completely discontinue medication use. To the authors' knowledge, there are no studies specifically comparing the success of different taper strategies. However, a clinical trial is currently underway that will compare different taper strategies among hypnotic-dependent subjects.[31]

Many practitioners find it helpful to switch from a short-acting to a long-acting BZD before initiating a taper.[27,32] This is done by switching to an equivalent dose of a long-acting BZD, commonly

Table 1	
Approximate equivalent doses of benzodiazepines to 5 mg diazepam	
BZD	**Equivalent Dose (mg)**
Alprazolam	0.25–0.5
Bromazepam	3–6
Lorazepam	0.5–1
Nitrazepam	5
Oxazepam	15
Temazepam	10
Triazolam	0.25

diazepam (**Table 1**). It is notable that a Cochrane Review published in 2006 noted higher dropout rates when tapering short half-life compounds compared with long-acting BZDs.[33] However, there was no difference in withdrawal symptoms between the groups, so switching from a short-acting to a long-acting BZD before a gradual taper was not supported. The authors are unaware of any studies specifically comparing the practice of switching to a long-acting BZD before gradual withdrawal versus a gradual withdrawal directly from a short-acting BZD.

ADJUNCT THERAPIES

Regardless of the taper strategy, several adjunct therapies have been studied to assist in hypnotic discontinuation. These include various degrees of patient education, psychological therapies, and medications.

Written Patient Education

There is some evidence that simply providing written information to patients can lead to hypnotic discontinuation. In 1 study, chronic BZD users were randomized to receive either routine care or advice during a single consultation supplemented by a self-help booklet.[34] The intervention resulted in a significant reduction in BDZ prescriptions compared with routine care alone (18% vs 5%). Several other studies used a letter sent to BZD users encouraging BZD reduction, with complete BZD cessation rates ranging from 14% to 27%.[23,24,35–37]

Psychological Therapies

Many studies have used psychological therapies to aid in medication discontinuation. A brief description of the different types of therapy is provided in **Table 2**.

Table 2
Psychological therapies for insomnia

Therapy	Description
Sleep hygiene education	Guidelines about practices and habits that support or interfere with sleep (eg, obtaining regular exercise, avoid electronics before bed)
Relaxation therapy	Techniques used to reduce muscular tension and intrusive thought processes interfering with sleep
Stimulus control therapy	Reinforcing the association of the bed with sleep by getting out of bed when unable to fall asleep, only going to bed when sleepy, keeping a strict rise time, and avoiding napping
Sleep restriction therapy	Reducing the amount of time spent in bed to match actual sleep time, with periodic adjustments as necessary
Cognitive therapy	A method of challenging false beliefs about sleep that contribute to insomnia
Cognitive behavioral therapy	Combining cognitive therapy with another behavioral treatment (eg, sleep restriction or stimulus control)
Self-efficacy enhancement	Improving perceived coping capabilities by providing positive vicarious experiences, discussing obstacles from prior failed attempts, and social persuasion

Sleep hygiene education

Sleep hygiene education is routinely provided to patients with insomnia. However, there is insufficient evidence to recommend sleep hygiene as a stand-alone therapy regardless of the presence or absence of hypnotic use.[38] Additionally, the authors are unaware of any studies that used sleep hygiene alone as an intervention to assist in hypnotic discontinuation.

Relaxation therapy

Relaxation therapy is a technique used to reduce muscular tension and intrusive thought processes interfering with sleep, and involves tensing and relaxing major muscle groups. Giblin and Clift[39] studied the effects of relaxation therapy on hypnotic discontinuation in 20 subjects. Notably, their intervention also included a discussion about sleep and insomnia, hypnotics and their effects on sleep, and general advice about problem-solving and optimism. There was a significant decrease in the number of subjects who resumed nightly hypnotic use at 12 weeks in the treatment group (2 of 10) compared with the control group (8 of 10), without any significant difference between the groups in reported sleep onset latency and overall sleep quality.

Lichstein and Johnson[40] used relaxation therapy for hypnotic cessation, resulting in a substantial reduction (47%) in sleep medication use. Lichstein and colleagues[41] assessed the usefulness of progressive relaxation techniques in addition to a standard drug withdrawal program in a randomized trial. All subjects had a 79% reduction in hypnotic consumption, without any significant difference between the groups. However, those assigned to the relaxation group had fewer withdrawal symptoms, greater sleep efficiency, and higher reported quality of sleep.

Stimulus control therapy

Stimulus control therapy is a method pioneered by Bootzin[42] and is used to reestablish the association between the bed and sleep. Patients are encouraged to remove themselves from the bed when unable to fall asleep, and only go to bed when sleepy rather than at a designated bedtime. They are also encouraged to keep a strict rise time and to avoid napping. A study of 7 long-term hypnotic users found that most (6 of 7) were able to reduce or stop their medication when stimulus control therapy was used.[43] Riedel and colleagues[44] randomized 21 subjects to either a medication withdrawal program, or the withdrawal program and stimulus control therapy. Both groups had significant reductions in the amount of sleep medication use but the stimulus control group also had significant improvements in total sleep time, sleep efficiency, sleep quality, and daytime sleepiness. Several other studies included stimulus control therapy as part of their intervention (see later discussion).

Sleep restriction therapy

Sleep restriction therapy is used to curtail the amount of time spent awake in bed. This is done by determining the amount of sleep a patient is regularly getting and limiting the total allowable time in bed to the same amount. For example, if a patient is currently spending 10 hours in bed per night but only sleeps 6 hours, then the amount of time in bed per night would be limited to 6 to 6.5 hours, depending on the specific sleep restriction protocol used.

Although sleep restriction is a well-established therapy for insomnia in general,[45] Taylor and colleagues[46] performed the only known study examining the effectiveness of sleep restriction in the setting of hypnotic discontinuation. Forty-six subjects were assigned to either sleep hygiene education or sleep restriction with medication withdrawal. In the sleep restriction group, 52.6% completely discontinued hypnotic medication use, compared with 15.4% in the sleep hygiene group. Additionally, there was improvement in sleep-onset latency and sleep efficiency, which was maintained through a 12-month follow-up period.

Cognitive behavioral therapy

Cognitive therapy is the method of challenging a patient's current beliefs about sleep that contribute to insomnia. Cognitive behavioral therapy (CBT) combines behavioral therapy (eg, relaxation, stimulus control, sleep restriction) with cognitive therapy to form a multicomponent and omnibus intervention. Therefore, CBT is a combination therapy with variation depending on the specific methods used. CBT has long been used for insomnia and an early study demonstrated its usefulness in hypnotic discontinuation.[47] Several subsequent studies have been performed.

Many studies specifically evaluated BZD cessation. Baillargeon and colleagues[48] studied 65 subjects with chronic insomnia taking BZDs nightly, randomizing subjects to a gradual supervised taper alone or combined with 8 weeks of CBT. At treatment completion, more subjects had complete drug cessation in the combined group (77%) compared with the taper-alone group (38%), with similar results at a 12-month follow-up (70% vs 24%). Although several other studies reported no improvement in BZD discontinuation rates with CBT,[23,49,50] other measures of sleep quality were generally improved. Morin and colleagues[25] considered the differential effects of supervised BZD withdrawal and CBT in their randomized trial. Seventy-six subjects underwent supervised withdrawal, CBT, or both. Although all groups had a significant reduction in quantity (90%) and

frequency (80%) of BZD use, the combined treatment group was the most successful at achieving complete drug cessation (85%), with supervised withdrawal and CBT alone producing less-successful results (48% and 54% respectively). Interestingly, the subjects in both groups that received CBT reported greater improvement in subjective sleep quality when compared with the group who only had supervised drug withdrawal. When a 24-month follow-up was conducted, 42.6% of subjects had resumed BZDs, with greater relapse in the CBT-alone group (69.2%) when compared with the combined (33.3%) and supervised withdrawal (30.8%) groups.

BzRAs have also been studied. Zavesicka and colleagues[51] reported 15 zolpidem-dependent subjects who were successfully weaned while receiving CBT, with associated improved sleep efficiency and decreased wakefulness after sleep onset. An 8-week hypnotic taper program, including 53 subjects taking either BZDs or BzRAs, found that those randomized to receive CBT had improved sleep efficiency and decreased total wake time when compared with the control group.[52] However, both groups successfully reduced hypnotic use, with no significant additional reduction in the CBT group. In contrast, Morgan and colleagues[53] found that CBT greatly reduced hypnotic drug use while improving sleep efficiency and reducing sleep onset latency in a cohort of 209 chronic hypnotic users. Lichstein and colleagues[54] further validated the usefulness of CBT in hypnotic-dependent insomnia patients using BZDs, BzRAs, or sedating antidepressants by randomizing subjects to CBT with drug withdrawal, placebo biofeedback with drug withdrawal, or drug withdrawal alone. There were no significant differences between groups in medication reduction, which decreased by 84% post-treatment, and 66% at a 12-month follow-up. However, only the CBT group had significant improvement in sleep onset latency and subjective sleep measures.

Self-efficacy enhancement

In some analyses of factors leading to success in hypnotic cessation, an individual's perceived self-efficacy has been positively correlated with medication cessation.[50,55] To further pursue the effect of self-efficacy on patient outcomes, Yang and colleagues[56] randomized 48 long-term hypnotic users (BZDs or BzRAs) to a standard drug taper alone or a self-efficacy educational program followed by the same drug taper. Those in the treatment group had a higher percentage of dose reduction than those in the taper-alone group, suggesting that self-efficacy can be learned and can improve hypnotic cessation outcomes.

Pharmacologic Therapies

Several studies have evaluated the usefulness of medications to assist in BZD discontinuation, though generally in the setting of anxiety or other psychological disorders. These have included ondansetron,[57] imipramine,[58,59] buspirone,[58–60] paroxetine,[61] carbamazepine,[62] pregabalin,[63] progesterone,[64] antihistamines,[65] and propranolol.[66] Only a few have examined the usefulness of medications to assist in BZDs cessation specifically for insomnia. There have also been some reports of other supplements to aid in hypnotic discontinuation.

Zopiclone

Withdrawal symptoms and rebound insomnia have been shown to be less severe with BzRAs compared with some BZDs.[18] Therefore, some investigators have proposed using a BzRA as a bridge to BZD discontinuation. Pat-Horenczyk and colleagues[67] studied 24 subjects taking flunitrazepam for insomnia. All underwent a 5-week withdrawal protocol and were followed with nightly actigraphy and serial polysomnograms during the withdrawal period. One group was transitioned to zopiclone and then weaned off, whereas the other was weaned off flunitrazepam directly. Both objective (polysomnogram and actigraphy) and subjective (sleep diaries) measures were improved in the zopiclone group compared with the flunitrazepam group. Similar positive findings were found in other reports.[68–70] Two studies indicated that abrupt medication substitution yielded better results than gradual substitution.[68,70]

Melatonin

Some have postulated that melatonin therapy could aid in the discontinuation of hypnotics. In a large retrospective study of prolonged-release melatonin, 31% discontinued hypnotic use (BZDs or BzRAs) after the melatonin was started.[71] Several randomized trials have also considered the usefulness of melatonin in hypnotic discontinuation, specifically BZDs. Although 2 of these trials showed some effectiveness,[72,73] most found that melatonin did not enhance BZD discontinuation.[74–78] A meta-analysis also concluded that melatonin supplementation did not affect rates of BZD discontinuation.[79]

Valerian

The evidence for the use of the herbal supplement valerian in insomnia to date has been inconclusive.[80] However, Poyares and colleagues[81] reported some positive outcomes with the use of valerian in BZD discontinuation. Subjects treated with valerian had better subjective sleep quality than the placebo group, with decreased wakefulness after sleep onset at a 2-week polysomnogram, though with a longer sleep onset latency.

SUMMARY

Discontinuation of hypnotic medications is often challenging. The current evidence suggests that a gradual taper is preferred over abrupt discontinuation owing to both rebound insomnia and withdrawal symptoms. However, an ideal taper schedule has not been well-established. A clinical trial is currently underway in an effort to improve understanding of the ideal wean schedule.[31] In addition to tapering hypnotics, providing patients with educational handouts may provide some benefit. Psychological therapies are also beneficial, with the most evidence supporting CBT in conjunction with a hypnotic taper. Some patients taking BZD hypnotics may benefit from bridging drug cessation with a BzRA. In those cases, an immediate switch to a BzRA was more beneficial than a gradual switch. Other medical therapies have not uniformly demonstrated benefit. Moreover, because most of the evidence for hypnotic discontinuation was done with BZDs, it is not clear that a similar approach can be made with sedating antidepressants, antihistamines, or other hypnotics. Furthermore, the discontinuation of hypnotics in the pediatric population is based only on the adult literature. Further research is needed to better establish optimal hypnotic discontinuation guidelines for both adults and children.

REFERENCES

1. Ohayon MM. Epidemiology of insomnia: what we know and what we still need to learn. Sleep Med Rev 2002;6(2):97–111.
2. Calhoun SL, Fernandez-Mendoza J, Vgontzas AN, et al. Prevalence of insomnia symptoms in a general population sample of young children and preadolescents: gender effects. Sleep Med 2014;15(1):91–5.
3. Chung KF, Yeung WF, Ho FY, et al. Cross-cultural and comparative epidemiology of insomnia: the Diagnostic and Statistical Manual (DSM), International Classification of Diseases (ICD) and International Classification of Sleep Disorders (ICSD). Sleep Med 2015;16(4):477–82.
4. Kronholm E, Partonen T, Härmä M, et al. Prevalence of insomnia-related symptoms continues to increase in the Finnish working-age population. J Sleep Res 2016;25(4):454–7.

5. Seow LS, Subramaniam M, Abdin E, et al. Sleep disturbance among people with major depressive disorders (MDD) in Singapore. J Ment Health 2016;25(6):492–9.

6. Kim KW, Kang SH, Yoon IY, et al. Prevalence and clinical characteristics of insomnia and its subtypes in the Korean elderly. Arch Gerontol Geriatr 2017;68:68–75.

7. Walsh JK. Pharmacologic management of insomnia. J Clin Psychiatry 2004;65(Suppl 16):41–5.

8. Owens JA, Rosen CL, Mindell JA. Medication use in the treatment of pediatric insomnia: results of a survey of community-based pediatricians. Pediatrics 2003;111(5 Pt 1):e628–35.

9. Nguyen M, Tharani S, Rahmani M, et al. A review of the use of clonidine as a sleep aid in the child and adolescent population. Clin Pediatr (Phila) 2014; 53(3):211–6.

10. Schutte-Rodin S, Broch L, Buysse D, et al. Clinical guideline for the evaluation and management of chronic insomnia in adults. J Clin Sleep Med 2008; 4(5):487–504.

11. Ostini R, Jackson C, Hegney D, et al. How is medication prescribing ceased? A systematic review. Med Care 2011;49(1):24–36.

12. Kales A, Scharf MB, Kales JD. Rebound insomnia: a new clinical syndrome. Science 1978;201(4360): 1039–41.

13. Roehrs T. Rebound insomnia: its determinants and significance. Am J Med 1990;88(3A):39S–42S.

14. Soldatos CR, Dikeos DG, Whitehead A. Tolerance and rebound insomnia with rapidly eliminated hypnotics: a meta-analysis of sleep laboratory studies. Int Clin Psychopharmacol 1999;14(5):287–303.

15. Staner L, Kerkhofs M, Detroux D, et al. Acute, subchronic and withdrawal sleep EEG changes during treatment with paroxetine and amitriptyline: a double-blind randomized trial in major depression. Sleep 1995;18(6):470–7.

16. Montgomery I, Oswald I, Morgan K, et al. Trazodone enhances sleep in subjective quality but not in objective duration. Br J Clin Pharmacol 1983;16(2): 139–44.

17. Monti JM, Attali P, Monti D, et al. Zolpidem and rebound insomnia–a double-blind, controlled polysomnographic study in chronic insomniac patients. Pharmacopsychiatry 1994;27(4):166–75.

18. Silvestri R, Ferrillo F, Murri L, et al. Rebound insomnia after abrupt discontinuation of hypnotic treatment: double-blind randomized comparison of zolpidem versus triazolam. Hum Psychopharmacol 1996;11(3):225–33.

19. Voshaar RC, van Balkom AJ, Zitman FG. Zolpidem is not superior to temazepam with respect to rebound insomnia: a controlled study. Eur Neuropsychopharmacol 2004;14(4):301–6.

20. Rickels K, Schweizer E, Case WG, et al. Long-term therapeutic use of benzodiazepines. I. Effects of abrupt discontinuation. Arch Gen Psychiatry 1990; 47(10):899–907.

21. Hopkins DR, Sethi KB, Mucklow JC. Benzodiazepine withdrawal in general practice. J R Coll Gen Pract 1982;32(245):758–62.

22. Murphy SM, Tyrer P. A double-blind comparison of the effects of gradual withdrawal of lorazepam, diazepam and bromazepam in benzodiazepine dependence. Br J Psychiatry 1991;158:511–6.

23. Voshaar RC, Gorgels WJ, Mol AJ, et al. Tapering off long-term benzodiazepine use with or without group cognitive-behavioural therapy: three-condition, randomised controlled trial. Br J Psychiatry 2003;182:498–504.

24. Gorgels WJ, Oude Voshaar RC, Mol AJ, et al. Discontinuation of long-term benzodiazepine use by sending a letter to users in family practice: a prospective controlled intervention study. Drug Alcohol Depend 2005;78(1):49–56.

25. Morin CM, Bastien CH, Guay B, et al. Randomized clinical trial of supervised tapering and cognitive-behavior therapy to facilitate benzodiazepine discontinuation in older adults with chronic insomnia. Am J Psychiatry 2004;161:332–42.

26. Lopez-Peig C, Mundet X, Casabella B, et al. Analysis of benzodiazepine withdrawal program managed by primary care nurses in Spain. BMC Res Notes 2012;5:684.

27. Vicens C, Sempere E, Bejarano F, et al. Efficacy of two interventions on the discontinuation of benzodiazepines in long-term users: 36-month follow-up of a cluster randomised trial in primary care. Br J Gen Pract 2016;66(643):e85–91.

28. Drake J. Temazepam 'Planpak': a multicentre general practice trial in planned benzodiazepine hypnotic withdrawal. Curr Med Res Opin 1991;12(6):390–3.

29. Lemoine P, Allain H, Janus C, et al. Gradual withdrawal of zopiclone (7.5 mg) and zolpidem (10 mg) in insomniacs treated for at least 3 months. Eur Psychiatry 1995;10(Suppl 3):161s–5s.

30. Raju B, Meagher D. Patient-controlled benzodiazepine dose reduction in a community mental health service. Ir J Psychol Med 2005;22:42–5.

31. ClinicalTrials.gov. The role of tapering pace and selected traits on hypnotic discontinuation. Bethesda (MD): National Library of Medicine (US); 2016. Identifier NCT02831894, Available at: https://clinicaltrials.gov/ct2/show/NCT02831894. Accessed August 17, 2017.

32. Lader M, Tylee A, Donoghue J. Withdrawing benzodiazepines in primary care. CNS Drugs 2009;23(1):19–34.

33. Denis C, Fatséas M, Lavie E, et al. Pharmacological interventions for benzodiazepine mono-dependence management in outpatient settings. Cochrane Database Syst Rev 2006;(3):CD005194.

34. Bashir K, King M, Ashworth M. Controlled evaluation of brief intervention by general practitioners to

reduce chronic use of benzodiazepines. Br J Gen Pract 1994;44(386):408–12.

35. Cormack MA, Sweeney KG, Hughes-Jones H, et al. Evaluation of an easy, cost-effective strategy for cutting benzodiazepine use in general practice. Br J Gen Pract 1994;44(378):5–8.

36. Stewart R, Niessen WJ, Broer J, et al. General Practitioners reduced benzodiazepine prescriptions in an intervention study: a multilevel application. J Clin Epidemiol 2007;60(10):1076–84.

37. Tannenbaum C, Martin P, Tamblyn R, et al. Reduction of inappropriate benzodiazepine prescriptions among older adults through direct patient education: the EMPOWER cluster randomized trial. JAMA Intern Med 2014;174(6):890–8.

38. Morgenthaler T, Kramer M, Alessi C, et al, American Academy of Sleep Medicine. Practice parameters for the psychological and behavioral treatment of insomnia: an update. An american academy of sleep medicine report. Sleep 2006;29(11):1415–9.

39. Giblin MJ, Clift AD. Sleep without drugs. J R Coll Gen Pract 1983;33(255):628–33.

40. Lichstein KL, Johnson RS. Relaxation for insomnia and hypnotic medication use in older women. Psychol Aging 1993;8(1):103–11.

41. Lichstein KL, Peterson BA, Riedel BW, et al. Relaxation to assist sleep medication withdrawal. Behav Modif 1999;23(3):379–402.

42. Bootzin RR. Stimulus control treatment for insomnia. Am Psychol Ass Proc 1972;7:395–6.

43. Baillargeon L, Demers M, Ladouceur R. Stimulus-control: nonpharmacologic treatment for insomnia. Can Fam Physician 1998;44:73–9.

44. Riedel B, Lichstein K, Peterson BA, et al. A comparison of the efficacy of stimulus control for medicated and nonmedicated insomniacs. Behav Modif 1998;22(1):3–28.

45. Morin CM, Bootzin RR, Buysse DJ, et al. Psychological and behavioral treatment of insomnia: update of the recent evidence (1998-2004). Sleep 2006;29(11):1398–414.

46. Taylor DJ, Schmidt-Nowara W, Jessop CA, et al. Sleep restriction therapy and hypnotic withdrawal versus sleep hygiene education in hypnotic using patients with insomnia. J Clin Sleep Med 2010;6(2):169–75.

47. Morin CM, Colecchi CA, Ling WD, et al. Cognitive behavior therapy to facilitate benzodiazepine discontinuation among hypnotic-dependent patients with insomnia. Behav Ther 1995;26(4):733–45.

48. Baillargeon L, Landreville P, Verreault R, et al. Discontinuation of benzodiazepines among older insomniac adults treated with cognitive-behavioural therapy combined with gradual tapering: a randomized trial. CMAJ 2003;169(10):1015–20.

49. Vorma H, Naukkarinen H, Sarna S, et al. Treatment of out-patients with complicated benzodiazepine dependence: comparison of two approaches. Addiction 2002;97(7):851–9.

50. O'Connor K, Marchand A, Brousseau L, et al. Cognitive-behavioural, pharmacological and psychosocial predictors of outcome during tapered discontinuation of benzodiazepine. Clin Psychol Psychother 2008;15(1):1–14.

51. Zavesicka L, Brunovsky M, Matousek M, et al. Discontinuation of hypnotics during cognitive behavioural therapy for insomnia. BMC psychiatry 2008;8(1):80.

52. Belleville G, Guay C, Guay B, et al. Hypnotic taper with or without self-help of insomnia: a randomized clinical trial. J Consult Clin Psychol 2007;75:325–35.

53. Morgan K, Dixon S, Mathers N, et al. Psychological treatment for insomnia in the management of long-term hypnotic drug use: a pragmatic randomised controlled trial. Br J Gen Pract 2003;53(497):923–8.

54. Lichstein KL, Nau SD, Wilson NM, et al. Psychological treatment of hypnotic-dependent insomnia in a primarily older adult sample. Behav Res Ther 2013;51(12):787–96.

55. Bélanger L, Morin CM, Bastien C, et al. Self-efficacy and compliance with benzodiazepine taper in older adults with chronic insomnia. Health Psychol 2005;24(3):281–7.

56. Yang CM, Tseng CH, Lai YS, et al. Self-efficacy enhancement can facilitate hypnotic tapering in patients with primary insomnia. Sleep Biol Rhythms 2015;13(3):242–51.

57. Romach MK, Kaplan HL, Busto UE, et al. A controlled trial of ondansetron, a 5-HT3 antagonist, in benzodiazepine discontinuation. J Clin Psychopharmacol 1998;18(2):121–31.

58. Rickels K, DeMartinis N, García-España F, et al. Imipramine and buspirone in treatment of patients with generalized anxiety disorder who are discontinuing long-term benzodiazepine therapy. Am J Psychiatry 2000;157(12):1973–9.

59. Rynn M, García-España F, Greenblatt DJ, et al. Imipramine and buspirone in patients with panic disorder who are discontinuing long-term benzodiazepine therapy. J Clin Psychopharmacol 2003;23(5):505–8.

60. Ashton CH, Rawlins MD, Tyrer SP. A double-blind placebo-controlled study of buspirone in diazepam withdrawal in chronic benzodiazepine users. Br J Psychiatry 1990;157:232–8.

61. Nakao M, Takeuchi T, Nomura K, et al. Clinical application of paroxetine for tapering benzodiazepine use in non-major-depressive outpatients visiting an internal medicine clinic. Psychiatry Clin Neurosci 2006;60(5):605–10.

62. Schweizer E, Rickels K, Case WG, et al. Carbamazepine treatment in patients discontinuing long-term benzodiazepine therapy. Effects on withdrawal severity and outcome. Arch Gen Psychiatry 1991;48(5):448–52.

63. Bobes J, Rubio G, Terán A, et al. Pregabalin for the discontinuation of long-term benzodiazepines use: an assessment of its effectiveness in daily clinical practice. Eur Psychiatry 2012;27(4):301–7.

64. Schweizer E, Case WG, Garcia-Espana F, et al. Progesterone co-administration in patients discontinuing long-term benzodiazepine therapy: effects on withdrawal severity and taper outcome. Psychopharmacology (Berl) 1995;117(4):424–9.

65. Gilhooly TC, Webster MG, Poole NW, et al. What happens when doctors stop prescribing temazepam? Use of alternative therapies. Br J Gen Pract 1998;48(434):1601–2.

66. Hallström C, Crouch G, Robson M, et al. The treatment of tranquilizer dependence by propranolol. Postgrad Med J 1988;64(Suppl 2):40–4.

67. Pat-Horenczyk R, Hacohen D, Herer P, et al. The effects of substituting zopiclone in withdrawal from chronic use of benzodiazepine hypnotics. Psychopharmacology (Berl) 1998;140(4):450–7.

68. Shapiro CM, MacFarlane JG, MacLean AW. Alleviating sleep-related discontinuance symptoms associated with benzodiazepine withdrawal: a new approach. J Psychosom Res 1993;37(Suppl 1):55–7.

69. Shapiro C, Sherman D, Peck D. Withdrawal from benzodiazepines by initially switching to zopiclone. Eur Psychiatry 1995;10(Suppl 3):145s–51s.

70. Lemoine P, Ohayon MM. Is hypnotic withdrawal facilitated by the transitory use of a substitute drug? Prog Neuropsychopharmacol Biol Psychiatry 1997;21(1):111–24.

71. Kunz D, Bineau S, Maman K, et al. Benzodiazepine discontinuation with prolonged-release melatonin: hints from a German longitudinal prescription database. Expert Opin Pharmacother 2012;13(1):9–16.

72. Garfinkel D, Zisapel N, Wainstein J, et al. Facilitation of benzodiazepine discontinuation by melatonin: a new clinical approach. Arch Intern Med 1999;159(20):2456–60.

73. Garzón C, Guerrero JM, Aramburu O, et al. Effect of melatonin administration on sleep, behavioral disorders and hypnotic drug discontinuation in the elderly: a randomized, double-blind, placebo-controlled study. Aging Clin Exp Res 2009;21(1):38–42.

74. Cardinali DP, Gvozdenovich E, Kaplan MR, et al. A double blind-placebo controlled study on melatonin efficacy to reduce anxiolytic benzodiazepine use in the elderly. Neuroendocrinol Lett 2002;23:55–60.

75. Peles E, Hetzroni T, Bar-Hamburger R, et al. Melatonin for perceived sleep disturbances associated with benzodiazepine withdrawal among patients in methadone maintenance treatment: a double-blind randomized clinical trial. Addiction 2007;102(12):1947–53.

76. Vissers FH, Knipschild PG, Crebolder HF. Is melatonin helpful in stopping the long-term use of hypnotics? A discontinuation trial. Pharm World Sci 2007;29(6):641–6.

77. Lähteenmäki R, Puustinen J, Vahlberg T, et al. Melatonin for sedative withdrawal in older patients with primary insomnia: a randomized double-blind placebo-controlled trial. Br J Clin Pharmacol 2014;77(6):975–85.

78. Baandrup L, Lindschou J, Winkel P, et al. Prolonged-release melatonin versus placebo for benzodiazepine discontinuation in patients with schizophrenia or bipolar disorder: a randomised, placebo-controlled, blinded trial. World J Biol Psychiatry 2016;17(7):514–24.

79. Wright A, Diebold J, Otal J, et al. The effect of melatonin on benzodiazepine discontinuation and sleep quality in adults attempting to discontinue benzodiazepines: a systematic review and meta-analysis. Drugs Aging 2015;32(12):1009–18.

80. Fernández-San-Martín MI, Masa-Font R, Palacios-Soler L, et al. Effectiveness of Valerian on insomnia: a meta-analysis of randomized placebo-controlled trials. Sleep Med 2010;11(6):505–11.

81. Poyares DR, Guilleminault C, Ohayon MM, et al. Can valerian improve the sleep of insomniacs after benzodiazepine withdrawal? Prog Neuropsychopharmacol Biol Psychiatry 2002;26(3):539–45.

Evaluation of the Sleepy Patient: Differential Diagnosis

Renee Monderer, MD*, Imran M. Ahmed, MD, Michael Thorpy, MD

KEYWORDS

- Excessive daytime sleepiness • Hypersomnolence • Evaluation • Sleep disorders

KEY POINTS

- Excessive daytime sleepiness is defined as the inability to maintain wakefulness during waking hours, resulting in unintended lapses into sleep. It is important to distinguish sleepiness from fatigue.
- The evaluation of a sleep patient begins with a careful clinical assessment that includes a detailed sleep history, medical and psychiatric history, a review of medications, as well as a social and family history.
- Physical examination should include a general medical examination with careful attention to the upper airway and the neurological examination.
- Appropriate objective testing with a polysomnogram and a multiple sleep latency test if needed will help confirm the diagnosis and direct the appropriate treatment plan.

INTRODUCTION

Excessive daytime sleepiness (EDS) is defined as the inability to maintain wakefulness during waking hours, resulting in unintended lapses into sleep.[1] Patients often describe their sleepiness using vague terms such as tired, fatigue, or lack of energy. It is important to distinguish sleepiness from fatigue. Fatigue is a physical or psychological feeling that may occur in a variety of other disorders, such as depression or Parkinson disease.[2,3] Unlike sleepiness, fatigued patients do not fall asleep when sedentary, such as while watching television or reading. This distinction is important because sleepiness indicates the presence of a sleep disorder or a problem with nighttime sleep. In a study of 190 obstructive sleep apnea (OSA) patients, approximately 47% used the term sleepiness to describe their symptoms. In contrast, 62% reported a lack of energy, 61% described themselves as feeling tiredness, and 57% used the term fatigue. When these patients were asked to select the most prominent symptom, only about 22% chose sleepiness, whereas more than 40% chose lack of energy.[4]

Patients may or may not be aware of their sleepiness before falling asleep, but it often significantly affects quality of life. EDS has many implications, including increased risk of injury at work or home, decreased alertness, car accidents, and lower productivity overall. EDS may also lead to heightened tension with family, friends, and co-workers, who may attribute the patient's symptoms to laziness or poor work ethic.

Driving while sleepy is perhaps the most worrisome behavior associated with EDS. This may take the form of dozing at a red light, while in stop-and-go traffic, or while traveling at higher speeds on a highway. Approximately 52% of drivers have driven while drowsy, with 50% reporting doing so within the last month.[5] Sleepiness while driving should be considered a medical emergency, and immediate evaluation and treatment should be initiated.[6,7]

Sleepiness can manifest in many different forms. For some patients, sleepiness is associated

This article originally appeared in September, 2017 issue of *Sleep Medicine Clinics* (Volume 12, Issue 3).
Sleep-Wake Disorders Center, Department of Neurology, Montefiore Medical Center, Albert Einstein College of Medicine, 111 East 210th Street, Bronx, NY 10467, USA
* Corresponding author.
E-mail address: rmondere@montefiore.org

sleep.theclinics.com

with more hours of sleep per day without feeling refreshed. For others, naps can be refreshing but sleepiness recurs. Children can paradoxically present with symptoms of hyperactivity or poor attention.

Many of the sleep disorders listed in the International Classifications of Sleep Disorders, 3rd edition (ICSD-3) can present with excessive sleepiness (**Box 1**). These disorders result in daytime sleepiness either because of shortened sleep time, fragmentation of the major sleep period, or central nervous system (CNS) dysfunction. Several studies of patients with OSA have demonstrated a significant correlation between the total number of arousals on a polysomnogram with the severity of sleepiness.[8–10] Other disorders, such as narcolepsy type 1 (with cataplexy) or type 2 (without cataplexy), idiopathic hypersomnia, or Kleine-Levin syndrome, are caused by a suspected CNS abnormality.[11–14] In contrast, insufficient sleep syndrome is caused by patients sleeping less than their biologic sleep requirement. Sleepiness in shift work disorder often results from insufficient sleep time because patients cannot sleep on their hours off due to noise, family, or social obligations. Medications, alcohol, substance abuse, and certain medical, neurologic, and psychiatric disorders can cause excessive sleepiness either by disturbing CNS sleep-wake mechanisms or by fragmenting the major sleep period (**Box 2**).

Box 1
Common sleep disorders associated with excessive daytime somnolence

1. Hypersomnia due to medical or psychiatric disorder or drug or substance
2. Narcolepsy type 1 or 2
3. Idiopathic hypersomnia
4. Kleine-Levin syndrome
5. Insufficient sleep syndrome (sleep deprivation)
6. OSA
7. Central sleep apnea
8. Shift work disorder
9. Delayed sleep phase type
10. Advanced sleep phase type
11. Long sleeper
12. Periodic limb movement disorder
13. Hypersomnia due to a medical disorder
14. Hypersomnia due to a medication or substance

Box 2
Common medical and psychiatric disorders that can cause excessive sleepiness

Brain tumors

Strokes

Head trauma

Seizures

Congestive heart failure

Bronchial asthma

Endocrine abnormalities (eg, excessive growth hormone, hypothyroidism, diabetes mellitus)

Chronic renal insufficiency

Infectious diseases (eg, human immunodeficiency virus, CNS Lyme disease)

Metabolic or infectious encephalopathies

Fibromyalgia

Chronic fatigue syndrome

Schizophrenia

Mood (depressive) disorders

Seasonal affective disorder

Conversion disorder

Factitious disorder

Malingering

Drug intoxication or withdrawal

Approximately 14% of the population report EDS at least a few days per week.[15] The prevalence seems to be higher among subjects age 65 years and older, ranging from 15% to 20%.[16,17] Although exact statistics are not known, the most common causes of daytime sleepiness are insufficient sleep syndrome, shift work disorder, and OSA. Central causes of daytime sleepiness, such as narcolepsy and idiopathic hypersomnia, are less prevalent but important to screen for as well.[15,18]

A systematic approach to the sleepy patient is needed to be able to distinguish between the many causes of daytime sleepiness. A thorough sleep history from the patient and, preferably, the patient's bed partner or caregiver, is needed. In addition, past medical, psychiatric history, surgical history, family history, physical examination, and appropriate laboratory tests are needed to form a complete differential diagnosis.

SLEEP EVALUATION

A thorough sleep evaluation begins with taking a careful history to determine the chief complaint; a detailed sleep history; and a medical, psychiatric, social, and family history. This should be followed by a focused physical examination; an appropriate sleep questionnaire; possible laboratory testing; and, if necessary, a sleep study.

History

As previously discussed, many patients with excessive sleepiness do not report sleepiness but rather describe their symptoms as fatigue, tiredness, lethargy, moodiness, or difficulty concentrating. If sleepiness is present, it is important to determine how that sleepiness affects daily activities. Many patients will report difficulty staying awake at work or completing tasks at home. Others will report negative effects on education, recreation, or personal relationships.[7] Discerning the effect that sleepiness has on a person's quality of life helps guide the evaluation and treatment to alleviate those symptoms.

Occasionally, patients, such as those with Parkinson disease or Alzheimer dementia, may not be aware of their sleepiness. It is helpful to have a bed partner or caretaker present to determine whether patients are unaware of episodes of falling asleep.[19]

To determine the severity of sleepiness, it is important to identify those situations in which a person experiences sleepiness. Mild sleepiness will manifest as falling asleep when sedentary and inactive, such as while watching television or reading. Moderate sleepiness is present when patients fall asleep during activities that require some attention, for instance during a meeting for work. Severe sleepiness is defined as sleepiness occurring during active situations, such as while driving.[20] The Epworth Sleepiness Scale (ESS) is an important tool that addresses the likelihood of falling asleep in these and other daily situations

The Epworth Sleepiness Scale (ESS) has 8 routine daytime situations that you rate on a scale from 0 to 3, based on your likelihood of dozing off or falling asleep in each situation. Write the number that corresponds with your answer for each situation in the "My score" box. Then add up your score, and share the results with your doctor.

SITUATION	Would Never Doze / Nunca se Queda Dormido (a)	Slight Chance Of Dozing / Posibilidad minina de Dormirse	Moderate Chance of Dozing / Posibilidad Moderada de Dormirse	High Chance Of Dozing / Major Posibilidad de Dormirse
Sitting and reading / Sentando(a) y leyendo	0	1	2	3
Watching television / Mirando television	0	1	2	3
Sitting inactive in a public place- for example, a theater or meeting / Sentado,(a) sin hacer nada en un lugar public por ejemplo, en el cine o en una reunion.	0	1	2	3
As a passenger in a car for an hour without a break / Como un pasajero en un carro for una hora sin ningun descanso.	0	1	2	3
Lying down to rest in the afternoon when circumstances permit / Recostado (a) en la tarde para descansar cuando sea permitido.	0	1	2	3
Sitting and talking to someone / Setando (a) hablando con alguien	0	1	2	3
Sitting quietly after lunch without alcohol / Setando (a) en silencio despues del almuerzo sin haber tomado alcohol	0	1	2	3
In a car, while stopped for a few minutes in traffic / En un carro detenido mientras espera por el trafico.	0	1	2	3
	TOTAL SCORE:			

Fig. 1. Epworth sleepiness scale.

(Fig. 1). The patient reports on a score from 0 to 3 the chance of dozing in 8 typical daytime activities. A score of 10 or more is considered significant daytime sleepiness, and above 15 is considered severe daytime sleepiness.

To discern if sleepiness while driving is present, it is important to inquire whether a person is using techniques such as rolling down the windows, turning up the volume on the radio, or talking to a passenger to keep themselves awake. Additionally, drivers should be asked about near-miss accidents to determine the level of sleepiness while driving. Sleepy near-miss accidents may be precursors to driving accidents.[21]

Sleep history

Obtaining a sleep history is essential to identifying a sleep disorder. Symptoms during the 24-hour cycle, rather than only those that occur at night, should be evaluated. The sleep history consists of the patient's bedtime, the length of time it takes to fall asleep, wake time, number of awakenings, naps, periods of dozing off, and any additional time spent in bed awake. It is often helpful to obtain a sleep log over a 2-week period to determine if there is sufficient amount of sleep per night or whether a circadian rhythm disorder, such as advanced or delayed sleep phase disorder, is present (Fig. 2). A person with delayed sleep phase may report sleepiness on awakening in the morning, whereas a person with advanced sleep phase

may complain of sleepiness in the evening hours. A sleep log may help a shift worker recognize lost sleep and formulate a strategy for how to obtain more hours of sleep. The sleep log can also help identify behaviors that disrupt the major sleep period and lead to daytime sleepiness.

Other sleep features

The diagnosis of a primary sleep disorder causing EDS needs to be considered. Sleep disorders such as narcolepsy, OSA, recurrent hypersomnia, insufficient sleep time, and circadian rhythm disorders can often be determined by the patient's history.

Obstructive sleep apnea

The presence of snoring, episodes of choking or gasping for air, or witnessed apnea may be reported by the patient or bed partner and often indicate sleep-related breathing disorders. Occasionally, only snoring is reported because the patient is unaware that she or he has trouble breathing while asleep. Additional signs of sleep apnea include awakening with a dry mouth, nasal congestion, nighttime cough, nocturnal enuresis, and morning headaches. It is helpful to have a bed partner present to identify variations in the quality of snoring, because apnea may present as episodes of loud snoring that alternate with quiet episodes of pauses in breathing.[22] The presence of a bed partner can also be helpful in

SLEEP DIARY

Fatigue Rating Scale	0 extremely fatigued	25 moderately fatigued	50 mildly fatigued	75 somewhat fatigued	100 very energetic

COMPLETE AT NIGHT in reference to today | | | | | | | | COMPLETE IN MORNING in reference to night before

Day and Date	Unusual daytime stressors	Fatigue rating (use rating scale on top of page)	Naps (time & length)	Exercise (Y/N, time of day and how long)	Caffeine (note type and time) Cigarettes	Sleep meds or alcohol (name & dose)	Time you went to bed and turned out the lights	How long it took you to fall asleep for the first time	Number of times you woke falling asleep	How long you were awake in total after falling asleep	Time you finally woke up	Time you finally got out of bed
Mon. 9/14	Pain/ Stress	68	2–4 pm	No	Coffee, 8oz at noon	Ambien 10mg	12:00	60 min.	3	60 min.	6:30	8:00

Fig. 2. Sleep diary.

identifying the deleterious effects of snoring on interpersonal relationships, a possibility that is often a key motivating factor in seeking out a sleep evaluation.

Obesity is an established risk factor for sleep apnea. The weight and height of each patient should be documented, as well as any weight changes over the past few years or attempts at weight loss.[23]

Menopause, independent of age and body mass index, is also a risk factor for sleep apnea.[24] Determining if a woman is premenopausal or postmenopausal can help determine if she is at risk for sleep apnea.

Narcolepsy

Daytime sleepiness is the hallmark of narcolepsy. Cataplexy, characterized by sudden loss of muscle tone brought on by emotions, is pathognomonic for narcolepsy. Additional features, such as hypnogogic hallucinations and sleep paralysis, can also help establish a diagnosis of narcolepsy; however, neither is specific to narcolepsy and both can be seen in disorders of sleep fragmentation.[25,26] Narcolepsy patients often report fragmented sleep and automatic behaviors. A detailed history of excessive, frequent, and bizarre dreams, as well as out-of-body experiences, delusional or lucid dreams, and dreams in naps can be consistent with a diagnosis of narcolepsy. A diagnosis of narcolepsy without cataplexy (narcolepsy type 2) is appropriate when EDS is present with rapid eye movement (REM) phenomenology (hypnogogic hallucinations and sleep paralysis) but without cataplexy.

Idiopathic hypersomnia

EDS without the presence of REM phenomena, such as cataplexy and hypnagogic hallucinations, that has persisted for more than 3 months may indicate idiopathic hypersomnia if all other causes of hypersomnia have been ruled out by polysomnography. This is often a diagnosis of exclusion.

Kleine-Levin syndrome

A history of relapsing and remitting episodes of sleepiness that occur at least once a year, lasting 2 days to 4 weeks, and that are associated with cognitive and behavioral disturbances, might suggest Kleine-Levin Syndrome. Normal levels of alertness, behavior, and cognition are present in between episodes.

Circadian rhythm disorders

Obtaining a detailed sleep history, as well as a sleep log, can help diagnose circadian rhythm disorders. Sleepiness in these disorders is caused by a misalignment between the endogenous circadian clock and the schedules imposed by society. In shift work disorder it is essential to determine the patient's work schedule. Rotating shifts that alternate schedules every few weeks can make patients particularly vulnerable to work-related injuries resulting from sleepiness.[27] Night shifts are usually the most disruptive to circadian rhythms; however, early morning shifts, especially when traveling to work is involved, can also present a problem and result in excessive sleepiness.

Other sleep disorders

It is important to differentiate fatigue and lack of energy from daytime sleepiness in insomnia patients. Insomnia patients do not generally report a propensity to fall asleep when sedentary. If EDS is present in the setting of insomnia, a suspicion for an underlying sleep disorder, such as sleep apnea, should be raised.[28]

Although restless leg syndrome (RLS) and periodic limb movement disorder are not a common cause of EDS, an inquiry into the presence of unpleasant sensations in the legs, an urge to move the limbs, or jerking of the legs in bed should be done.

Medical History

A comprehensive medical history should be performed with particular focus on cardiovascular, cerebrovascular, and nasopharyngeal disease. Hypertension, type II diabetes, ischemic heart disease, heart failure, atrial fibrillation, and pulmonary hypertension have all been linked to OSA.[29–36] Congestive heart failure is also a risk factor for central sleep apnea.[37] Sleep apnea and stroke have also been linked in a bidirectional manner, with sleep apnea, increasing the risk for stroke and the incidence of sleep apnea being increased following a stroke.[38–41]

Chronic nasal congestion is associated with fragmented sleep and sleep-disordered breathing.[42,43] It is helpful to inquire about the presence of nasal allergies, postnasal drip, sinus disease, and rhinitis. Additionally, any prior history of adenoid or tonsil surgery or upper airway surgery should be documented.

The association of sleep and pain is bidirectional.[44] Pain syndromes, such as neuropathy or arthritis, can fragment sleep, leading to daytime sleepiness.[45,46] Conversely, newer studies have shown that disrupted sleep can reliably predict new occurrence and worsening of chronic pain.[47,48]

Metabolic disorders, such as thyroid dysfunction or diabetes, can cause EDS and should be inquired about in a medical history.[49–51]

Many prescription medications can cause either daytime sleepiness or impair nighttime sleep.[52] Pain medications, such as opioids, have been linked with an increase in sleep-disordered breathing.[53,54] Methadone has been linked to an increase in both central sleep apnea and OSA.[55,56]

Psychiatric History

It is prudent to inquire about mood disorders, such as depression or bipolar disorder, because these disorders can manifest as excessive sleepiness. Sleepiness can be due to a psychiatric condition, psychiatric medications, or a comorbid sleep disorder. Prolonged nocturnal sleep or EDS can be a presenting symptom in atypical depression or some bipolar depression.[57,58] Nocturnal panic attacks, which can present as part of an anxiety disorder, can cause fragmented nocturnal sleep and result in daytime sleepiness.[59]

Tricyclic antidepressants, antipsychotic medications, benzodiazepines, and certain serotonin reuptake inhibitors can lead to daytime sleepiness.[60,61] Additionally, many mood stabilizing medications can lead to weight gain, which is a risk factor for OSA.[62]

Social and Family History

The social history should focus on any personal stressors that may disrupt nighttime sleep. The frequency and timing of exercise should also be determined because it can also have an effect on nighttime sleep.[63]

Caffeine consumption should be inquired about because of its disruptive effects on sleep.[64] Furthermore, excessive caffeine consumption can indicate a need to self-medicate to combat daytime sleepiness.

Smoking tobacco, both during consumption and withdrawal, has been associated with fragmented sleep. Additionally, it may be a risk factor for sleep-disordered breathing.[65,66]

Alcohol decreases sleep latency and consolidates sleep in the first part of the night, but it disrupts the second half of sleep.[67,68] Alcoholics, both during binge drinking and withdrawal, experience excessive sleepiness, insomnia, and fragmented nighttime sleep.[69,70] Illicit drugs, such as cocaine, methylenedioxymethamphetamine (ecstasy), and ketamine, can also cause severe sleep disruption both during consumption and withdrawal.[71,72]

A family history is found in many sleep disorders, such as narcolepsy, RLS, and OSA with or without obesity, and should be inquired about.[1]

Physical Examination

The physical examination should include an evaluation of the nose, throat, neck, heart, lungs, abdomen, extremities, and neurologic system. Vital signs, including blood pressure, heart rate, weight, height, body mass index, and neck circumference, should be collected. Evaluation of the upper airway should focus on size and shape of the soft palate, tongue, uvula, airway, pharyngeal tissue, and tongue. Nasal examination should look for the presence of a deviated nasal septum and/or turbinate hypertrophy. The cervicofacial angle should be examined for possible retrognathia or micrognathia, both of which can be associated with OSA.[73,74] A patient can be referred to an otolaryngologist for upper airway endoscopy to establish the location and severity of obstruction in the nasopharynx and/or oropharynx. Thyroid size should be determined because enlargement can obstruct the upper airway.[75,76] For a patient suspected of having narcolepsy and cataplexy, observing the patients face during the interview may reveal facial muscle weakness or twitching during emotion that can indicate cataplexy.

A neurologic examination should be performed to look for secondary causes of narcolepsy, idiopathic hypersomnia, and RLS. Additionally, a neurologic examination to evaluate the possibility of Parkinson disease or a previous stroke can help with differentiating causes of excessive sleepiness. A vascular examination, including assessing for distal pulses and for the presence of peripheral edema, is also helpful in ruling out secondary causes of leg symptoms that disturb sleep.

Sleep Questionnaires

Sleep questionnaires can be valuable tools for obtaining information regarding sleep complaints, sleep pattern, sleep hygiene, and medical and social history. The ESS is widely used to assess the degree of daytime sleepiness (see **Fig. 1**). Other sleep questionnaires that can be useful in assessing sleepiness include the Stanford Sleepiness Scale, the Pittsburgh Sleep Quality Index, the Ullanlinna Narcolepsy Scale, or the Karolinska Sleepiness Scale. The Swiss Narcolepsy Scale can be helpful to detect cataplexy. When positive, it is consistent with a diagnosis of narcolepsy type 1 (**Box 3**).

A sleep log kept over a 2-week period that documents time of sleep onset, awakenings during the night, wake time, naps, and other sleep-related habits can be helpful in monitoring sleep patterns and determining what factors are contributing to daytime sleepiness.

Box 3
Swiss narcolepsy scale

1. How often are you unable to fall asleep?
   a. Never
   b. Rarely (less than once a month)
   c. Sometimes (1–3 times a month)
   d. Often (1–2 times a week)
   e. Almost always

2. How often do you feel bad or not well rested in the morning?
   a. Never
   b. Rarely (less than once a month)
   c. Sometimes (1–3 times a month)
   d. Often (1–2 times a week)
   e. Almost always

3. How often do you take a nap during the day?
   a. Never
   b. I would like to but cannot
   c. 1 to 2 times a week
   d. 3 to 5 times a week
   e. Almost daily

4. How often have you experienced weak knees or buckling of the knees during emotions like laughing, happiness, or anger?
   a. Never
   b. Rarely (less than once a month)
   c. Sometimes (1–3 times a month)
   d. Often (1–2 times a week)
   e. Almost always

5. How often have you experienced sagging of the jaw during emotions like laughing, happiness, or anger?
   a. Never
   b. Rarely (less than once a month)
   c. Sometimes (1–3 times a month)
   d. Often (1–2 times a week)
   e. Almost always

Each question (Q) is weighted by a positive or negative factor, with the score calculated using the following equation: $(6 \times Q1 + 9 \times Q2 - 5 \times Q3 - 11 \times Q4 - 13 \times Q5 + 20)$.[101,102] Interpretation: A Swiss Narcolepsy Scale (SNS) score less than 0 is suggestive of narcolepsy with cataplexy.[101,102] Validation: In patients with narcolepsy with cataplexy, an SNS score less than 0 was shown to have a sensitivity of 96% and specificity of 98%.[102]

Blood and Urine Tests

Screening blood work is usually done by the primary care physician before referral to the sleep physician for EDS. If signs of thyroid dysfunction are present, the patient should be sent for thyroid function tests. However, this is not recommended routinely unless the patient is in a high-risk group for the development of hypothyroidism, such as women over age 60 years.[77,78]

Blood work should be done as part of the evaluation of patients with RLS. These tests should include a complete blood count, chemistry panel, iron studies, and serum ferritin levels. An iron saturation below 16% or a serum ferritin below 50 μg/L indicates a need for iron supplementation.[79]

Serum and urine drug screening can be an important part of the evaluation for EDS. Recent studies suggest that use of opioids, cannabis, and/or amphetamines can mimic the findings of idiopathic hypersomnia and/or narcolepsy on a multiple sleep latency test (MSLT).[80,81] In these studies, substance use was not reported on initial interview and most physicians did not suspect drug use.[80] Undetected drug or substance abuse could lead to over-diagnosing central causes of hypersomnia and inappropriate treatment. A genetic blood test for the HLA antigen HLA-DQB1*0602 can be helpful in the diagnosis of narcolepsy because it is nearly 100% positive in narcolepsy type 1.

Polysomnography

Polysomnography is an objective measure of sleep that is indicated in evaluating a patient with EDS, unless a circadian rhythm disorder or insufficient sleep disorder is suspected by history. The amount of sleep, percentage of time in each sleep stage, sleep fragmentation, as well as the possible cause of sleep fragmentation is recorded. Causes of sleep fragmentation on polysomnography include respiratory events, such as apneas or hypopneas; abnormal movements in sleep, such as periodic limb movements; and/or other disruptive behaviors, such as parasomnias or epileptiform activity.

An overnight attended polysomnogram in the sleep laboratory monitors sleep parameters and stages via electroencephalogram (EEG), body movements via electromyography (EMG) applied to the lower limbs and chin, eye movement to differentiate sleep stages via electrooculogram, and cardiac tracing via electrocardiogram (EKG). Respiratory parameters are measured with respiratory effort belts that monitor movement of the chest and abdomen, airflow and air pressure sensors applied to the nose and mouth, and oxygen saturation using an infrared oximeter. Other sensors that can be placed when appropriate are upper-extremity EMG to record arm movements, sensors to record end-tidal carbon dioxide concentration, body position, snoring sounds, or gastroesophageal pH. The information is stored digitally on a computer that is later analyzed. Recording speed is typically at 15 mm per second, but this can be adjusted when needed, such as when epileptiform activity is suspected.[82]

The attended polysomnogram is invaluable in providing the information needed to elucidate most causes of sleep fragmentation and resultant daytime sleepiness. An unattended ambulatory polysomnogram done at the patient's home can be used when there is a high suspicion for OSA as the cause of daytime sleepiness.[83–85] However, technical difficulties associated with an unattended recording often limit its value. Additionally, other causes of daytime sleepiness can be missed on home polysomnogram because it routinely only monitors respiratory parameters and EKG without capturing sleep stages and awakenings via EEG.

An in-laboratory, attended, polysomnography is needed in the diagnosing of parasomnias, such as REM sleep behavior disorder; abnormal movements in sleep, such as periodic limb movements; and central causes of sleepiness, such as narcolepsy. Video monitoring, extra EEG leads, and additional EMG leads on the arms are needed to capture abnormal activity in sleep and to help differentiate parasomnias from epileptic disorders.[86] In-laboratory polysomnography can also help confirm the presence of narcolepsy by documenting a short REM latency and by ruling out other causes of sleepiness on the polysomnogram, such as OSA. When narcolepsy is suspected, the polysomnogram is followed by a MSLT. A diagnosis of narcolepsy can be made when the MSLT demonstrates 2 or more sleep-onset REM periods (SOREMPs) with a mean sleep latency of 8 minutes or less.[1] The presence of a SOREMP within 15 minutes on a polysomnogram is highly suggestive of narcolepsy and can count as 1 of the 2 required for a diagnosis of narcolepsy[1]

Polysomnography is not indicated in the diagnosis of insomnia, unless a second sleep disorder is suspected. If EDS, defined as the tendency to fall asleep in the daytime, is present in a patient with insomnia, then a second sleep disorder, such as OSA, should be considered. Older patients with OSA often present with symptoms of insomnia because of their disturbed nighttime sleep. Often these patients report symptoms of insomnia as well as EDS, and a polysomnogram should be done.[87]

Multiple Sleep Latency Test

The MSLT is used to document the degree of daytime sleepiness. It is performed 2 hours after waking from an overnight polysomnogram and consists of 4 or 5 naps, each 2 hours apart. Twenty minutes are allotted to achieve sleep, and the average time to fall asleep on each of the naps is documented. Additionally, the presence of REM sleep in the daytime naps is also documented. Multiple studies have determined that a mean sleep latency of 11.1 minutes or greater with 1 episode of REM sleep is normal for the general population.[88–94] Narcolepsy is suspected when there is a mean sleep latency of less than 8 minutes and 2 SOREMPs, 1 of which may be seen during the preceding night's polysomnogram.[1] Idiopathic hypersomnia patients have a similar mean sleep latency without the presence of REM sleep in daytime naps.[1] Studies of shift workers have documented an average mean sleep latency of less than 5 minutes, which indicates severe sleepiness.[95,96]

Maintenance of Wakefulness Test

The maintenance of wakefulness test (MWT) is used to measure the ability to stay awake. It consists of 4 40-minute intervals in which a patient is asked to sit still and not engage in any stimulating activities. It is often used to measure the effects of alerting medication on daytime functioning. Additionally, it can be used to assess a person's ability to remain awake during work as a commercial driver, a pilot, or other occupations. The Federal Aviation Administration requires an annual MWT to determine the fitness for work in pilots (www.faa.gov). Some employers use the MWT to document response to continuous positive airway pressure in OSA patients.

Performance Testing

Research studies often use performance tests, such as the psychomotor vigilance test (PVT), to assess the behavioral consequences of EDS. The PVT measures reaction time to tasks with high stimulus density to measure attention and performance. Reliable performance changes have been demonstrated on the PVT even with moderate levels of sleepiness due to sleep deprivation.[97] Memory and executive functioning can also be assessed using various cognitive assessment tests when needed.[98]

The Oxford Sleepiness Resistance Test (OSLER) is an alternative test that combines elements of the MWT and psychomotor testing. The OSLER tracks continuing behavioral responses to the activation of a light turning on. A failure to respond to 7 consecutive presentations suggests sleep onset. Multiple studies have shown the OSLER to be a reliable tool for determining a patient's ability to stay awake and vigilant.[99,100]

Electroencephalogram

The EEG is used to investigate possible seizures and to differentiate seizures from other abnormal activity in sleep, such as parasomnias. If seizures are suspected, extra EEG leads are placed in addition to the standard number of leads used for a routine polysomnogram. If epileptiform activity is captured, a more detailed seizure work up should be done.

Neuroimaging

Neuroimaging is needed when an underlying neurologic disorder is being considered as a cause of daytime sleepiness. It can be used to rule out structural lesions in the brainstem that may cause sleepiness. It is usually not required in narcolepsy but may be indicated in patients with idiopathic hypersomnia and patients with REM sleep behavior disorder.

Other Studies

EMG and nerve conduction studies may be used when underlying neuropathy is a possible cause of symptoms of RLS. Upper airway endoscopy can be used in patients with OSA to determine the location of obstruction and guide possible intervention. Pulmonary function tests can be used when an underlying respiratory disorder is suspected in patients with sleep-related breathing disorders. An EKG or echocardiogram is needed when underlying ischemic heart disease or congestive heart failure is suspected, such as in patients with central sleep apnea.

SUMMARY

This article outlines the approach to a patient presenting with excessive sleepiness. The evaluation begins with a careful clinical assessment that includes a detailed sleep history, medical, psychiatric, medications, and social and family history. Physical examination should include a general medical examination, as well as an examination of the upper airway and a neurologic examination. A sleep log can often be very helpful. The patient's history and physical examination will often reveal the suspected cause of daytime sleepiness. Appropriate objective testing with a polysomnogram and possibly an MSLT will help confirm the diagnosis and direct the appropriate treatment plan.

REFERENCES

1. ICSD-3. International classification of sleep disorders. 3rd edition. Chicago: American Academy of Sleep Medicine; 2014.
2. Neu D, Linkowski P, le Bon O. Clinical complaints of daytime sleepiness and fatigue: how to distinguish and treat them, especially when they become 'excessive' or 'chronic'? Acta Neurol Belg 2010;110(1):15–25.
3. Chaudhuri KR. Nocturnal symptom complex in PD and its management. Neurology 2003;61(6 Suppl 3):S17–23.
4. Chervin RD. Sleepiness, fatigue, tiredness, and lack of energy in obstructive sleep apnea. Chest 2000;118(2):372–9.
5. Gradisar M, Wolfson AR, Harvey AG, et al. The sleep and technology use of Americans: findings from the National Sleep Foundation's 2011 Sleep in America poll. J Clin Sleep Med 2013;9(12):1291–9.
6. Thorpy M. Current concepts in the etiology, diagnosis and treatment of narcolepsy. Sleep Med 2001;2(1):5–17.
7. Broughton R, Ghanem Q, Hishikawa Y, et al. Life effects of narcolepsy in 180 patients from North America, Asia and Europe compared to matched controls. Can J Neurol Sci 1981;8(4):299–304.
8. Stepanski E, Lamphere J, Badia P, et al. Sleep fragmentation and daytime sleepiness. Sleep 1984;7(1):18–26.
9. McKenna JT, Tartar JL, Ward CP, et al. Sleep fragmentation elevates behavioral, electrographic and neurochemical measures of sleepiness. Neuroscience 2007;146(4):1462–73.
10. Oksenberg A, Arons E, Nasser K, et al. Severe obstructive sleep apnea: sleepy versus non sleepy patients. Laryngoscope 2010;120(3):643–8.
11. Frenette E, Kushida CA. Primary hypersomnias of central origin. Semin Neurol 2009;29(4):354–67.
12. Bove A, Culebras A, Moore JT, et al. Relationship between sleep spindles and hypersomnia. Sleep 1994;17(5):449–55.
13. Sforza E, Gaudreau H, Petit D, et al. Homeostatic sleep regulation in patients with idiopathic hypersomnia. Clin Neurophysiol 2000;111(2):277–82.
14. Nishino S, Kanbayashi T. Symptomatic narcolepsy, cataplexy and hypersomnia, and their implications in the hypothalamic hypocretin/orexin system. Sleep Med Rev 2005;9(4):269–310.
15. Swanson LM, Arned JT, Rosekind MR, et al. Sleep disorders and work performance: findings from the 2008 National Sleep Foundation Sleep in America poll. J Sleep Res 2011;20(3):487–94.
16. Enright P, Newman A, Wahl P, et al. Prevalence and correlates of snoring and observes apneas in 5,201 older adults. Sleep 1996;19:531–8.

17. Whitney C, Enright P, Newman A, et al. Correlates of daytime sleepiness in 4578 elderly persons: the Cardiovascular Health Study. Sleep 1998;21:27–36.

18. Ohayon M. Epidemiology of excessive sleepiness. In: Thorpy M, Billiard M, editors. Sleepiness causes, consequences and treatment. New York: Cambridge University Press; 2011. p. 3–13.

19. Merino-Andreu M, Arnulf I, Konofal E, et al. Unawareness of naps in Parkinson disease and in disorders with excessive daytime sleepiness. Neurology 2003;60(9):1553–4.

20. Sleep-related breathing disorders in adults: recommendations for syndrome definition and measurement techniques in clinical research. The Report of an American Academy of Sleep Medicine Task Force. Sleep 1999;22(5):667–89.

21. Powell N, Schechtman K, Riley R, et al. Sleepy driver near-misses may predict accident risks. Sleep 2007;30(3):331–42.

22. Takegami M, Hayashino Y, Chin K, et al. Simple four-variable screening tool for identification of patients with sleep-disordered breathing. Sleep 2009; 32(7):939–48.

23. Tuomilehto H, Seppä J, Uusitupa M. Obesity and obstructive sleep apnea–clinical significance of weight loss. Sleep Med Rev 2013;17(5):321–9.

24. Young T, Peppard P, Gottlieb D. The epidemiology of obstructive sleep apnea: a population health perspective. Am J Respir Crit Care Med 2002; 165:1217–39.

25. Sharpless BA, Barber JP. Lifetime prevalence rates of sleep paralysis: a systematic review. Sleep Med Rev 2011;15(5):311–5.

26. Ohayon MM, Priest RG, Caulet M, et al. Hypnagogic and hypnopompic hallucinations: pathological phenomena? Br J Psychiatry 1996;169(4):459–67.

27. Wong I, Smith P, Mustard C, et al. For better or worse? Changing shift schedules and the risk of work injury among men and women. Scand J Work Environ Health 2014;40(6):621–30.

28. Fung C, Martin J, Dzierzewski J, et al. Prevalence and symptoms of occult sleep disordered breathing among older veterans with insomnia. J Clin Sleep Med 2013;9(11):1173–8.

29. Wang Y, Li C, Feng L, et al. Prevalence of hypertension and circadian blood pressure variations in patients with obstructive sleep apnoea-hypopnoea syndrome. J Int Med Res 2014;42(3):773–80.

30. Herrscher TE, Akre H, Overland B, et al. High prevalence of sleep apnea in heart failure outpatients: even in patients with preserved systolic function. J Card Fail 2011;17:420–5.

31. Levy P, Ryan S, Oldenburg O, et al. Sleep apnoea and the heart. Eur Respir Rev 2013;22(129):333–52.

32. Bradley TD, Floras JS. Obstructive sleep apnoea and its cardiovascular consequences. Lancet 2009;373(9657):82–93.

33. Dumitrascu R, Tiede H, Eckermann J, et al. Sleep apnea in precapillary pulmonary hypertension. Sleep Med 2013;14:247–51.

34. Reichmuth KJ, Austin D, Skatrud JB, et al. Association of sleep apnea and type II diabetes: a population-based study. Am J Respir Crit Care Med 2005;172(12):1590–5.

35. Botros N, Concato J, Mohsenin V, et al. Obstructive sleep apnea as a risk factor for type 2 diabetes. Am J Med 2009;122(12):1122–7.

36. Gami AS, Hodge DO, Herges RM, et al. Obstructive sleep apnea, obesity, and the risk of incident atrial fibrillation. J Am Coll Cardiol 2007;49(5):565–71.

37. Garcia-Touchard A, Somers VK, Olson LJ, et al. Central sleep apnea: implications for congestive heart failure. Chest 2008;133:1495–504.

38. Redline S, Yenokyan G, Gottlieb DJ, et al. Obstructive sleep apnea-hypopnea and incident stroke: the sleep heart health study. Am J Respir Crit Care Med 2010;182:269–77.

39. Yaggi HK, Concato J, Kernan WN, et al. Obstructive sleep apnea as a risk factor for stroke and death. N Engl J Med 2005;353:2034–41.

40. Broadley SA, Jorgensen L, Cheek A, et al. Early investigation and treatment of obstructive sleep apnea after stroke. J Clin Neurosci 2007;14(4):328–33.

41. Noradina AT, Hamidon BB, Roslan H, et al. Risk factors for developing sleep-disordered breathing in patients with recent ischaemic stroke. Singapore Med J 2006;47(5):392–9.

42. Lunn M, Craig T. Rhinitis and sleep. Sleep Med Rev 2011;15(5):293–9.

43. Sardana N, Craig TJ. Congestion and sleep impairment in allergic rhinitis. Asian Pac J Allergy Immunol 2011;29(4):297–306.

44. Finan P, Goodin B, Smith M. The association of sleep and pain: an update and a path forward. J Pain 2013;14(12):1539–52.

45. Allen KD, Renner JB, Devellis B, et al. Osteoarthritis and sleep: the Johnston county osteoarthritis project. J Rheumatol 2008;35(6):1102–7.

46. Palermo TM, Kiska R. Subjective sleep disturbances in adolescents with chronic pain: relationship to daily functioning and quality of life. J Pain 2005;6(3):201–7.

47. Odegard S, Sand T, Engstrom M, et al. The long-term effect of insomnia on primary headaches: a prospective population-based cohort study (HUNT-2 and HUNT-3) headache. Headache 2011;51:570–80.

48. Mork PJ, Nilsen TI. Sleep problems and risk of fibromyalgia: longitudinal data on an adult female population in Norway. Arthritis Rheum 2012;64:281–4.

49. Misiolek M, Marek B, Namyslowski G, et al. Sleep apnea syndrome and snoring in patients with

hypothyroidism with relation to overweight. J Physiol Pharmacol 2007;58(Suppl 1):77–85.

50. Chasens ER, Umlauf MG, Weaver TE. Sleepiness, physical activity, and functional outcomes in veterans with type 2 diabetes. Appl Nurs Res 2009; 22(3):176–82.

51. Saaresranta T, Irjala K, Aittokallio T, et al. Sleep quality, daytime sleepiness and fasting insulin levels in women with chronic obstructive pulmonary disease. Respir Med 2005;99(7):856–63.

52. Obermeyer WH, Benca RM. Effects of drugs on sleep. Neurol Clin 1996;14(4):827–40.

53. Morasco B, O'Hearn D, Turk D, et al. Associations between prescription opioid use and sleep impairment among veterans with chronic pain. Pain Med 2014;15(11):1902–10.

54. Cheatle MD, Webster LR. Opioid therapy and sleep disorders: risks and mitigation strategies. Pain Med 2015;16(Suppl 1):S22–6.

55. Wang D, Teichtahl H, Drummer O. Central sleep apnea in stable methadone maintenance treatment patients. Chest 2005;128(3):1348–56.

56. Sharkey K, Kurth M, Anderson B. Obstructive sleep apnea is more common than central sleep apnea in methadone maintenance patients with subjective sleep complaints. Drug Alcohol Depend 2010; 108(1–2):77–83.

57. Posternak MA, Zimmerman M. Symptoms of atypical depression. Psychiatry Res 2001;104(2): 175–81.

58. Mitchell PB, Wilhelm K, Parker G, et al. The clinical features of bipolar depression: a comparison with matched major depressive disorder patients. J Clin Psychiatry 2001;62(3):212–6.

59. Vgontzas AN, Bixler EO, Kales A, et al. Differences in nocturnal and daytime sleep between primary and psychiatric hypersomnia: diagnostic and treatment implications. Psychosom Med 2000;62(2): 220–6.

60. Wichniak A, Wierzbicka A, Jernajczyk W. Sleep and antidepressant treatment. Curr Pharm Des 2012; 18(36):5802–17.

61. Waters F, Faulkner D, Naik N, et al. Effects of polypharmacy on sleep in psychiatric inpatients. Schizophr Res 2012;139(1–3):225–8.

62. Rishi MA, Shetty M, Wolff A, et al. Atypical antipsychotic medications are independently associated with severe obstructive sleep apnea. Clin Neuropharmacol 2010;33(3):109–13.

63. Youngstedt SD, Kline CE. Epidemiology of exercise and sleep. Sleep Biol Rhythms 2006;4(3):215–21.

64. Drake C, Roehrs T, Shambroom J, et al. Caffeine effects on sleep taken 0, 3, or 6 hours before going to bed. J Clin Sleep Med 2013;9(11):1195–2000.

65. Deleanu OC, Pocora D, Mihălcuţă S, et al. Influence of smoking on sleep and obstructive sleep apnea syndrome. Pneumologia 2016;65(1):28–35.

66. Balaguer C, Palou A, Alonso-Fernández A. Smoking and sleep disorders. Arch Bronconeumol 2009;45(9):449–58.

67. Thakkar MM, Sharma R, Sahota P. Alcohol disrupts sleep homeostasis. Alcohol 2015;49(4):299–310.

68. Ebrahim IO, Shapiro CM, Williams AJ, et al. Alcohol and sleep I: effects on normal sleep. Alcohol Clin Exp Res 2013;37(4):539–49.

69. Colrain IM, Turlington S, Baker FC. Impact of alcoholism on sleep architecture and EEG power spectra in men and women. Sleep 2009;32: 1341–52.

70. Brower KJ, Perron BE. Sleep disturbance as a universal risk factor for relapse in addictions to psychoactive substances. Med Hypotheses 2010;74: 928–33.

71. Schierenbeck T, Riemann D, Berger M, et al. Effect of illicit recreational drugs upon sleep: cocaine, ecstasy and marijuana. Sleep Med Rev 2008;12(5): 381–9.

72. Tang J, Liao Y, He H, et al. Sleeping problems in Chinese illicit drug dependent subjects. BMC Psychiatry 2015;15:28.

73. Lowe AA, Fleetham JA, Adachi S, et al. Cephalometric and computed tomographic predictors of obstructive sleep apnea severity. Am J Orthod Dentofacial Orthop 1995;107(6):589–95.

74. Johns FR, Strollo PJ Jr, Buckley M, et al. The influence of craniofacial structure on obstructive sleep apnea in young adults. J Oral Maxillofac Surg 1998;56(5):596–602.

75. Lin WN, Lee LA, Wang CC, et al. Obstructive sleep apnea syndrome in an adolescent girl with hypertrophic lingual thyroid. Pediatr Pulmonol 2009; 44(1):93–5.

76. Barnes TW, Olsen KD, Morgenthaler TI. Obstructive lingual thyroid causing sleep apnea: a case report and review of the literature. Sleep Med 2004;5(6):605–7.

77. Mickelson SA, Lian T, Rosenthal L. Thyroid testing and thyroid hormone replacement in patients with sleep disordered breathing. Ear Nose Throat J 1999;78(10):768–71, 774-5.

78. Winkelman JW, Goldman H, Piscatelli N, et al. Are thyroid function tests necessary in patients with suspected sleep apnea? Sleep 1996;19(10):790–3.

79. Kryger MH, Otake K, Foerster J. Low body stores of iron and restless legs syndrome: a correctable cause of insomnia in adolescents and teenagers. Sleep Med 2002;3(2):127–32.

80. Kosky CA, Bonakis A, Yogendran A, et al. Urine toxicology in adults evaluated for a central hypersomnia and how the results modify the Physician's diagnosis. J Clin Sleep Med 2016;12(11): 1499–505.

81. Dzodzomenyo S, Stolfi A, Splaingard D, et al. Urine toxicology screen in multiple sleep latency test: the

correlation of positive tetrahydrocannabinol, drug negative patients, and narcolepsy. J Clin Sleep Med 2015;11(2):93–9.

82. Berry RB, Gamaldo CE, Harding SM, et al. AASM Scoring Manual Version 2.2 Updates: new chapters for scoring infant sleep staging and home sleep apnea testing. J Clin Sleep Med 2015;11(11):1253–4.

83. Garg N, Rolle AJ, Lee TA, et al. Home-based diagnosis of obstructive sleep apnea in an urban population. J Clin Sleep Med 2014;10(8):879–85.

84. Dawson A, Loving RT, Gordon RM, et al. Type III home sleep testing versus pulse oximetry: is the respiratory disturbance index better than the oxygen desaturation index to predict the apnoea-hypopnoea index measured during laboratory polysomnography? BMJ Open 2015;5(6):e007956.

85. Tedeschi E, Carratù P, Damiani MF, et al. Home unattended portable monitoring and automatic CPAP titration in patients with high risk for moderate to severe obstructive sleep apnea. Respir Care 2013; 58(7):1178–83.

86. Aldrich M, Jahnke B. Diagnostic value of video-EEG polysomnography. Neurology 1991;41:1060–6.

87. Littner M, Hirshkowitz M, Kramer M, et al. Practice parameters for using polysomnography to evaluate insomnia: an update. Sleep 2003;26(6):754–60.

88. Levine B, Roehrs T, Zorick F, et al. Daytime sleepiness in young adults. Sleep 1988;11(1):39–46.

89. Johns MW. Sensitivity and specificity of the multiple latency test (MSLT), the maintenance of wakefulness test and the Epworth sleepiness scale: failure of the MSLT as a gold standard. J Sleep Res 2000;9(1):5–11.

90. Bliwise DL, Carskadon MA, Seidel WF, et al. MSLT-defined sleepiness and neuropsychological test performance do not correlate in the elderly. Neurobiol Aging 1991;12(5):463–8.

91. Steinberg R, Schonberg C, Weess HG, et al. The validity of the multiple sleep latency test. J Sleep Res 1996;5(Suppl 1):220.

92. Hartse KM, Zorick F, Sicklesteel J, et al. Nap recordings in the diagnosis of daytime somnolence. J Sleep Res 1979;8:190.

93. Van den Hoed J, Kraemer H, Guilleminault C, et al. Disorders of excessive daytime somnolence: polygraphic and clinical data for 100 patients. Sleep 1981;4(1):23–37.

94. Carskadon MA, Dement WC, Mitler MM, et al. Guidelines for the multiple sleep latency test (MSLT): standard measure of sleepiness. Sleep 1986;9(4):519–24.

95. Roehrs T, Roth T. Multiple sleep latency test: technical aspects of normal values. J Clin Neuropsychol 1992;9:63–7.

96. Czeisler CA, Walsh JK, Roth T, et al. Modafinil for excessive sleepiness associated with shift-work sleep disorder. N Engl J Med 2005;353:476–86.

97. Lim J, Dinges DF. Sleep deprivation and vigilant attention. Ann N Y Acad Sci 2008;1129:305–22.

98. Dubois B, Slachevsky A, Litvan I, et al. The FAB:a frontal assessment battery at bedside. Neurology 2000;55(11):1621–6.

99. Mazza S, Pepin JL, Deschaux C, et al. Analysis of error profiles occurring during the OSLER test: a sensitive means of detecting fluctuation in vigilance in patients with obstructive sleep apnea syndrome. Am J Respir Crit Care Med 2002;166(4): 474–8.

100. Priest B, Brichard C, Aubert G, et al. Microsleep during a simplified maintenance of wakefulness test. A validation study of the OSLER test. Am J Respir Crit Care Med 2001;163(7):1619–25.

101. Bassetti CL. Spectrum of narcolepsy. In: Baumann CR, Bassetti CL, Scammell TE, editors. Narcolepsy: pathophysiology, diagnosis, and treatment. New York: Springer Science+Business Media; 2011. p. 309–19.

102. Sturzenegger C, Bassetti CL. The clinical spectrum of narcolepsy with cataplexy: a reappraisal. J Sleep Res 2004;13(4):395–406.

Subjective and Objective Assessment of Hypersomnolence

Brian James Murray, MD, FRCPC, D,ABSM

KEYWORDS

- Sleepiness • Hypersomnia • Multiple sleep latency test • Maintenance of wakefulness test
- Epworth Sleepiness Scale • Subjective sleepiness • Objective sleepiness

KEY POINTS

- Subjective measures of sleepiness are prone to bias.
- Objective measures of sleepiness should be used where possible.
- The multiple sleep latency test (MSLT) is most appropriate for assessment of narcolepsy.
- The maintenance of wakefulness test (MWT) has better conceptual validity for safety assessments.
- Better tests are needed and under development.

INTRODUCTION

Sleep is important for general health. Lack of sleep and sleep disorders are associated with several psychological[1,2] and medical complications.[3–5] Impaired alertness can lead to accidents.[6] Recent studies have suggested that the financial impact of sleep loss is dramatic in society.[7] Sleepiness can be operationalized in terms of the inability to remain awake for various activities. Lack of sleep itself does not correlate with sleepiness[8] because genetic differences and underlying sleep disorders can affect propensity to sleepiness, and circadian factors[9] can significantly influence moment-to-moment alertness. Subjective report of daytime sleepiness is composed of several characteristic components, including perceived sleepiness and the tendency to fall asleep in passive and active situations.[10]

Appropriate selection of a subjective or objective scale for the assessment of sleepiness should take into account several factors. No test is perfect, but careful consideration of the goals of a tool can help identify techniques that may be able to address particular clinical needs.[11]

Considerations include whether a tool is for clinical or research purposes; whether a tool is for assessment of a trait, such as a diagnosis, or a state, such as current alertness; the practicality of an assessment; and implications of an assessment, such as the commonly queried clinical assessment of driving safety. Repeatability of the assessment, such as assessing circadian variations in alertness or assessing the response to therapies over time, is also a consideration. This article outlines some of the most common instruments and suggests situations where particular tools may be most appropriate.

Ontogeny

Sleep needs change over the course of a life span. The National Sleep Foundation recently published guidelines for suggested sleep times across various age ranges. School-aged children were suggested as requiring 9 hours to 11 hours and young adults 7 hours to 9 hours.[12] Because most of the assessment tools have been developed for adults, special consideration for groups such as children need to be made.

This article originally appeared in September, 2017 issue of *Sleep Medicine Clinics* (Volume 12, Issue 3).
Disclosures: Dr B.J. Murray has written for UpToDate.
Neurology and Sleep Medicine, Sunnybrook Health Sciences Centre, University of Toronto, Room M1-600, 2075 Bayview Avenue, Toronto, Ontario M4N 3M5, Canada
E-mail address: brian.murray@sunnybrook.ca

Sleep Med Clin 15 (2020) 167–176
https://doi.org/10.1016/j.jsmc.2020.02.005

Shift Work

Separate consideration should also be made for patients who adopt atypical sleep patterns, such as sleep during the light period. Patients who engage in shift work have sleepiness for a variety of reasons. There are natural periods of vulnerability[13] throughout the day and participants with shift work often become progressively sleep deprived. One problem in interpreting sleepiness in this context is that studies routinely used for the assessment of sleepiness, such as the MSLT, are not standardized at alternate times of day.

PATIENT EVALUATION OVERVIEW

The clinical assessment of patients often starts with subjective assessments. Objective neurophysiologic assessments are subsequently arranged if appropriate.

SUBJECTIVE ASSESSMENT

To understand the clinical presentation of patients with sleepiness, it is important to understand the motivation for the visit. Sometimes sleepiness is identified as a separate issue in the investigation of a clinical problem, such as investigation for obstructive sleep apnea. Frequently in hypersomnia there is a concern about safety. Rarely there are concerns about drug-seeking behaviors in patients looking for stimulant therapy. It is important to interview others familiar with a patient. Family and friends may be more likely to report excessive daytime sleepiness than the patient. Some patients may lack insight into the degree of their sleepiness and under-report the problem. It is not uncommon for patients with daytime sleepiness to deny difficulties but family members bring them to medical attention because they may fall asleep in traffic, for example. In other situations, patients may fall asleep in inappropriate social situations. In children, poor school performance is sometimes a trigger for assessment.

Sleep Log

Patients should keep track of bedtimes and rise times on a calendar and track degree of sleepiness. This can lead to insights, such as individuals reporting excessive sleepiness throughout the week suddenly becoming less sleepy on the weekend, where sleep extended due to increased sleep opportunity might be seen.

Interpretation of sleepiness at any given time point should also consider the effects of medication administration as well as common substances, such as caffeine, which are known to alter alertness.[14]

Epworth Sleepiness Scale

The Epworth Sleepiness Scale (ESS) is a commonly administered scale where subjects indicate how likely they would be to fall asleep or doze in 8 common situations, such as watching television.[15] This scale asks a patient to reflect over a period of time rather than assessing sleepiness at any specific point in time and yields a score from 0 to 24 (least–highest likelihood of falling asleep). This is, therefore, more of a trait measure, although it can clearly be influenced by treatments. One American study looked at a group of persons renewing their driver's licenses in the general population and found a mean score of 7.5, with 26.2% of the populations having a score of 10 of higher, which has typically been used as a cutoff to identify sleepiness.[16] A German study of 9710 people noted 23% of the sample had a score greater than 10.[17] A systematic review of the ESS revealed that this instrument could be used for research group assessments but was not recommended for individual-level comparisons.[18] Although the total score is commonly used, some items are of clinical concern, such as falling asleep while sitting and talking to someone, presumably suggesting a significant degree of impairment.

Barcelona Sleepiness Index

Based on focus groups in patients with sleep-disordered breathing, a set of items was generated and assessed against objective measures, such as the Sustained Attention to Response Task (SART), MWT, and MSLT. Two items on this interviewer-administered scale, ranging from 0 to 6, produced the highest predictive value for the MWT and were sensitive to treatment changes with continuous positive airway pressure.[19] This is, therefore, a simple instrument that can be used for a common clinical problem but validation is required in English.

Observation and Interview Based Diurnal Sleepiness Inventory

The recently developed Observation and Interview Based Diurnal Sleepiness Inventory is a 3-item instrument tested in elderly subjects that was able to quickly screen for daytime sleepiness among elderly patients with obstructive sleep apnea but has so far only been assessed against another subjective scale—the ESS.[20] Again this is more of a trait measure.

Stanford Sleepiness Scale

Other scales are more focused on clinical state. The Stanford Sleepiness Scale (SSS) addresses sleepiness at any given moment in time and ranges over 7 descriptions, from "feeling active, vital, alert, wide awake" to "almost in reverie, cannot stay awake, sleep onset appears imminent." The scale was developed in 5 students over the course of several days and after sleep deprivation[21] but has been extensively used. Psychometric properties of this scale have suggested that descriptors at each level of the scale are not equivalent and that the test does not assess a unidimensional construct. Furthermore, studies comparing the SSS to MSLT and pupillographic assessment of sleepiness suggest that the SSS does not correlate well with physiologic measures of sleepiness.[22]

Karolinska Sleepiness Scale

The Karolinska Sleepiness Scale is a 9-point scale ranging from "extremely alert" to "extremely sleepy, fighting sleep" based on subjective assessment of drowsiness at a given point in time.[23] The scale has been noted to correlate with physiologic variables, such as electroencephalography (EEG) and the psychomotor vigilance task, suggesting high validity at specific time points.[24] Some investigators have adapted this scale to assess longer more trait-like periods of time, such as shift work.[25]

Sleepiness-Wakefulness Inability and Fatigue Test

Another scale called the Sleepiness-Wakefulness Inability and Fatigue Test[26] has been developed to focus less on the tendency to fall asleep and more on the inability to maintain wakefulness and capture associated tiredness. This 12-item scale was assessed in several hundred patients with a variety of sleep disorders, including sleep apnea specifically, was reliable and valid, and had a better discriminant ability than the ESS with factors specific to driving.

Time of Day Sleepiness Scale

Because there are variations in the circadian tendency to be alert, this new scale, The Time of Day Sleepiness Scale, addresses sleepiness in light of circadian variation.[27] The scale takes approximately 5 minutes to complete and assesses sleepiness across morning, afternoon, and evening. There is a need to have further normative data across other times of day, particularly for shift workers.

Pittsburgh Sleep Quality Index

Many general psychiatric or psychological scales, such as the Profile of Mood States,[28] have

subscales components that reflect fatigue or sleepiness and could be used if already collected but were not specifically designed with sleepiness as a focus. The Pittsburgh Sleep Quality Index is commonly used for self-reported general sleep characteristics and reflects a broader set of sleep pathologies aside from alertness, such as insomnia.[29] Nonetheless, a component of the scale, daytime dysfunction, can reflect daytime alertness and may correlate with alertness measures.

Leeds Sleep Evaluation Questionnaire

Similarly, the Leeds Sleep Evaluation Questionnaire is a 10-item linear analog scale based on questions across several domains of sleep. Three questions can be extracted from this tool reflect alertness[30] and have been geared toward the assessment of psychoactive drug responses.[31] This scale may be helpful for assessing treatment responses within an individual and has been widely used in pharmacologic studies.

Pediatric Scales

Several pediatric scales have been developed given the specific needs of this population. The ESS is most directed toward adults and, therefore, children may not commonly experience all 8 clinical situations. An extensive evidence-based review of pediatric sleep measures has recently been published.[32] One scale that focused on alertness was well- established with respect to evidence base—the Pediatric Daytime Sleepiness Scale. This is an 8-item self-report scale developed for 11 to 15 years olds that assesses sleepiness, such as how often individuals fall asleep or get drowsy during classes, and has excellent psychometric properties.[33] Importantly, the scale also correlates with academic performance. Other scales include a modified ESS with pediatric appropriate clinical scenarios[34] and the Cleveland Adolescent Sleepiness Questionnaire, which is a 16-item scale developed for ages 11 years to 17 years[35] and includes items, such as "I feel sleepy when I ride in a bus to a school event like a field trip or sports game."

Problems with Subjective Measures

Patients with subjective sleepiness may not be aware of the degree of their impairment. There can be a disconnect between subjective ratings of sleepiness, such as the ESS, and objective measures, such as the MSLT.[36] Some participants may be prone to underestimate their sleepiness to preserve driving privileges. Others may be prone to exaggerate their symptoms if they are seeking stimulant medications. As such, interpretation of subjective scales is probably best done when a clinician can gauge the reliability of the participant and the participant's insight into the problem. Tracking changes on subjective scales may be more useful than using absolute values for establishing a diagnosis, for example. Some individuals may be nonverbal or unable to participate in daily activities that are assessed in many subjective scales. There may also be language or cultural differences in the scales necessitating that validation be done for specific patient populations. Given some of these concerns, objective scales are frequently essential.

OBJECTIVE MEASURES
Clinical Observation

Clinical impression of sleepiness might be evident from the initial presentation. Observing patients in a waiting room can sometimes identify napping during daytime hours. Patients may have yawning or eyelid drooping or even manifest slow roving eye movements during an interview. Sleepiness can be observed in meetings with a drop in neck muscle tone and quick postural correction.

Clinical Neurophysiology

Often, when sleepiness is of medical concern, objective information should be collected in the form of several standardized neurophysiologic tests. Some recent developments in objective assessment of alertness have been outlined.[37] Polysomnography does not provide for measurement of sleepiness, but limited information may be available in an overnight study. For example, prolonged sleep-onset latency is not typically expected in a patient with narcolepsy. Perhaps the most important feature of polysomnography is ensuring that underlying sleep disorders are not

present, such as obstructive sleep apnea. Polysomnography is also required prior to the MSLT to ensure adequate sleep time has been obtained.

Practice parameters have been published for the use of the MSLT and MWT.[38] The tests are widely used but have problems in interpretation outside the laboratory setting.[39,40] Standardization of the tests and appropriate use help in their interpretation but some investigators have noted that normative values remain limited, particularly for the MWT, and that these tests are limited in terms of their implications in the real world.[41] Although these tests are not perfect, they are the best standardized tests currently available and provide useful objective information, particularly when there is a clear clinical question.[42] All clinical decisions require an appropriate clinical context and these tests should not be seen as absolute without appropriate interpretation. The selection of the appropriate test depends on several factors. See **Table 1** for some considerations in test selection.

Multiple Sleep Latency Test

The MSLT is predominantly a test for narcolepsy. Patients have 4 to 5 nap opportunities of 20 minutes' duration spaced 2 hours apart throughout the day, for example 09:00, 11:00, 13:00, 15:00, and 17:00. A fifth nap is often added if there is 1 sleep-onset rapid eye movement (REM) period (SOREMP) in the first 4 naps to help establish a neurophysiologic diagnosis of narcolepsy. The study is done in darkness in a comfortable bed at an acceptable temperature. Patients are instructed to try to fall asleep. If patients fall asleep, they are allowed to sleep for further 15 minutes to see if they enter REM sleep. Sleep latency on this test can suggest a degree of sleep propensity, for example, the ability to willingly initiate asleep. If a patient achieves REM sleep on 2 of

Table 1
Considerations in neurophysiological assessment of sleepiness

	Multiple Sleep Latency Test	Maintenance of Wakefulness Test
General goal of the test	Assesses the ability to fall asleep	Assesses the ability to remain awake
Preceding polysomnography	Required	Not required
Narcolepsy diagnosis	Useful in the diagnosis of narcolepsy	
Assessment of safety		Better conceptual validity
Stimulant-seeking behaviors	Less prone to exaggerating abnormalities—although toxicology screen should be obtained	Highly prone to motivation and may be problematic in interpretation
Medications	Formally interpreted off medications	Can be used to assess response to alerting medications

the naps or at least 1 nap and falls into REM early on the preceding night's polysomnography, this study can also help support a diagnosis of narcolepsy. Patients are supposed to remain awake between naps but sleepy patients commonly do not, although this does not seem to significantly affect the eventual diagnosis.[43]

Patients must have routine sleep in the week prior to the recording, and the preceding night's polysomnogram ensures that at least 6 hours of good-quality sleep has been recorded for appropriate interpretation. The polysomnogram ensures that certain common intrinsic sleep disorders, such as sleep apnea, are not contributing to daytime sleepiness. Psychoactive medications should be held for several weeks prior to the study. This can be problematic in some participants with, for example, significant psychiatric conditions.

Normative values have been published.[44,45] Subtle differences in test interpretation can provide different interpretations. For example, sleep onset, as defined by the first epoch of stage N1, can suggest diagnostic differences in different disorders compared with a definition of sleep onset constituting consecutive epochs of N1 or another stage of sleep.[46]

It is problematic to use the MSLT in the general population without some pretest probability of an abnormality. One study looked at the prevalence and correlates of SOREMPs in a large community-based sleep group.[47] The study looked at 556 predominantly white participants and noted that there was sleep latency less than 8 minutes and 2 or more SOREMPs in approximately 6% of men and 1% of women. In men, SOREMPs were increased in shift workers and individuals with suggestions of sleep restriction. Another study looking at cross-sectional and longitudinal studies of sleep in the general community noted, in a sample of 1725 polysomnography/MSLT participants, including approximately half who had repeated the test, that the prevalence of a mean sleep latency less than 8 minutes was 22%. A sleep latency less than 8 minutes and 2 or more SOREMPs was noted in 3.4% of the population. The study also noted that the value of the MSLT was significantly altered by shift work and sleep deprivation.[48]

In the context of the repeated MSLTs, there can be variations, particularly with respect to sleepiness.[43] One recent study commented on problems in the test–retest reliability of the MSLT in patients with narcolepsy without cataplexy and idiopathic hypersomnia. Of 36 individuals tested approximately 4 years apart, the mean sleep latency on the first and second tests were 5.5 minutes and 7.3 minutes, respectively, with no significant correlation. Change in diagnosis occurred in 53% of patients, predominantly via change in the mean sleep latency. As such, the investigators concluded the MSLT demonstrates poor test-retest reliability for diagnostic purposes in a clinical population of patients with central nervous system hypersomnia.[49] The diagnosis of narcolepsy can also be aided by a clinical history of cataplexy, HLA typing, or low cerebrospinal fluid orexin/hypocretin levels. Again, no one sleep tool should be used independent of the clinical interpretation.

Practice parameters for use of the MSLT in children have recently been published.[50] This publication notes concerns about the technical capacity for the study and problems with limited age-adjusted normative values. Diagnostic criteria are not available for patients under age 6.[51] It was also noted that patients in early pubertal stages or earlier were less likely to fall asleep than older adolescents. Some clinicians have consequently used 30-minute nap opportunities to have a higher chance of detecting SOREMPs but this has not been validated in large samples. There are also concerns in children with napping behaviors because it is hard to standardize and interpret in the context of the MSLT where adults are typically asked to remain awake between tests. Toxicology screens are required even in children, given that they may have habits unknown to their parents or there may be features of Munchausen syndrome by proxy.

Although the MSLT and MWT are frequently used for the assessment of driving safety, there is a paucity of evidence linking the predictive abilities of these tests. One recent important study looked at MSLT values and 10-year crash rate with records from a Department of Motor Vehicles.[52] In this study of 618 participants who were recruited using random digit dialing, 3 MSLT groups were identified: excessively sleepy, moderately sleepy, and alert. The accident rates for the groups were 59.4%, 52.5%, and 47.3%, respectively. The investigators concluded that the MSLT was predictive of an increased risk of documented automotive crashes. Perhaps this effect would have even been more significant had they assessed the MWT.

Maintenance of Wakefulness Test

The MWT has more conceptual validity for assessing the ability to resist sleep in the day. This could be helpful for patients where safety is a concern.

In this test, patients have 20-minute to 40-minute sessions that are spread 2 hours apart throughout the day for typically 4 sessions, for example, 09:00, 11:00, 13:00, and 15:00. Patients sit in a comfortable chair in a dimly lit room of comfortable temperature and attempt to maintain alertness. Participants are specifically instructed to stay awake as long as possible. They are not allowed to vocalize or make excessive movements. Patients can demonstrate abnormalities on the MWT in a variety of sleep conditions, such as the upper airway resistance syndrome.[53] Normative values have been published[45,54] although there is some controversy about what constitutes a normal MWT. Some experts have noted that with appropriate motivation, patients remain awake longer and clinicians consider no sleep on this test or a value of 40 minutes to be normal.

The 40-minute test is recommended over shorter duration assessments, because this is more sensitive for picking up sleepiness. In 1 study of patients using the MWT for driving safety, participants were instructed that if they failed the test, their driver's license would be revoked.[55] In 39 patients with severe obstructive sleep apnea with a respiratory disturbance index over 40, 48.7% fell asleep. On a 20-minute test, only 7% of patients with severe sleep apnea fell asleep once. The investigators concluded that the MWT for 40 minutes' duration was superior to the 20-minute test for detecting difficulties in remaining alert. One study noted differences in a driving simulator when drivers had a mean sleep latency under 34 minutes,[56] and other studies have noted differences in driving abilities based on level of impairment in several conditions.[57]

Deeper analysis of physiologic data may provide more information than is seen on visual inspection. For example, digital signal interpretation with Fourier analysis is a simple consideration to extract hidden information in an EEG that may be a better marker of sleepiness.[58] Again, definition of sleep onset may be a factor in conditions where there is instability of sleep onset.

Ambulatory Electroencephalogram

Devices that track EEG over prolonged periods of time can also help detect lapses in attention. Consumer purchasable portable EEG headbands are available. Automated computerized scoring of large volumes of data helps facilitate monitoring over prolonged periods.

Actigraphy

There has been rapid development in the use of consumer technologies to track sleep-wake behaviors. Common devices for assessing fitness include activity trackers, which can suggest sleep

in the context of absence of movement. Although this relation is not perfect, it can estimate sleep and periods of inactivity in the day that may also reflect a tendency toward sleepiness. Current protocols for assessment of actigraphy in daytime napping are limited,[59] but the tool can be helpful for unobtrusively tracking sleep-wake activity over long periods of time.

Psychomotor Vigilance Test

Several devices track performance metrics to help infer inattention or drowsiness. One commercially available device for assessing state alertness is the psychomotor vigilance task.[60] This paradigm measures reaction time typically over the course of 10 minutes with 2-second to 10-second variable stimulus presentation rates. The reaction time to these signals is recorded and this reaction time can correlate with sleepiness. Perhaps more importantly, lapses are identified that are periods of nonresponse to the target stimulus. A nonresponse of greater than 500 milliseconds has traditionally been reported in the literature, although this is somewhat arbitrary. The lack of response to the stimulus likely represents the first movement of the sleep switch from alert to asleep and implicates a change in brain activation patterns.[61] This device can be used in clinical settings easily, requires little training, and has virtually no learning curve. As such, the test can be repeated multiple times throughout the day for longer duration assessments. The test is sensitive to sleep deprivation as well as circadian variations in alertness.

Oxford Sleep Resistance Test

The Oxford Sleep Resistance Test is another commercially available device available based on a task where subjects are asked to press a switch in response to a light.[62] This is a behavioral variant of the MWT but has the advantage of simplified administration compared with the MWT in that EEG is not required. Sleep latencies on this tool correlate well with the MWT.[63] This assessment has sensitivity of 85% and specificity of 94% in the detection of 3 seconds of sleep.[64] The test was also comparable to a shorter reaction time task presented by visual or auditory means and demonstrated an improvement with treatment of sleep apnea.[65]

Sustained Attention to Response Task

Another variation on this theme is the simple neuropsychological test, the SART, which involves inhibiting response to 1/9 of 225 target stimuli. The test has been assessed in conjunction with the MSLT in patients with narcolepsy and controls and was noted to have good sensitivity and specificity for predicting a mean sleep latency of 5 minutes[66] but did not correlate with the MSLT or ESS. The test has been used to assess treatment responses in pharmacologic treatment of narcolepsy.[67] The task is short and easy to administer, which provides advantages over conventional neurophysiologic assessments and has been tested in a variety of patient groups.[68]

Eyelid Movement

One of the most common features of drowsiness is eyelid closure. Eyelid closure can be detected with new technologies given advances in computing power and new devices. A variety of eyelid closure characteristics, such as the velocity of closure and duration of eye closure, can be analyzed to assess real-time drowsiness.[69] One recent study used an infrared modified glasses frame to track sleepiness in nurses doing shift work and was able to demonstrate inattention in a naturalistic setting—the drive home from work.[70]

Eye Movements

Roving eye movements are also a feature of sleepiness and can be monitored with ambulatory recordings to assess momentary sleepiness. One study of 8 subjects looked at continuous EEG and electrooculogram recordings to detect slow eye movements; these were most readily detected when subjects reported significant sleepiness.[23]

Pupillography

Another eye tool to track sleepiness is pupillography—measurements of pupil size and variability in size changes. These are best detected in the dark where there is maximal pupillary dilation. Pupillary size oscillations have been used to track level of arousal in medical personnel, although this requires a dark room and specialized equipment currently.[71] One study compared pupillometric studies to the MSLT and noted correlation in some measures but pointed out concerns that need to be addressed before using this as a screening tool.[72]

Driving Simulators

Several driving simulators have been tested as an operationalization of sleepiness and with some conceptual validity for interpretation of a common clinical problem.[73] Unfortunately, there is no standard device because they are often developed for a variety of other driving safety considerations, and they may be large and expensive for better lifelike assessments. Medications may contribute

to sleepiness and with deviation of road position is a likely marker for lapses in attention with incipient sleep.[74] Monotonous driving conditions showed correlations with the MSLT and subjective sleepiness as assessed by the SSS and a visual analog scale in normal individuals after sleep deprivation.[75]

FUTURE DIRECTIONS

Again, the increase in wearable technologies should help identify better tools to track variations in alertness. Eye movement tracking characteristics are of interest given the prominence of ptosis and slow-moving eye movements with drowsiness. Measures of gait stability have been used to assess alertness.[76] Auditory evoked potentials have been found to change under conditions of sleepiness[77] and could even be incorporated in devices that record EEG. A few studies have noted changes in autonomic function, such as heart rate variability monitoring that correlated with lapses on the psychomotor vigilance task in normal persons undergoing sleep deprivation conditions,[78,79] suggesting that even less conspicuous recording devices, such as cardiac monitors, could track information over time and eventually even provide real-time feedback to individuals about their safety.

SUMMARY

Given the clinical significance of sleepiness, having ways to track sleepiness is important for clinicians and patients. Subjective scales have some advantages in terms of ease of administration and expense but are prone to bias and have to be interpreted with this potential confound. The use of subjective scales can be helpful when a patient has insight into the degree of the problem and is reporting openly. When there are concerns about reliability of reporting and when there are significant implications of abnormal test results, a reliance on objective measures may be needed. Although the MSLT and MWT have problems, they continue to be used as the best standardized tests to date. Refinements of objective scales are required. Many reaction time–type tasks provide objective information and are easy to use. Further standardization of these tests in clinical scenarios is warranted. Newer devices will provide accurate real world measurement of alertness and may even be adapted to provide real-time feedback. Combinations of physiologic measures may also provide further information.[80] Often, subjective scales and objective scales should be used together in a multicomponent assessment of sleepiness.[81]

REFERENCES

1. Winokur A. The relationship between sleep disturbances and psychiatric disorders: introduction and overview. Psychiatr Clin North Am 2015;38(4):603–14.
2. Pilcher JJ, Huffcutt AI. Effects of sleep deprivation on performance: a meta-analysis. Sleep 1996;19(4):318–26.
3. Badran M, Yassin BA, Fox N, et al. Epidemiology of sleep disturbances and cardiovascular consequences. Can J Cardiol 2015;31(7):873–9.
4. Newman AB, Spiekerman CF, Enright P, et al. Daytime sleepiness predicts mortality and cardiovascular disease in older adults. The Cardiovascular Health Study Research Group. J Am Geriatr Soc 2000;48(2):115–23.
5. Al Lawati NM, Patel SR, Ayas NT. Epidemiology, risk factors, and consequences of obstructive sleep apnea and short sleep duration. Prog Cardiovasc Dis 2009;51(4):285–93.
6. American Academy of Sleep Medicine Board of Directors, Watson NF, Morgenthaler T, et al. Confronting drowsy driving: the American Academy of sleep medicine perspective. J Clin Sleep Med 2015;11(11):1335–6.
7. Hafner M, Stepanek M, Taylor J, et al. Why sleep matters — the economic costs of insufficient sleep: a cross-country comparative analysis. Santa Monica (CA): RAND Corporation; 2016.
8. Czeisler CA. Impact of sleepiness and sleep deficiency on public health–utility of biomarkers. J Clin Sleep Med 2011;7(5 Suppl):S6–8.
9. Mitler MM, Miller JC. Methods of testing for sleepiness [corrected]. Behav Med 1996;21(4):171–83.
10. Kim H, Young T. Subjective daytime sleepiness: dimensions and correlates in the general population. Sleep 2005;28(5):625–34.
11. Carskadon MA. Evaluation of excessive daytime sleepiness. Neurophysiol Clin 1993;23(1):91–100.
12. Watson NF, Badr MS, Belenky G, et al. Recommended amount of sleep for a healthy adult: a joint consensus statement of the American Academy of sleep medicine and sleep research society. Sleep 2015;38(6):843–4.
13. Akerstedt T, Wright KP Jr. Sleep loss and fatigue in shift work and shift work disorder. Sleep Med Clin 2009;4(2):257–71.
14. Roehrs T, Roth T. Caffeine: sleep and daytime sleepiness. Sleep Med Rev 2008;12(2):153–62.
15. Johns MW. A new method for measuring daytime sleepiness: the Epworth sleepiness scale. Sleep 1991;14(6):540–5.
16. Benbadis SR, Perry MC, Sundstad LS, et al. Prevalence of daytime sleepiness in a population of drivers. Neurology 1999;52(1):209–10.
17. Sander C, Hegerl U, Wirkner K, et al. Normative values of the Epworth Sleepiness Scale (ESS), derived from a large German sample. Sleep Breath 2016;20(4):1337–45.
18. Kendzerska TB, Smith PM, Brignardello-Petersen R, et al. Evaluation of the measurement properties of the Epworth sleepiness scale: a systematic review. Sleep Med Rev 2014;18(4):321–31.
19. Guaita M, Salamero M, Vilaseca I, et al. The barcelona sleepiness Index: a new instrument to assess excessive daytime sleepiness in sleep disordered breathing. J Clin Sleep Med 2015;11(11):1289–98.
20. Onen F, Lalanne C, Pak VM, et al. A three-item instrument for measuring daytime sleepiness: the observation and interview based diurnal sleepiness inventory (ODSI). J Clin Sleep Med 2016;12(4):505–12.
21. Hoddes E, Zarcone V, Smythe H, et al. Quantification of sleepiness: a new approach. Psychophysiology 1973;10(4):431–6.
22. Danker-Hopfe H, Kraemer S, Dorn H, et al. Time-of-day variations in different measures of sleepiness (MSLT, pupillography, and SSS) and their interrelations. Psychophysiology 2001;38(5):828–35.
23. Akerstedt T, Gillberg M. Subjective and objective sleepiness in the active individual. Int J Neurosci 1990;52(1–2):29–37.
24. Kaida K, Takahashi M, Akerstedt T, et al. Validation of the Karolinska sleepiness scale against performance and EEG variables. Clin Neurophysiol 2006;117(7):1574–81.
25. Geiger Brown J, Wieroney M, Blair L, et al. Measuring subjective sleepiness at work in hospital nurses: validation of a modified delivery format of the Karolinska Sleepiness Scale. Sleep Breath 2014;18(4):731–9.
26. Sangal RB. Evaluating sleepiness-related daytime function by querying wakefulness inability and fatigue: sleepiness-Wakefulness Inability and Fatigue Test (SWIFT). J Clin Sleep Med 2012;8(6):701–11.
27. Dolan DC, Taylor DJ, Okonkwo R, et al. The Time of Day Sleepiness Scale to assess differential levels of sleepiness across the day. J Psychosom Res 2009;67(2):127–33.
28. McNair DM, Lorr M, Droppelman LF. Manual for the profile of mood states. San Diego (CA): Educational and Industrial Testing Service; 1971. p. 27.
29. Buysse DJ, Reynolds CF 3rd, Monk TH, et al. The Pittsburgh Sleep Quality Index: a new instrument for psychiatric practice and research. Psychiatry Res 1989;28(2):193–213.
30. Parrott AC, Hindmarch I. Factor analysis of a sleep evaluation questionnaire. Psychol Med 1978;8(2):325–9.
31. Zisapel N, Laudon M. Subjective assessment of the effects of CNS-active drugs on sleep by the Leeds

sleep evaluation questionnaire: a review. Hum Psychopharmacol 2003;18(1):1–20.

32. Lewandowski AS, Toliver-Sokol M, Palermo TM. Evidence-based review of subjective pediatric sleep measures. J Pediatr Psychol 2011;36(7):780–93.

33. Drake C, Nickel C, Burduvali E, et al. The pediatric daytime sleepiness scale (PDSS): sleep habits and school outcomes in middle-school children. Sleep 2003;26(4):455–8.

34. Melendres MC, Lutz JM, Rubin ED, et al. Daytime sleepiness and hyperactivity in children with suspected sleep-disordered breathing. Pediatrics 2004;114(3):768–75.

35. Spilsbury JC, Drotar D, Rosen CL, et al. The Cleveland adolescent sleepiness questionnaire: a new measure to assess excessive daytime sleepiness in adolescents. J Clin Sleep Med 2007;3(6):603–12.

36. Benbadis SR, Mascha E, Perry MC, et al. Association between the Epworth sleepiness scale and the multiple sleep latency test in a clinical population. Ann Intern Med 1999;130(4 Pt 1):289–92.

37. Coelho FM, Narayansingh M, Murray BJ. Testing sleepiness and vigilance in the sleep laboratory. Curr Opin Pulm Med 2011;17(6):406–11.

38. Littner MR, Kushida C, Wise M, et al. Practice parameters for clinical use of the multiple sleep latency test and the maintenance of wakefulness test. Sleep 2005;28(1):113–21.

39. Lammers GJ, van Dijk JG. The multiple sleep latency test: a paradoxical test? Clin Neurol Neurosurg 1992;94(Suppl):S108–10.

40. Bonnet MH. ACNS clinical controversy: MSLT and MWT have limited clinical utility. J Clin Neurophysiol 2006;23(1):50–8.

41. Sullivan SS, Kushida CA. Multiple sleep latency test and maintenance of wakefulness test. Chest 2008; 134(4):854–61.

42. Wise MS. Objective measures of sleepiness and wakefulness: application to the real world? J Clin Neurophysiol 2006;23(1):39–49.

43. Kasravi N, Legault G, Jewell D, et al. Minimal impact of inadvertent sleep between naps on the MSLT and MWT. J Clin Neurophysiol 2007;24(4):363–5.

44. Roehrs T, Roth T. Multiple Sleep Latency Test: technical aspects and normal values. J Clin Neurophysiol 1992;9(1):63–7.

45. Arand D, Bonnet M, Hurwitz T, et al. The clinical use of the MSLT and MWT. Sleep 2005;28(1):123–44.

46. Pizza F, Vandi S, Detto S, et al. Different sleep onset criteria at the multiple sleep latency test (MSLT): an additional marker to differentiate central nervous system (CNS) hypersomnias. J Sleep Res 2011; 20(1 Pt 2):250–6.

47. Mignot E, Lin L, Finn L, et al. Correlates of sleep-onset REM periods during the multiple sleep latency test in community adults. Brain 2006;129(Pt 6): 1609–23.

48. Goldbart A, Peppard P, Finn L, et al. Narcolepsy and predictors of positive MSLTs in the Wisconsin sleep cohort. Sleep 2014;37(6):1043–51.

49. Trotti LM, Staab BA, Rye DB. Test-retest reliability of the multiple sleep latency test in narcolepsy without cataplexy and idiopathic hypersomnia. J Clin Sleep Med 2013;9(8):789–95.

50. Aurora RN, Lamm CI, Zak RS, et al. Practice parameters for the non-respiratory indications for polysomnography and multiple sleep latency testing for children. Sleep 2012;35(11):1467–73.

51. Nevsimalova S. The diagnosis and treatment of pediatric narcolepsy. Curr Neurol Neurosci Rep 2014; 14(8):469.

52. Drake C, Roehrs T, Breslau N, et al. The 10-year risk of verified motor vehicle crashes in relation to physiologic sleepiness. Sleep 2010;33(6):745–52.

53. Powers CR, Frey WC. Maintenance of wakefulness test in military personnel with upper airway resistance syndrome and mild to moderate obstructive sleep apnea. Sleep Breath 2009;13(3):253–8.

54. Doghramji K, Mitler MM, Sangal RB, et al. A normative study of the maintenance of wakefulness test (MWT). Electroencephalogr Clin Neurophysiol 1997;103(5):554–62.

55. Arzi L, Shreter R, El-Ad B, et al. Forty- versus 20-minute trials of the maintenance of wakefulness test regimen for licensing of drivers. J Clin Sleep Med 2009;5(1):57–62.

56. Philip P, Sagaspe P, Taillard J, et al. Maintenance of Wakefulness Test, obstructive sleep apnea syndrome, and driving risk. Ann Neurol 2008;64(4): 410–6.

57. Philip P, Chaufton C, Taillard J, et al. Maintenance of Wakefulness Test scores and driving performance in sleep disorder patients and controls. Int J Psychophysiol 2013;89(2):195–202.

58. Gast H, Schindler K, Rummel C, et al. EEG correlation and power during maintenance of wakefulness test after sleep-deprivation. Clin Neurophysiol 2011;122(10):2025–31.

59. Martin JL, Hakim AD. Wrist actigraphy. Chest 2011; 139(6):1514–27.

60. Dinges DF, Pack F, Williams K, et al. Cumulative sleepiness, mood disturbance, and psychomotor vigilance performance decrements during a week of sleep restricted to 4-5 hours per night. Sleep 1997;20(4):267–77.

61. Drummond SP, Bischoff-Grethe A, Dinges DF, et al. The neural basis of the psychomotor vigilance task. Sleep 2005;28(9):1059–68.

62. Bennett LS, Stradling JR, Davies RJ. A behavioural test to assess daytime sleepiness in obstructive sleep apnoea. J Sleep Res 1997;6(2):142–5.

63. Krieger AC, Ayappa I, Norman RG, et al. Comparison of the maintenance of wakefulness test (MWT) to a modified behavioral test (OSLER) in the

evaluation of daytime sleepiness. J Sleep Res 2004; 13(4):407–11.

64. Priest B, Brichard C, Aubert G, et al. Microsleep during a simplified maintenance of wakefulness test. A validation study of the OSLER test. Am J Respir Crit Care Med 2001;163(7):1619–25.

65. Alakuijala A, Maasilta P, Bachour A. The oxford sleep resistance test (OSLER) and the multiple unprepared reaction time test (MURT) detect vigilance modifications in sleep apnea patients. J Clin Sleep Med 2014;10(10):1075–82.

66. Fronczek R, Middelkoop HA, van Dijk JG, et al. Focusing on vigilance instead of sleepiness in the assessment of narcolepsy: high sensitivity of the Sustained Attention to Response Task (SART). Sleep 2006;29(2):187–91.

67. van der Heide A, van Schie MK, Lammers GJ, et al. Comparing treatment effect measurements in narcolepsy: the sustained attention to response task, Epworth sleepiness scale and maintenance of wakefulness test. Sleep 2015;38(7):1051–8.

68. Van Schie MK, Thijs RD, Fronczek R, et al. Sustained attention to response task (SART) shows impaired vigilance in a spectrum of disorders of excessive daytime sleepiness. J Sleep Res 2012;21(4):390–5.

69. Wilkinson VE, Jackson ML, Westlake J, et al. The accuracy of eyelid movement parameters for drowsiness detection. J Clin Sleep Med 2013;9(12):1315–24.

70. Ftouni S, Sletten TL, Howard M, et al. Objective and subjective measures of sleepiness, and their associations with on-road driving events in shift workers. J Sleep Res 2013;22(1):58–69.

71. Wilhelm BJ, Widmann A, Durst W, et al. Objective and quantitative analysis of daytime sleepiness in physicians after night duties. Int J Psychophysiol 2009;72(3):307–13.

72. Yamamoto K, Kobayashi F, Hori R, et al. Association between pupillometric sleepiness measures and sleep latency derived by MSLT in clinically sleepy patients. Environ Health Prev Med 2013;18(5):361–7.

73. George CF. Driving simulators in clinical practice. Sleep Med Rev 2003;7(4):311–20.

74. Rapoport MJ, Lanctot KL, Streiner DL, et al. Benzodiazepine use and driving: a meta-analysis. J Clin Psychiatry 2009;70(5):663–73.

75. Pizza F, Contardi S, Mostacci B, et al. A driving simulation task: correlations with Multiple Sleep Latency Test. Brain Res Bull 2004;63(5):423–6.

76. Forsman P, Wallin A, Tietavainen A, et al. Posturographic sleepiness monitoring. J Sleep Res 2007;16(3):259–61.

77. Dorokhov VB, Verbitskaya YS, Lavrova TP. Auditory evoked potentials and impairments to psychomotor activity evoked by falling asleep. Neurosci Behav Physiol 2010;40(4):411–9.

78. Chua EC, Tan WQ, Yeo SC, et al. Heart rate variability can be used to estimate sleepiness-related decrements in psychomotor vigilance during total sleep deprivation. Sleep 2012;35(3):325–34.

79. Henelius A, Sallinen M, Huotilainen M, et al. Heart rate variability for evaluating vigilant attention in partial chronic sleep restriction. Sleep 2014;37(7):1257–67.

80. Borghini G, Astolfi L, Vecchiato G, et al. Measuring neurophysiological signals in aircraft pilots and car drivers for the assessment of mental workload, fatigue and drowsiness. Neurosci Biobehav Rev 2014;44:58–75.

81. Mathis J, Hess CW. Sleepiness and vigilance tests. Swiss Med Wkly 2009;139(15–16):214–9.

Pharmacologic Management of Excessive Daytime Sleepiness

Shinichi Takenoshita, MD, MPH, Seiji Nishino, MD, PhD*

KEYWORDS

- Stimulants • Excessive daytime sleepiness • Narcolepsy • Idiopathic hypersomnia

KEY POINTS

- Excessive daytime sleepiness (EDS) is related to medical and social problems, including mental disorders, physical diseases, poor quality of life, and so forth.
- Several different types of stimulants (or wake-promoting compounds) are available to treat EDS, and a variety of new drugs are under development.
- The side effects of some of the stimulants are potent, and careful selection and management is required.

INTRODUCTION

EDS is defined as "irresistible sleepiness in a situation when an individual would be expected to be awake, and alert."[1] EDS has been a big concern not only from a medical but also from a public health point of view. According to recently published articles, the prevalence of patients who suffer from EDS is approximately 20% in the world.[2-4] Patients with EDS have the possibility of falling asleep even when they should wake up and concentrate, for example, when they drive, play sports, or walk outside. Subjects who have EDS encounter a lower quality of life and have a higher odds ratio of developing a mental disorder, cognitive impairment, and motor vehicle accidents.[5-8]

Although nonpharmacologic treatments (ie, napping and work accommodations) are often helpful, a large majority of the diagnosed patients reported using pharmacologic therapies, mostly stimulant medications.[9]

Historically, EDS was also a large concern in the military. Many countries let soldiers take stimulants when they were engaged in military service in World War II. Currently, preventing sleepiness caused by sleep deprivation is still a major research project by the Defense Advanced Research Projects Agency in the United States.

In 1931, the first stimulant (ie, amphetamine) was applied to treat EDS associated with narcolepsy.[10] Since then, many new stimulants have developed to treat EDS, and many patients received benefits. Stimulants, however, are drugs with strong side effects (ie, sympathomimetic) and addiction potential and these treatments are mostly symptomatic; they improve the level of alertness by simply suppressing sleepiness.

Abuse potential of stimulants is a problem especially when diagnoses of hypersomomnias are loosely made, and this is particularly true for narcolepsy, where stimulant abuse is rare among patients with well-defined narcolepsy.[11-14] In this article, clinical characteristics of common hypersomnias and pharmacologic treatments of each hypersomnia are described. New treatment options under development for treating EDS associated with these hypersomnias are also

This article originally appeared in September, 2017 issue of *Sleep Medicine Clinics* (Volume 12, Issue 3).
Disclosure Statement: S. Nishino had a sponsored research contract (SPO#50970) with Ono Pharmacutical Co. Ltd.
Sleep and Circadian Neurobiology Laboratory, Department of Psychiatry and Behavioral Sciences, Stanford University School of Medicine, Stanford University, Palo Alto, CA, USA
* Corresponding author. 3155 Porter Drive, Room 2141, Palo Alto, CA 94304.
E-mail address: nishino@stanford.edu

discussed. The hypersomnias focused on in this article are narcolepsy type 1, narcolepsy type 2, idiopathic hypersomnia, and hypersomnia due to a medical disorder, defined in the *International Classification of Sleep Disorders, Third Edition* (*ICSD-3*).

TYPES OF HYPERSOMNIAS

According to the *ICDS-3*, published in 2014, diseases that result from EDS are listed as narcolepsy type 1, narcolepsy type 2, idiopathic hypersomnia, Kleine-Levin syndrome, hypersomnia due to a medical disorder, hypersomnia due to a medication or substance, hypersomnia associated with a psychiatric disorder, and insufficient sleep syndrome.[15]

This review covers the pharmacologic treatments of EDS associated with narcolepsy type 1, narcolepsy type 2, idiopathic hypersomnia, and hypersomnia due to a medical disorder, because relatively consistent guidelines for the pharmacotherapy of these diseases are available. The *ICSD-3* diagnostic criteria of these hypersomnias are summarized in **Table 1**. For the treatment of Kleine-Levin syndrome and other hypersomnias, see the article by Arnulf.[16]

NARCOLEPSY
Symptoms of Narcolepsy

Narcolepsy is a syndrome characterized by "EDS that is typically associated with cataplexy and other [rapid eye movement] REM sleep phenomena such as sleep paralysis and hypnagogic hallucinations."[17] The prevalence of narcolepsy with cataplexy has been examined in many studies and falls between 25 and 50 per 100,000 people

Table 1
Diagnostic criteria, *International Classification of Sleep Disorders, Third Edition*

Narcolepsy Type 1	Narcolepsy Type 2	Idiopathic Hypersomnia	Hypersomnia due to a Medical Disorder
Criteria A and B	All Criteria A–E	All Criteria A–F	All Criteria A–D

A. Daily periods of irrepressible need to sleep or daytime lapses into sleep, present for at least 3 mo
B. Either 1 or 2 or both
  1. Cataplexy and mean sleep latency ≤8 min and 2 or more SOREM periods on MSLT. REM within 15 min of sleep onset on the preceding nocturnal polysomnogram may replace one of SOREM periods.
  2. Low CSF hypocretin-1 concentration (<110 pg/mL or less than one-third of control values)
	A. Daily periods of irrepressible need to sleep or daytime lapses into sleep, present for at least 3 mo
	B. Mean sleep latency ≤8 min and 2 or more SOREM periods on MSLT. REM within 15 min of sleep onset on the preceding nocturnal polysomnogram may replace one of the SOREM periods.
	C. No cataplexy
	D. CSF hypocretin-1 concentration has not been measured or CSF hypocretin-1 concentration is ≥110 pg/mL or greater than one-third of control values.
	E. The hypersomnolence and/or MSLT findings are not better explained by other causes.
		A. Daily periods of irrepressible need to sleep or daytime lapses into sleep, present for at least 3 mo
		B. Fewer than 2 SOREM periods on MSLT (or fewer than one of nocturnal REM latency was ≤15 min)
		C. No cataplexy
		D. Either 1 or 2 or both
		  1. Mean sleep latency ≤8 min on MSLT
		  2. Total 24-h sleep time ≥660 min on 24-h polysomnographic monitoring or wrist actigraphy (averaged over ≥7 d)
		E. Insufficient sleep syndrome is ruled out.
		F. The hypersomnolence and/or MSLT findings are not better explained by other causes.
			A. Daily periods of irrepressible need to sleep or daytime lapses into sleep, present for at least 3 mo
			B. The daytime sleepiness occurs as a consequence of a significant underlying medical or neurologic condition.
			C. Mean sleep latency is ≤8 min, and fewer than 2 SOREM periods are observed.
			D. The symptoms are not better explained by another untreated sleep disorder, a mental disorder, or the effects of medications or drugs.

From International classification of sleep disorders: diagnostic and coding manual, 3rd edition. Westchester (IL): American Academy of Sleep Medicine; 2014; with permission.

(0.025%–0.05%).[18,19] The onset of the disease is most often seen during adolescence around puberty.[20] As with the sleepiness of other sleep disorders, sleepiness or EDS of narcolepsy presents with an increased propensity to fall asleep, nodding, or easily dozing in relaxed or sedentary situations or a need to exert extra effort to avoid sleeping in these situations.[21] Additionally, irresistible or overwhelming urges to sleep commonly occur from time to time during wakeful periods in untreated narcolepsy patients. These so-called sleep attacks are not instantaneous lapses into sleep, as is often thought by the general public, but represent episodes of profound sleepiness experienced by those with marked sleep deprivation or other severe sleep disorders. This feeling is most often relieved by short naps (15–30 minutes), but in most cases the refreshed sensation only lasts a short time after awaking. The refreshing value of short naps is of considerable diagnostic value for EDS associated with narcolepsy.

EDS can be objectively measured with the standardized multiple sleep latency test (MSLT), and the MSLT findings (mean sleep latency <8 minutes) were included in the diagnostic criteria of EDS associated with narcolepsy and other hypersomnias (see **Table 1**).[17] The maintenance of wakefulness test (MWT) was also developed to measure how alert patients are when they are set in a boring situation during the day.[22] Although the MWT is not included in the diagnostic criteria of any hypersomnias, many researchers believe that the MWT is more sensitive in evaluating effects of treatments, such as by pharmacotherapy with wake-promoting compounds. One of the reasons for this is the floor effects seen with MSLT; when the EDS is sever, it is often difficult to detect the therapeutic effects (to sleep vs to stay awake with MWT) with the MSLT protocol. Therefore, the MWT is often used to examine the therapeutic effects of wake-promoting compounds. There is not enough evidence, however, to set the cutoff value even when the MWT is used to measure the effect of the treatment of diseases.[23,24]

In addition to EDS, narcoleptic patients exhibit cataplexy and other abnormal manifestations of REM sleep, such as hypnagogic hallucinations and sleep paralysis.[25] Cataplexy, the sudden occurrence of muscle weakness in association with emotions, such as laughing, joking, or anger, has long been considered a pathognomonic symptom of the syndrome.[21,26,27] Cataplectic events usually last from a few seconds to 2 or 3 minutes but occasionally continue longer.[28] Patients are usually alert and oriented during the event despite their inability to respond. Positive emotions, such as laughter, more commonly trigger cataplexy than negative emotions; however, any strong emotion is a potential trigger.[29]

Hypnagogic or hypnopompic hallucinations may be visual, tactile, auditory, or multisensory events, usually brief but occasionally continuing for a few minutes, that occur at transitions from wakefulness to sleep (hypnagogic) or from sleep to wakefulness (hypnopompic).[21] Hallucinations may contain combined elements of dream sleep and consciousness and are often bizarre or disturbing to patients.

Sleep paralysis is the inability to move, lasting from a few seconds to a few minutes, during the transition from sleep to wakefulness or from wakefulness to sleep. Episodes of sleep paralysis may alarm patients, particularly those who experience the sensation of being unable to breathe. Although accessory respiratory muscles may not be active during these episodes, diaphragmatic activity continues, and air exchange remains adequate.

One of the most frequently associated symptoms is insomnia, best characterized as a difficulty to maintain nighttime sleep. Typically, narcoleptic patients fall asleep easily, only to wake up after a short nap and are unable to return to sleep for another hour or so. Narcoleptic patients do not usually sleep more than normal individuals over the 24-hour cycle[30–32] but frequently have disrupted nighttime sleep.[30–32] Frequently associated problems are periodic leg movements,[33,34] REM behavior disorder, other parasomnias,[35,36] and obstructive sleep apnea.[34,37,38]

Other commonly reported symptoms include automatic behavior — absent-minded behavior or speech that is often nonsensical that the patient does not remember. Hypnagogic hallucinations, sleep paralysis, and automatic behavior are nonspecific to narcolepsy and occur in other sleep disorders (as well as in healthy individuals); however, these symptoms are far more common and occur with much greater frequency in narcolepsy.[39]

Hypocretin/Orexin Deficiency in Type 1 Narcolepsy

In most patients with cataplexy, a deficiency in the hypocretin neuropeptide system is involved in the pathophysiology of human narcolepsy.[40] The observation that cerebrospinal fluid (CSF) hypocretin-1 levels are decreased in patients with narcolepsy provides a new diagnostic tool and refines the nosologic considerations for narcolepsy.

Using a large sample of patients and controls, the authors determined that 110 pg/mL (30% of mean control values) was the most specific and sensitive cutoff value for diagnosing narcolepsy.[41] Most samples had undetectable levels (<40 pg/mL), and a few had detectable but very diminished levels. None of the patients with idiopathic hypersomnia, sleep apnea, restless legs syndrome, or insomnia had abnormal hypocretin levels. Because the specificity of the CSF finding is also high, low CSF hypocretin-1 levels were included in the *International Classifications of Sleep Disorder, Second Edition*, as a positive diagnosis for narcolepsy-cataplexy.[42] In the most recent revision of the *ICSD*, *ICSD-3*, published in 2014,[15] narcolepsy-cataplexy was renamed narcolepsy type 1, or hypocretin deficiency syndrome, whereas narcolepsy without cataplexy was renamed narcolepsy type 2 (hypocretin nondeficient) to emphasize the pathophysiologic basis of the diseases.

Immune System and Narcolepsy

It has been reported that a large majority people with narcolepsy have the tissue-type HLA DR2.[21,28] High-resolution typing revealed that narcolepsy has the closest association with HLA-DQB1*0602, which is found in 95% of narcoleptic patients with cataplexy and 41% of patients with narcolepsy without cataplexy but only 18% to 35% of the general population.[21,43] The tight association between narcolepsy and an antigen-presenting class II HLA type suggests that autoimmune processes may play a critical role in type 1 narcolepsy because many autoimmune diseases exhibit tight associations with class II HLA haplotypes. Type 1 narcolepsy cases could thus involve an autoimmune alteration of hypocretin-containing cells in the central nervous system (CNS), but the antigen for this pathologic process has not yet been identified. Dauvilliers and colleagues[44] reported an HLA-DQB1*0602–positive monozygotic twin pair discordant for narcolepsy and CSF hypocretin-1 (only the affected subject had a low hypocretin-1 level), suggesting that altered CSF hypocretin levels are state dependent and not trait dependent and likely an acquired deficit. In other words, the genetic background is likely not sufficient to develop an abnormality in the hypocretin system. This finding is also complementary to the autoimmune hypothesis.

Considerations for the Pathophysiology of Type 2 Narcolepsy

There are debates about the pathophysiology of narcolepsy with normal hypocretin levels (ie, type 2 narcolepsy). More than 90% of the patients with narcolepsy without cataplexy show normal CSF hypocretin levels, yet they show apparent REM sleep abnormalities (ie, sleep-onset REMs [SOREMs]). Furthermore, even if the strict criteria for narcolepsy-cataplexy are applied, up to 10% of patients with narcolepsy-cataplexy show normal CSF hypocretin levels. Considering that occurrence of cataplexy is tightly associated with hypocretin deficiency, impaired hypocretin neurotransmission is still likely involved in narcolepsy-cataplexy with normal CSF hypocretin levels. Conceptually, there are 2 possibilities to explain these mechanisms: (1) specific impairment of hypocretin receptor and their downstream pathway and (2) partial/localized loss of hypocretin ligand (yet normal CSF levels exhibited). A good example for the former is Hcrtr 2-mutated narcoleptic dogs; they exhibit normal CSF hypocretin-1 levels[45] while having full-blown narcolepsy. Thannickal and colleagues[46] reported 1 narcolepsy without cataplexy patient (HLA typing was unknown) who had an overall loss of 33% of hypocretin cells compared with normal, with maximal cell loss in the posterior hypothalamus. This result favors the second hypothesis, but studies with more cases are needed.

Treatment of Excessive Daytime Sleepiness Associated with Narcolepsy Types 1 and 2

Nonpharmacologic treatments (ie, behavioral modification, such as regular napping and work accommodations) are often helpful. In a survey by a patient group organization,[47–49] however, 94% of all patients reported using pharmacologic therapies, mostly stimulant medications.[50]

Sleepiness is usually treated using amphetamine-like CNS stimulants (ie, methylphenidate) or modafinil (ie, 2-[(diphenylmethy)sulfinyl] acetamide) and its R-enantiomer, armodafinil, which are wake-promoting compounds unrelated to amphetamines (**Table 2**[51]). More recently, the American Academy of Sleep Medicine (AASM) recommended the use of sodium oxybate, a short-lasting sedative of unknown mechanisms, as first-line treatment of EDS and cataplexy, The most commonly used amphetamine-like compounds are methylphenidate, methamphetamine, D-amphetamine (all schedule II compounds), and mazindol (a schedule IV compound) (**Fig. 1**; see **Table 2**). The clinical use of stimulants in narcolepsy often has been the subject of standards of practice published by AASM.[52] Typically, a patient is started on a low dose, which is then increased progressively to obtain satisfactory results. Studies have shown that daytime sleepiness can be greatly improved subjectively, but sleep variables are never completely normalized by stimulant treatments.[53] Milder stimulants with low

Table 2
Current pharmacologic treatment of excessive daytime sleepiness associated with narcolepsy

Compound	Scheduled Class[a]	Usual Daily Doses	Half-Life (h)	Side Effects/Notes
Modafinil	IV	100–400 mg	9–14[b]	No peripheral sympathomimetic action, headaches, nausea
Armodafinil	IV	100–300 mg	10–15[b]	Similar to those of modafinil
Mazindol	IV	2–8 mg	10–13	Reduction of appetite or increase in blood pressure
Methylphenidate hydrochloride	II	≤80 mg	2–4	Same as amphetamines; less reduction of appetite or increase in blood pressure
Methamphetamine	II	5–80 mg	9–12	Irritability, mood changes, headache, palpitations, tremors, excessive sweating, insomnia
D-Amphetamine sulfate	II	≤60 mg	10–28	Irritability, mood changes, headache, palpitations, tremors, excessive sweating, insomnia
Sodium oxybate	III	4.5–9 g	0.5–1	Overdoses (a single dose of 60–100 mg/kg) induce dizziness, nausea, vomiting, confusion, agitation, epileptic seizures, hallucinations, coma with bradycardia, and respiratory depression; evidence of withdrawal syndrome

[a] All compounds in the list are scheduled and the class is listed.
[b] The half-life of the S-enantiomer of modafinil is short (approximately 3–4 h), so the half-life of racemic modafinil mostly reflects the R-enantiomer (armodafinil).

efficacy and potency, such as modafinil or armodafinil, are usually tried first (see **Fig. 1**). More effective amphetamine-like stimulants (methylphenidate, D-amphetamine, and methamphetamine) are then used if needed (see **Fig. 1**). Stimulant compounds are generally well tolerated in patients with narcolepsy. Minor adverse effects, such as headaches, irritability, nervousness, tremors, anorexia, palpitations, sweating, and gastric discomfort, are common. Cardiovascular impact, such as increased blood pressure, is possible, considering that sympathomimetic effects of these classes of compounds have been established in animals, although they have been remarkably difficult to document in human studies. Surprisingly, tolerance rarely occurs in this patient population and drug holidays are not recommended by the AASM.[52] Stimulant abuse is rare among patients with well-defined narcolepsy.[11–14] A compliance study has shown that approximately 50% of patients who receive stimulants reduce or withdraw stimulant medications by themselves.[54]

Exceptionally, psychotic complications may be observed, most often when the medications are used at high doses and chronically disrupt nocturnal sleep.[55]

Modafinil/armodafinil

Modafinil (2-[(diphenylmethyl)sulfinyl]acetamide) is a chemically unique compound developed in France. Modafinil has been available in France since 1984 on a compassionate mode and was officially approved in France in 1992. Modafinil (and its R-enantiomer) has been approved in 1998 in the United States for the treatment of narcolepsy, shift-work disorder, and residual sleepiness in treated patients with sleep apnea syndrome.

Armodafinil, the R-enantiomer of racemic modafinil, with a longer half-life, was also recently approved by the Food and Drug Administration (FDA) for EDS associated with narcolepsy as well as for residual sleepiness in nasal continuous positive airway pressure–treated individuals and

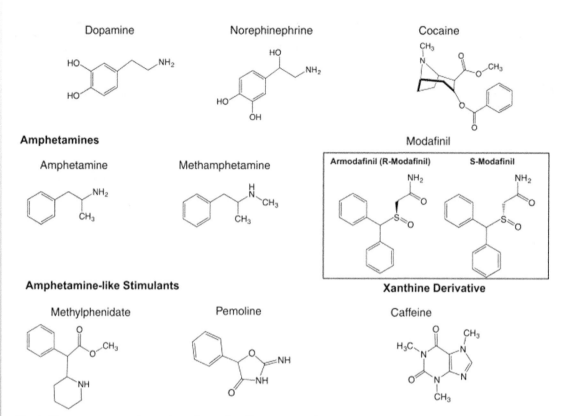

Fig. 1. The most commonly used amphetamine-like compounds.

sleepiness in shift work sleep disorder. Importantly, the R-enantiomer of modafinil has a half-life of 10 hours to 15 hours, which is longer than that of the S-enantiomer of modafinil (3–4 hours).[56] The dual pharmacokinetic properties of the racemic mixture may explain why modafinil is often more potent when taken twice per day at the beginning of therapy, during the period of drug accumulation. In terms of plasma concentrations, armodafinil is higher than modafinil late in the day on a milligram-to-milligram basis.[57] That is the reason why modafinil is given twice a day at the beginning of therapy, and armodafinil is given once a day.

Several randomized trials have shown that modafinil is effective against EDS in narcolepsy compared with placebo.[58,59] Armodafinil improves the MWT compared with placebo among narcolepsy patients.[60] Both modafinil and armodafinil are classified as schedule IV (defined as drugs with low potential for abuse and low risk of dependence) (see **Table 2**).[61]

The prevalence of side effects of modafinil/armodafinil is not high, and headache, nausea, dry mouth, and anorexia are the known side effects.[62] Modafinil can cause a serious rash in children, although rarely.[63]

In clinical practice, modafinil is given once a day in the morning on an empty stomach in bed to maximize the effect of the drug. The starting dose is usually 200 mg, and the dose range can vary between 100 mg and 400 mg, as needed, depending on the effect.[64] If the maximum dose (400 mg/d) is not sufficient to treat EDS among narcolepsy patients, then it is recommended to increase the dose up to 600 mg per day.

As discussed previously, armodafinil is usually given once a day in the early morning, and the dose range of armodafinil is 100 mg to 300 mg each morning.

The mechanism of action of modafinil/armodafinil is highly debated. There are few studies addressing the mode of action of armodafinil, and this review mostly discusses the action of racemic modafinil. Modafinil/armodafinil has not been shown to bind to or inhibit any receptors or enzymes of known neurotransmitters.[65,66] In vitro, modafinil/armodafinil binds to the dopamine transporter [DAT] and inhibits dopamine (DA) reuptake.[66,67] These binding inhibitory effects have been shown associated with increased extracellular DA levels in the striatum in rats and dog brain.[68,69]

The most striking finding was that DAT knockout mice were completely unresponsive to the wake-promoting effects of methamphetamine, GBR12909 (a selective DAT blocker), and modafinil. These results further confirm the critical role of DAT in mediating the wake-promoting effects of amphetamines and modafinil and that an intact DAT molecule is required for mediating the arousal effects of these compounds.[69] Qu and colleagues[70] further demonstrated that wake-promoting effects of modafinil were attenuated in D2 receptor knockout mice and were completely abolished in D2 receptor knockout mice with D1 antagonist, confirming the importance of dopaminergic neurotransmission for the modes of the action of modafinil.

Furthermore, a recent human PET study in 10 healthy humans with [11C] cocaine (DAT radioligand) and [11C] raclopride (D2/D3 radioligand sensitive to changes in endogenous DA) also demonstrated that modafinil (200 mg and 400 mg given orally) decreased [11C] cocaine binding potential in the caudate (53.8%), putamen (47.2%), and nucleus accumbens (39.3%).[71] In addition, modafinil also reduced binding potential of [11C] raclopride in these structures, suggesting the increases in extracellular DA were caused by DAT blockades.[71] These results are highly consistent with the results of the animal studies, discussed previously; modafinil's effects on alertness are entirely abolished in mice without the DAT protein[69] and in animals lacking D1 and D2 receptor functions.[70]

Methylphenidate and amphetamines

In 1935, amphetamine was used for the first time for the treatment of narcolepsy. Narcolepsy was possibly the first condition for which amphetamine was used clinically. It revolutionized therapy for the condition, even though it was not curative. Methylphenidate, the piperazine derivative of amphetamine, was introduced for the treatment of narcolepsy in 1959, and both compounds share similar pharmacologic properties.[72] Phenylisopropylamine (amphetamine) has a simple chemical structure resembling endogenous catecholamines.

Amphetamine-like compounds, such as methylphenidate, pemoline, and fencamfamine, are structurally similar to amphetamines; all compounds include a benzene core with an ethylamine group side chain (phenethylamine derivatives). Methylphenidate has been commonly used for the treatment of EDS in narcolepsy, and a racemic mixture of both the D-enantiomer and L-enantiomer is used, but D-methylphenidate mainly contributes to clinical effects, especially after oral administration.

Molecular targets mediating amphetamine-like stimulant effects are complex and vary depending on the specific analog/isomer and the dose administered. Amphetamine per se increases catecholamine (DA and norepinephrine [NE]) release and inhibits reuptake. These effects are mediated by specific catecholamine transporters (ie, DAT and NE transporter).[73] Amphetamine derivatives inhibit the uptake and enhance the release of DA, NE, or both by interacting with these molecules. These mechanisms, as well as the reverse transport (ie, exchange diffusion) and the blocking of reuptake of DA/NE by amphetamine, all lead to an increase in NE and DA synaptic concentrations.[73]

Methylphenidate is now recommended for use as one of the second-line options. Because there are new medicines available, like sodium oxybate and modafinil/armodafinil, methylphenidate is used when patients do not response to these new classes of drugs.

The mechanism of action of methylphenidate is similar to that of amphetamines and mainly increases the extracellular concentration of DA by blockage of the DAT and also, to a lesser degree, increases DA release.[74,75]

The side effects of methylphenidate are reduced appetite, nausea, headache, insomnia, and psychosis, which are similar to that of amphetamine.[74] It has been said that methylphenidate increases the risk of cardiovascular events in children and adults[76]; however, a large cohort, including more than 1 million children and young adults, has shown that the cardiovascular events risk is not strongly associated with attention deficit-hyperactivity disorder drugs, which is mainly methylphenidate.[77]

In clinical practice, methylphenidate is initially prescribed 10 mg per day at first. The recommended maximum dose is up to 80 mg per day.

Sodium oxybate

Sodium oxybate, the sodium salt of γ-hydroxybutyrate (GHB), taken in the evening and once again during the night, reduces daytime sleepiness, cataplectic attacks, and other manifestations of REM sleep.[78–82] GHB has been used in Canada and European countries for the treatment of narcolepsy-cataplexy. The administration of GHB was followed by a significant decrease in number of stage shifts and awakenings, wakefulness after sleep onset, and percentage of sleep stage 1. Sleep efficiency and slow-wave sleep percentage increased REM latency decreased significantly.[83] Although improvement in sleepiness occurs relatively quickly, anticataplectic effects appear 1 week to 2 weeks after the initiation of the treatment. Due to its positive effects on mood and libido, its slow-wave sleep–enhancing properties, and a subsequent increase in growth hormone release, GHB is widely abused by athletes and other populations.[84,85] In addition, because of its euphorigenic, behavioral disinhibitive, and amnestic properties, coupled with simple administration (ie, high solubility, colorlessness, and tastelessness when mixed with a drink), the abuse/misuse of GHB as a recreational substance and as a date rape drug has risen sharply in recent years, leading to an increased number of overdoses and intoxications for which no specific antidote exists.[81,86] GHB was classified as a schedule I drug that currently has no accepted medical use for treatment in the United States. Recent large-scale, double-blind, placebo-controlled clinical trials in the United States, however, led to reestablish sodium oxybate (the sodium salt of GHB) as a first-line treatment of narcolepsy-cataplexy.[79–81,87] In the United States, sodium oxybate is the approved formula of GHB and is classified as a schedule III compound. The compound is especially useful in patients with severe insomnia and cataplexy who do not tolerate antidepressant medication well because of its side effects on sexual potency. Although improvement in sleepiness occurs quickly, anticataplectic effects appeared 1 week to 2 weeks after the initiation of the treatment. Sodium oxybate has demonstrated statistically significant improvements in both symptoms, EDS and cataplexy, either as a monotherapy or in combination with modafinil, in clinical trials.[88] According to the meta-analysis, sodium oxybate was superior to placebo in increasing MWT (5.18 minutes; 95% CI, 2.59–7.78) and reducing weekly sleep attacks (−9.65 times; 95% CI, −17.72–1.59).[89] From these wake-promoting effects (on the day after the intake of compound at night), some researchers try to classify sodium oxybate as a CNS stimulant, but the mode of action of wake-promoting effects of sodium oxybate is unknown. Patients first need to take liquid sodium oxybate before they go to bed, and then they need to take the second dose 2.5 hours to 4 hours after the first dose. This is because of the short half-life (0.5–1 hour in the body) and short duration of action (2–4 hours) of sodium oxybate.[90] The recommended starting dose is 4.5 g a night divided into 2 equal doses of 2.25 g, which may be adjusted up to a maximum of 9 g per night in increments of 1.5 g per night with 1-week to 2-week intervals. The benefit was significant after 4 weeks, highest after 8 weeks, and maintained during long-term therapy.[91] The side effects of sodium oxybate are nausea, insomnia, headache, dizziness, vomiting, weight loss, psychiatric complications, and sleep apnea[92] (see **Table 2**).

Because of the abuse potency of the compound, the Risk Evaluation and Mitigation Strategies program operated by the US FDA mandates prescriber/patient education for safe use and registration to prescribe sodium oxybate.[93] There are also economic drawbacks to using sodium oxybate for the treatment of narcolepsy. The cost of sodium oxybate is expensive, at up to $143,604 per 1 year.[94] The patent will expire in 2024, and the cost of sodium oxybate is likely to be more economical after 2024.

The mechanism of how sodium oxybate works has not been fully understood and it may have multiple mechanisms of action in the brain. A series of experimental evidence suggests that sodium oxybate may work as an agonist on γ-aminobutyric acid (GABA)$_B$ receptors.[95] Sodium oxybate is one of the precursors of GABA, and a portion of it may be converted to GABA and stimulate GABA receptors.[96] Several researchers also claimed that sodium oxybate has its own receptor (GHB receptor),[97] but functional roles of this receptor are still largely unknown (**Fig. 2**).

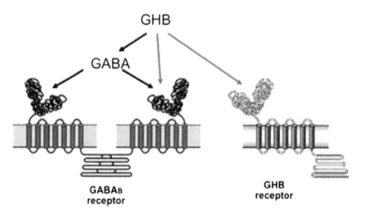

Fig. 2. The GHB receptor.

Despite these new findings, the physiologic significance of the brain GHB signaling pathway, especially for the therapeutic effects against EDS and cataplexy, is still unknown. One of the possible modes of action is mediating the regulation of activities of adrenergic locus coeruleus (LC) neurons. The activity of the LC is essential for the maintenance of muscle tone, and the LC ceases to fire during cataplectic attacks.[98] GHB may prevent a cataplectic attack by dampening the tone of LC neurons via the stimulation of inhibitory extrasynaptic GABA receptors in the LC, thus increasing the threshold for autoinhibition.[99] Worsening of periodic leg movements in narcoleptic patients by sodium oxybate may suggest dopaminergic involvements in the drug action.

Pitolisant (H₃ inverse agonist)

Histamine has long been implicated in the control of vigilance, and H_1 antagonists are strongly sedative. The downstream effects of hypocretins on the histaminergic system (hcrtr2 excitatory effects) are likely important in mediating the wake-promoting properties of hypocretin.[100] Although centrally injected histamine or histaminergic H_1 agonists promote wakefulness, systemic administrations of these compounds induce various unacceptable side effects via peripheral H_1 receptor stimulation. In contrast, the histaminergic H_3 receptors are regarded as inhibitory autoreceptors and are enriched in the CNS. H_3 antagonists or inverse agonist enhance wakefulness in normal rats and cats[101] and in narcoleptic mice models.[102] Histaminergic H_3 antagonists might be a useful as wake-promoting compounds for the treatment of EDS or as cognitive enhancers,[103] and several histaminergic H_3 receptor antagonists/inverse agonists are currently being investigated. Pitolisant (previously called BF2.649 and tiprolisant; Bioprojet, Wakix, Paris, France) was the first clinically used inverse agonist of the histamine H_3 autoreceptor and increases histamine release in the hypothalamus and cortex. In a pilot single-blind study on 22 patients with narcolepsy/cataplexy, pitolisant (40 mg in the morning) reduced EDS.[104] Recent double-blind phase III trials on 95 narcoleptic subjects in 32 sleep disorder centers in 5 European countries revealed that pitolisant (10 mg, 20 mg, or 40 mg) once a day was efficacious on the 2 major symptoms of narcolepsy, EDS and cataplexy, compared with placebo and was better tolerated compared with twice-a-day modafinil (100 mg, 200 mg, or 400 mg).[105] If these findings are substantiated in further ongoing studies, H₃-receptor inverse agonists, including pitolisant, could offer a new treatment option for patients with narcolepsy.

Pitolisant is currently only available in Europe. The side effects are gastrointestinal pain, increased appetite, weight gain, headache, insomnia, and anxiety.[106] The initial dose of pitolisant is 9 mg, taken as a single dose in the morning. The maximum dose is up to 36 mg.

Combination strategy

Combination therapy of some stimulants is also recommended when the administration of a single type of stimulant is not effective against EDS of narcolepsy patients.

The recommended combinations of stimulants are sodium oxybate + modafinil/armodafinil, pitolisant, or methylphenidate + sodium oxybate, and modafinil or methylphenidate + pitolisant.

Other stimulants

Amphetamine and dextroamphetamine (amphetamines, dose 5–60 mg/d), mazindol (a weak DA releaser with DA and NE reuptake inhibitor, dose 2–8 mg/d), pemoline (amphetamine-like stimulant, dose 37.5–112.5 mg/d), and bupropion (DA uptake inhibitor with wake-promotion, dose 150–300 mg/d) are occasionally used if the first-line and second-line medications turn out to be insufficient.

Pharmacotherapy of Rapid Eye Movement Sleep–Related Symptoms in Narcolepsy

The pharmacotherapy of REM sleep–related symptoms in narcolepsy is briefly discussed. Besides sodium oxybate, tricyclic antidepressants; serotonin–NE reuptake inhibitors, such as milnacipran; and selective serotonin reuptake inhibitors, such as paroxetine and fluvoxamine, are recommended for patients suffering from cataplexy, hypnagogic hallucinations, and sleep paralysis.[107] Side effects of these antidepressants include dry mouth, obesity, sexual dysfunction, type 2 diabetes, and suicidal tendencies.[108] Antidepressants suppress cataplexy, hypnagogic hallucinations, and sleep paralysis, and this effect seems due to suppression of REM sleep or prolongation of REM sleep latency.[21,109]

Idiopathic Hypersomnia

With the clear definition of narcolepsy (cataplexy and dissociated manifestations of REM sleep), it became apparent that some patients with hypersomnia suffer from a different disorder. In the late 1950s and early 1960s, Bedrich Roth[110] first described a syndrome characterized by EDS, prolonged sleep, and sleep drunkenness, and by the absence of sleep attacks, cataplexy, sleep paralysis, and hallucinations. The terms, *independent sleep drunkenness* and *hypersomnia with sleep drunkenness* were initially suggested, but now this syndrome is categorized as idiopathic hypersomnia with and without long sleep time.[42]

In the absence of systematic studies, the prevalence of idiopathic hypersomnia is unknown. Nosologic uncertainty causes difficulty in determining the epidemiology of the disorder. Recent reports from large sleep centers reported the ratio of idiopathic hypersomnia to narcolepsy to be 1:10.[111] The age of onset of symptoms varies, but it is frequently between 10 years and 30 years. The condition usually develops progressively over several weeks or months. Once established, symptoms are generally stable and long lasting, but spontaneous improvement in EDS may be observed in up to one-quarter of patients.[111]

The pathogenesis of idiopathic hypersomnia is unknown. Hypersomnia usually starts insidiously. Occasionally, EDS is first experienced after transient insomnia, abrupt changes in sleep-wake habits, overexertion, general anesthesia, viral illness, or mild head trauma.[111] Despite reports of an increase in HLA-DQ1, DQ11, DR5, Cw2, and DQ3 and decrease in Cw3, no consistent findings have emerged.[111]

The most recent attempts to understand the pathophysiology of idiopathic hypersomnia relate to the investigation of potential role of the hypocretins. Most studies suggest, however, normal CSF levels of hypocretin-1 in idiopathic hypersomnia.[41,112]

Patients of idiopathic hypersomnia have less sleep paralysis (20% of patients with idiopathic hypersomnia) and sleep hallucinations (25%) than narcolepsy. Among idiopathic hypersomnia patients, sleep drunkenness and long nocturnal sleep times without fragmentation are common, and the effects and duration of naps are unrefreshing and long compared with narcolepsy patients.[15,113,114]

There is no FDA-approved medicine to treat EDS caused by idiopathic hypersomnia. In the clinical setting, modafinil is used off-label to treat EDS in idiopathic hypersomnia, as in narcolepsy.[115,116] If EDS is irresistible and resistant to modafinil, methylphenidate and amphetamine-like compounds are also used. A recent article has shown that sodium oxybate improves the sleepiness of idiopathic patients as much as it improves sleepiness in narcolepsy type 1; however, sodium oxybate has strong side effects and dependency, as discussed preivously.[116,117]

Hypersomnia due to a Medical Disorder

The prevalence of symptomatic narcolepsy (ie, narcolepsy due to a medical disorder) is likely small, and only approximately 120 of such cases have been reported in the literature in the past 30 years.[118] The prevalence of symptomatic (ie, hypersomnia due to a medical disorder) hypersomnia, however, may be much higher. For example, several million subjects in the United States suffer from chronic brain injury; 75% of these patients have sleep problems and approximately half of them claim sleepiness.[119] Patients with hypersomnia due to a medical disorder have EDS caused by coexisting medical or neurologic disorders. Daytime sleepiness of this disorder may be similar to that of narcolepsy or idiopathic hypersomnia.[15,114] Common disorders are discussed later, and in any secondary hypersomnia, it is important to treat the underlying disease besides providing symptomatic therapies.

Posttraumatic Hypersomnia

According to a meta-analysis research, the prevalence of EDS among posttraumatic brain injury patients is 27%.[120] CSF hypocretin-1 levels are low in most of patients with moderate to severe traumatic brain injury in their acute injury phase.[121] Regarding treatment, the effectiveness of modafinil is still under controversy. A randomized controlled trial (RCT) has shown that modafinil improves the Epworth Sleepiness Scale (ESS) score significantly compared with placebo at 6 treatment weeks.[122] Another RCT shows, however, that modafinil did not consistently improve the ESS score compared with the placebo at 10 treatment weeks.[123] Another RCT has demonstrated that armodafinil do not improve the ESS score compared with placebo at 12 treatment weeks.[124]

Hypersomnia Secondary to Parkinson Disease

Like narcolepsy and idiopathic hypersomnia, daytime sleepiness is measured by ESS and MSLT. Among Parkinson disease patients, 20% to 50% are said to have EDS.[125–127]

The effect of modafinil on this disorder is still controversial. There are some studies that have shown that modafinil improves the EDS in Parkinson disease patients,[128,129] whereas there are other articles that have shown that modafinil does not improve the EDS in Parkinson disease patients.[129,130] An article has also shown that sodium oxybate can improve the EDS in Parkinson disease patients.[131]

Common Stimulants in Daily Life

Caffeine is probably the most popular and widely consumed CNS stimulant in the world. Caffeine is digested from foods, drinks, and sometimes chocolate, coffee, energy drinks, soft drinks, and so forth. Caffeine is a xanthine derivative and acts as an adenosine A_1 and adenosine A_{2A} receptor agonist.[132] Adenosine content is increased in the basal forebrain after sleep deprivation. Adenosine has thus been proposed as a sleep-inducing substance accumulating in the brain during prolonged wakefulness.[133] Side effects of caffeine are often overlooked; however, sometimes they are crucial. A variety of side effects of caffeine are well known, which are headache, stomach upset, nervousness, and so forth. For the common side effects of caffeine in terms of sleep, caffeine typically prolongs sleep latency, reduces total sleep time and sleep efficiency, and worsens perceived sleep quality.[132] An average cup of coffee contains 50 mg to 150 mg of caffeine. Caffeine is also available over the counter (NoDoz, 200 mg caffeine [GlaxoSmithKline plc, Middlesex, United Kingdom]; Vivarin, 200 mg caffeine [Meda Consumer Healthcare Inc, NJ]). This suggests that stimulant effects of caffeine tablets are not strong enough to manage pathologic sleepiness, but narcoleptic patients often take caffeine before they are diagnosed. According to a recent review, moderate caffeine intake (400 mg/d) is not associated with adverse effects.[134] The average cup of ground roasted coffee contains 85 mg of caffeine, and instant coffee contains 60 mg of caffeine.[135] Drinking fewer than 5 cups of ground roasted coffee per day is better for health.

FUTURE TREATMENT OPTIONS
Hypocertin-Based Treatments

Because a large majority of human narcolepsy patients are hypocretin ligand deficient, hypocretin replacement therapy may be a new therapeutic option. This may be effective for both sleepiness (ie, fragmented sleep/wake pattern) and cataplexy. Animal experiments using ligand-deficient narcoleptic dogs suggest that stable and centrally active hypocretin analogs (possibly nonpeptide synthetic hypocretin ligands) need to be developed to be peripherally effective.[136,137] This is also substantiated by a mice study that found normalization of sleep/wake patterns and behavioral arrest episodes (equivalent to cataplexy and REM sleep onset) in hypocretin-deficient mice knockout models supplemented by central administration of hypocretin-1.[138] In addition, orexin gene therapy (injection of an aden-oassociated viral vector coding for prepro-orexin plus a red fluorescence protein into the mediobasal hypothalamus) markedly improved the MWT in orexin/ataxin-3 narcoleptic mice.[139] These results demonstrate that cell transplantations and gene therapy may be developed in the future. One of the concerns for this option is that the hypocretin

peptides do not cross the blood-brain barrier (BBB) well. Intranasal delivery is a noninvasive method of bypassing the BBB to deliver therapeutic agents to the brain and spinal cord. Although developments of small molecule nonpeptide hypocretin receptor agonists are in progress and shown effective in mouse models,[140] these are still not available for clinical use. The toxicity/side effects of systemic administration of hypocretin receptor agonists are also unknown.

Recent reports in both rhesus monkeys and humans show some effects using intranasal hypocretin-1 administration.[141,142] A recent double-blind, randomized, placebo-controlled crossover design study on 7 patients with narcolepsy/cataplexy and matched healthy controls showed that intranasal hypocretin-1 restores olfactory function in narcolepsy/cataplexy patients.[141] But unfortunately, no data exist concerning potential effects on daytime sleepiness and cataplexy at this time.

Immune-Based Treatments

Type 1 narcolepsy is currently thought to be an autoimmune disorder targeting hypothalamus hypocretin neurons. An autoimmune basis for the hypocretin cell loss in narcolepsy has been suspected due to its strong DQB1*0602 association and association with T-cell receptor polymorphisms.[143] Based on the autoimmune hypothesis of narcolepsy, immune-based therapy, such as steroids (in 1 patient), intravenous immunoglobulins, and plasmapheresis have been proposed, with some promising results in a few cases.[144,145] Recently, a case of narcolepsy with cataplexy with undetectable CSF hypocretin-1 level that completely reversed shortly after disease onset was reported.[144] Although needing replication in well-designed trials, these results suggest that immune-based therapy could become a new treatment option for patients with narcolepsy/cataplexy at disease onset.

Other Possible Treatments of Interests (Non–Hypocretin-Based Treatments)

In addition to hypocretin replacement, preclinical and clinical trials for new classes of compounds are also in progress.

More than a decade ago, Osamu Hayaishi[146] and his group claimed that prostaglandin (PG) D2 is an endogenous sleep substance, and a series of animal studies by his group reported that PGD2 or PGD2 receptor (DP1) agonists promote sleep in animals (see Huang and colleagues[147]). The same research group also reported that PG DP1 potently promotes wakefulness. This suggests the possibility use of PG DP1 antagonists as wake-promoting compounds. This may also be clinically important because it is reported that increased serum lipocalin-type PGD synthase (beta-trace) levels correlate with EDS associated with narcolepsy.[148] Wake-promoting effects of a DP1 antagonist, ONO-4127, were evaluated in a mouse model of narcolepsy (ie, orexin/ataxin-3 transgenic mice) and compared with effects of modafinil.[149] ONO-4127 perfused in the basal forebrain area potently promoted wakefulness in both wild-type and narcoleptic mice, and the wake-promoting effects of ONO-4127 at 2.93×10^{-4} M approximately corresponded to those of modafinil at 100 mg/kg, orally; ONO-4127 reduced DREM (direct transitions from wake to REM sleep), an electroencephalogram/electromyogram assessment of behavioral cataplexy, in narcoleptic mice, suggesting ONO-4127 is likely to have anticataplectic effects; DP1 antagonists may be a new class of compounds for the treatment of narcolepsy-cataplexy.

Another possible area that currently gathers less pharmaceutical interest is the use of thyrotropin-releasing hormone (TRH) direct or indirect agonists. TRH itself is a small peptide, which penetrates the BBB at very high doses. Small molecules with agonist properties and increased BBB penetration (ie, CG3703, CG3509, or TA0910) have been developed, partially thanks to the small nature of the starting peptide.[150] TRH (at a high dose of several milligrams/kilogram) and TRH agonists increase alertness and have been shown to be wake promoting and anticataplectic in the narcoleptic canine model,[151,152] and these effects might be related to the excitatory effects of TRH on motoneurons.[153] Initial studies had demonstrated that TRH enhances DA and NE neurotransmission,[154,155] and these properties may partially contribute to the wake-promoting and anticataplectic effects of TRH. Recent studies have suggested that TRH may promote wakefulness by directly interacting with the thalamocortical network; TRH itself and TRH receptor type 2 are abundant in the reticular thalamic nucleus.[156] Local application of TRH in the thalamus abolishes spindle wave activity,[157] and in the slice preparations, TRH depolarized thalamocortical and reticular/perigenuculate neurons by inhibition of leak K+ conductance.[157]

Other pathways with possible applications in the development of novel stimulant medications include the adenosinergic system (more selective receptor antagonists than caffeine), the dopaminergic/adrenergic system (for example, DA/NE-reuptake inhibitors), the GABAergic system (for example, inverse benzodiazepine agonists), and the glutamatergic system (ampakines).[158]

SUMMARY

This article overviews pharmacotherapy of EDS associated with narcolepsy type 1, narcolepsy type 2, idiopathic hypersomnia, and hypersomnia due to a medical disorder.

Narcolepsy-cataplexy is most commonly caused by a loss of hypocretin-producing cells in the hypothalamus (ie, type 1 narcolepsy). Low CSF hypocretin-1 levels can be used to diagnose the condition. The disorder is tightly associated with HLA-DQB1*0602, suggesting that the cause in most patients may be autoimmune destruction of these cells. The treatment of EDS includes the use of amphetamine-like CNS stimulants, modafinil and its R-enantiomer armodafinil. Methylphenidate is the most commonly prescribed amphetamine-like stimulant in the United States, and this compound is efficacious and well tolerated by most narcoleptic patients. Because of its safety and low side-effect profile, modafinil became the first-line treatment of choice for EDS associated with narcolepsy. These wake-promoting compounds, however, do not improve cataplexy and dissociated manifestations of REM sleep, so antidepressants (monoamine uptake inhibitors) are additionally used to treat these aspects. Sodium oxybate (a sodium salt of GHB, available in the United States), when given at night, improves EDS and cataplexy, Therefore, the number of US patients treated with sodium oxybate is increasing, and it has become the first-line treatment of narcolepsy. Combination therapy with some stimulants is also recommended when the administration of single stimulant type is not effective against EDS of narcolepsy patients.

There is no FDA-approved medicine to treat EDS associated with idiopathic hypersomnia. In the clinical setting, modafinil is used off-label to treat EDS in idiopathic hypersomnia. If EDS is irresistible and resistant to modafinil, methylphenidate and amphaemine-like compounds are also used.

Treatments of EDS associated with symptomatic hypersomnia (ie, hypersomnias due to a medical disorder) are more complex because these conditions are heterogeneous, and hypocretin involvements are seen in some disease conditions but not in all. Specific brain structures that have been damaged and mechanisms involved in the EDS are likely varied. Unresponsiveness to stimulant treatments may occur depending on the underlying pathophysiologic mechanism. In this regard, development of new types of wake-promoting compounds would likely benefit these patients.

Emerging treatments undergoing investigation include histaminergic compounds (pitolisant, an

H_3 inverse agonist, is available in Europe), TRH agonists, DP1 antagonists, hypocretin replacement/supplement therapies, and immunomodulation as prevention.

There are many potential approaches for narcolepsy; compounds and new therapies, such as hypocretin transplant or gene technology, are being developed.[159] The development of small molecular synthetic hypocretin receptor agonists, however, is likely the next step for this therapeutic option in humans, because hypocretin peptides themselves do not penetrate the brain effectively. If ligand replacement therapy is demonstrated as effective in hypocretin-deficient narcolepsy, hypocretin cell transplant or gene therapy technology may also be applicable in the near future. These therapies, however, are many years away, and the efficacy of exogenously administered hypocretin analogs (nonpeptide agonists) in humans should be established first.

To prevent hypoceretin neuronal loss (ie, narcolepsy type 1), immune-based treatments is promising, but accumulation of much cases is needed to prove the efficacy of this approach.

REFERENCES

1. Arand D, Bonnet M, Hurwitz T, et al. The clinical use of the MSLT and MWT. Sleep 2005;28(1):123–44.
2. Pagnin D, de Queiroz V, Carvalho YT, et al. The relation between burnout and sleep disorders in medical students. Acad Psychiatry 2014;38(4): 438–44.
3. Swanson LM, Arnedt JT, Rosekind MR, et al. Sleep disorders and work performance: findings from the 2008 National Sleep Foundation Sleep in America poll. J Sleep Res 2011;20(3):487–94.
4. Young TB. Epidemiology of daytime sleepiness: definitions, symptomatology, and prevalence. J Clin Psychiatry 2004;65(Suppl 16):12–6.
5. Wu S, Wang R, Ma X, et al. Excessive daytime sleepiness assessed by the Epworth Sleepiness Scale and its association with health related quality of life: a population-based study in China. BMC Public Health 2012;12:849.
6. Plante DT, Finn LA, Hagen EW, et al. Longitudinal associations of hypersomnolence and depression in the Wisconsin sleep cohort study. J Affect Disord 2017;207:197–202.
7. Roth T. Effects of excessive daytime sleepiness and fatigue on overall health and cognitive function. J Clin Psychiatry 2015;76(9):e1145.
8. Garbarino S, Durando P, Guglielmi O, et al. Sleep apnea, sleep debt and daytime sleepiness are independently associated with road accidents. A cross-sectional study on truck drivers. PLoS One 2016;11(11):e0166262.
9. Murray BJ. A practical approach to excessive daytime sleepiness: a focused review. Can Respir J 2016;2016:4215938.
10. Doyle JB, Daniels LE. Symptomatic treatment for narcolepsy. J Am Med Assoc 1931;96(17):1370–2.
11. Akimoto H, Honda Y, Takahashi Y. Pharmacotherapy in narcolepsy. Dis Nerv Syst 1960;21: 704–6.
12. Guilleminault C, Carskadon M, Dement WC. On the treatment of rapid eye movement narcolepsy. Arch Neurol 1974;30(1):90–3.
13. Parkes JD, Baraitser M, Marsden CD, et al. Natural history, symptoms and treatment of the narcoleptic syndrome. Acta Neurol Scand 1975;52(5):337–53.
14. Passouant P, Billiard M. [Narcolepsy]. Rev Prat 1976;26(27):1917–23.
15. ICSD-3. International classification of sleep disorders. 3rd edition. Rochester (MN): American Sleep Disorders Association; 2014. Medicine AAoS.
16. Arnulf I. Kleine-levin syndrome. Sleep Med Clin 2015;10(2):151–61.
17. Medicine AAoS. International classification of sleep disorders. 3rd edition. Daren (IL): American Academy of Sleep Medicine; 2014.
18. Hublin C, Kaprio J, Partinene M, et al. The prevalence of narcolepsy: an epidemiological study of the Finnish twin cohort. Ann Neurol 1994;35: 709–16.
19. Tashiro T, Kanbayashi T, Hishikawa Y. An epidemiological study of narcolepsy in Japanese. Paper presented at: The 4th International Symposium on Narcolepsy. Tokyo, Japan, June 16–17, 1994. p. 13.
20. Dauvilliers Y, Montplaisir J, Molinari N, et al. Age at onset of narcolepsy in two large populations of patients in France and Quebec. Neurology 2001; 57(11):2029–33.
21. Nishino S, Mignot E. Pharmacological aspects of human and canine narcolepsy. Prog Neurobiol 1997;52(1):27–78.
22. Pizza F, Contardi S, Mondini S, et al. Daytime sleepiness and driving performance in patients with obstructive sleep apnea: comparison of the MSLT, the MWT, and a simulated driving task. Sleep 2009;32(3):382–91.
23. Littner MR, Kushida C, Wise M, et al. Practice parameters for clinical use of the multiple sleep latency test and the maintenance of wakefulness test. Sleep 2005;28(1):113–21.
24. Sullivan SS, Kushida CA. Multiple sleep latency test and maintenance of wakefulness test. Chest 2008;134(4):854–61.
25. Scammell TE. Narcolepsy. N Engl J Med 2015; 373(27):2654–62.
26. Dauvilliers Y, Billiard M, Montplaisir J. Clinical aspects and pathophysiology of narcolepsy. Clin Neurophysiol 2003;114(11):2000–17.

27. Guilleminault C, Kryger MH, Roth T, et al. Narco-lepsy syndrome. Principles and Practice of Sleep Medicine. 2nd edition. Philadelphia: WB Saunders; 1994. p. 549–61.

28. Juji T, Satake M, Honda Y, et al. HLA antigens in Japanese patients with narcolepsy. All the patients were DR2 positive. Tissue Antigens 1984;24(5): 316–9.

29. Gelb M, Guilleminault C, Kraemer H, et al. Stability of cataplexy over several months–information for the design of therapeutic trials. Sleep 1994;17(3): 265–73.

30. Hishikawa Y, Wakamatsu H, Furuya E, et al. Sleep satiation in narcoleptic patients. Electroencepha-logr Clin Neurophysiol 1976;41:1–18.

31. Broughton R, Dunham W, Newman J, et al. Ambu-latory 24 hour sleep-wake monitoring in narcolepsy-cataplexy compared to matched con-trol. Electroencephalogr Clin Neurophysiol 1988; 70:473–81.

32. Montplaisir J, Billard M, Takahashi S, et al. Twenty-four-hour recording in REM-narcoleptics with spe-cial reference to nocturnal sleep disruption. Biol Psychiatry 1978;13(1):78–89.

33. Godbout R, Montplaisir J. Comparison of sleep pa-rameters in narcoleptics with and without periodic movements of sleep. In: Koella WP, Ruther E, Schulz H, editors. Sleep '84. New York: Gustav Fischer Verlag; 1985. p. 380–2.

34. Mosko SS, Shampain DS, Sassin JF. Nocturnal REM latency and sleep disturbance in narcolepsy. Sleep 1984;7:115–25.

35. Mayer G, Pollmächer T, Meier-Ewert K, et al. Zur Einschätzung des Behinderungsgrades bei Narkolepsie. Gesundheitswesen 1993;55: 337–42.

36. Schenck CH, Mahowald MW. Motor dyscontrol in narcolepsy: Rapid-Eye-Movement (REM) sleep without atonia and REM sleep behavior disorder. Ann Neurol 1992;32(1):3–10.

37. Chokroverty S. Sleep apnea in narcolepsy. Sleep 1986;9(1):250–3.

38. Guilleminault C, Dement WC, Passouant P, editors. Narcolepsy. New York: Spectrum Publications; 1976. Advances in Sleep Research; No. 3.

39. Juji T, Matsuki K, Tokunaga K, et al. Narcolepsy and HLA in the Japanese. Ann N Y Acad Sci 1988;540:106–14.

40. Nishino S, Ripley B, Overeem S, et al. Hypocretin (orexin) deficiency in human narcolepsy. Lancet 2000;355(9197):39–40.

41. Mignot E, Lammers GJ, Ripley B, et al. The role of cerebrospinal fluid hypocretin measurement in the diagnosis of narcolepsy and other hypersomnias. Arch Neurol 2002;59(10):1553–62.

42. ICSD-2. ICSD-2-International classification of sleep disorders. In: Sateia MJ, editor. Diagnostic and

coding manual. 2nd edition. Westchester (IL): American Academy of Sleep Medicine; 2005. p. 38–43.

43. Mignot E, Hayduk R, Black J, et al. HLA DQB1*0602 is associated with cataplexy in 509 narcoleptic patients. Sleep 1997;20(11): 1012–20.

44. Dauvilliers Y, Maret S, Bassetti C, et al. A monozygotic twin pair discordant for narcolepsy and CSF hypocretin-1. Neurology 2004;62(11): 2137–8.

45. Ripley B, Fujiki N, Okura M, et al. Hypocretin levels in sporadic and familial cases of canine narco-lepsy. Neurobiol Dis 2001;8(3):525–34.

46. Thannickal TC, Nienhuis R, Siegel JM. Localized loss of hypocretin (orexin) cells in narcolepsy without cataplexy. Sleep 2009;32(8):993–8.

47. Garma L, Marchand F. Non-pharmacological ap-proaches to the treatment of narcolepsy. Sleep 1994;17(8 Suppl):S97–102.

48. Roehrs T, Zorick F, Wittig R, et al. Alerting effects of naps in patients with narcolepsy. Sleep 1986;9(1): 194–9.

49. Rogers AE. Problems and coping strategies identi-fied by narcoleptic patients. J Neurosurg Nurs 1984;16(6):326–34.

50. Morgenthaler TI, Kapur VK, Brown T, et al. Practice parameters for the treatment of narcolepsy and other hypersomnias of central origin. Sleep 2007; 30(12):1705–11.

51. Hirai N, Nishino S. Recent advances in the treat-ment of narcolepsy. Curr Treat Options Neurol 2011;13(5):437–57.

52. Mitler MM, Aldrich MS, Koob GF, et al. Narcolepsy and its treatment with stimulants. ASDA standards of practice. Sleep 1994;17(4):352–71.

53. Mitler MM, Hajdukovic R. Relative efficacy of drugs for the treatment of sleepiness in narcolepsy. Sleep 1991;14(3):218–20.

54. Rogers AE, Aldrich MS, Berrios AM, et al. Compli-ance with stimulant medications in patients with narcolepsy. Sleep 1997;20(1):28–33.

55. Auger RR, Goodman SH, Silber MH, et al. Risks of high-dose stimulants in the treatment of disorders of excessive somnolence: a case-control study. Sleep 2005;28(6):667–72.

56. Nishino S, Okuro M. Armodafinil for excessive day-time sleepiness. Drugs Today (Barc) 2008;44(6): 395–414.

57. Darwish M, Kirby M, Hellriegel ET, et al. Armodafinil and modafinil have substantially different pharma-cokinetic profiles despite having the same terminal half-lives: analysis of data from three randomized, single-dose, pharmacokinetic studies. Clin Drug Investig 2009;29(9):613–23.

58. Randomized trial of modafinil for the treatment of pathological somnolence in narcolepsy. US

Modafinil in Narcolepsy Multicenter Study Group. Ann Neurol 1998;43(1):88–97.

59. Randomized trial of modafinil as a treatment for the excessive daytime somnolence of narcolepsy: US Modafinil in Narcolepsy Multicenter Study Group. Neurology 2000;54(5):1166–75.

60. Harsh JR, Hayduk R, Rosenberg R, et al. The efficacy and safety of armodafinil as treatment for adults with excessive sleepiness associated with narcolepsy. Curr Med Res Opin 2006;22(4):761–74.

61. United States Department of Justice. Drug Enforcement Administration. Drug Scheduling. Available at: https://www.dea.gov/druginfo/ds.shtml. Accessed February 10, 2017.

62. Roth T, Schwartz JR, Hirshkowitz M, et al. Evaluation of the safety of modafinil for treatment of excessive sleepiness. J Clin Sleep Med 2007;3(6):595–602.

63. U.S. Food & Drug Administration. Drug Safety. Medication Guide. Available at: http://www.fda.gov/downloads/drugs/drugsafety/ucm231722.pdf. Accessed February 11, 2017.

64. Schwartz JR, Feldman NT, Bogan RK, et al. Dosing regimen effects of modafinil for improving daytime wakefulness in patients with narcolepsy. Clin Neuropharmacol 2003;26(5):252–7.

65. Cephalon, Inc. FDA approval of NUVIGIL. Available at: https://www.sec.gov/Archives/edgar/data/873364/000110465907048203/a07-16834_1ex99d1.htm. Accessed February 11, 2017.

66. Mignot E, Nishino S, Guilleminault C, et al. Modafinil binds to the dopamine uptake carrier site with low affinity. Sleep 1994;17(5):436–7.

67. Nishino S, Mao J, Sampathkumaran R, et al. Increased dopaminergic transmission mediates the wake-promoting effects of CNS stimulants. Sleep Res Online 1998;1(1):49–61.

68. Dopheide MM, Morgan RE, Rodvelt KR, et al. Modafinil evokes striatal [(3)H]dopamine release and alters the subjective properties of stimulants. Eur J Pharmacol 2007;568(1–3):112–23.

69. Wisor JP, Nishino S, Sora I, et al. Dopaminergic role in stimulant-induced wakefulness. J Neurosci 2001;21(5):1787–94.

70. Qu WM, Huang ZL, Xu XH, et al. Dopaminergic D1 and D2 receptors are essential for the arousal effect of modafinil. J Neurosci 2008;28(34):8462–9.

71. Volkow ND, Fowler JS, Logan J, et al. Effects of modafinil on dopamine and dopamine transporters in the male human brain: clinical implications. JAMA 2009;301(11):1148–54.

72. Yoss RE, Daly D. Treatment of narcolepsy with ritalin. Neurology 1959;9(3):171–3.

73. Kuczenski R, Segal DS. Neurochemistry of amphetamine, in psychopharmacology, toxicology and abuse. San Diego (CA): Academic Press; 1994. p. 81–113.

74. Leonard BE, McCartan D, White J, et al. Methylphenidate: a review of its neuropharmacological, neuropsychological and adverse clinical effects. Hum Psychopharmacol 2004;19(3):151–80.

75. Schenk JO. The functioning neuronal transporter for dopamine: kinetic mechanisms and effects of amphetamines, cocaine and methylphenidate. Prog Drug Res 2002;59:111–31.

76. Nissen SE. ADHD drugs and cardiovascular risk. N Engl J Med 2006;354(14):1445–8.

77. Cooper WO, Habel LA, Sox CM, et al. ADHD drugs and serious cardiovascular events in children and young adults. N Engl J Med 2011;365(20):1896–904.

78. Broughton R, Mamelak M. The treatment of narcolepsy-cataplexy with nocturnal gamma-hydroxybutyrate. Can J Neurol Sci 1979;6(1):1–6.

79. Group USXMS. A randomized, double blind, placebo-controlled multicenter trial comparing the effects of three doses of orally administered sodium oxybate with placebo for the treatment of narcolepsy. Sleep 2002;25(1):42–9.

80. Group USXMS. A 12-month, open-label, multicenter extension trial of orally administered sodium oxybate for the treatment of narcolepsy. Sleep 2003;26(1):31–5.

81. Group USXMS. Sodium oxybate demonstrates long-term efficacy for the treatment of cataplexy in patients with narcolepsy. Sleep Med 2004;5(2):119–23.

82. Mamelak M, Scharf MB, Woods M. Treatment of narcolepsy with gamma-hydroxybutyrate. A review of clinical and sleep laboratory findings. Sleep 1986;9(1 Pt 2):285–9.

83. Plazzi G, Pizza F, Vandi S, et al. Impact of acute administration of sodium oxybate on nocturnal sleep polysomnography and on multiple sleep latency test in narcolepsy with cataplexy. Sleep Med 2014;15(9):1046–54.

84. Mack RB. Love potion number 8 1/2. Gamma-hydroxybutyrate poisoning. N C Med J 1993;54(5):232–3.

85. Wong CG, Gibson KM, Snead OC 3rd. From the street to the brain: neurobiology of the recreational drug gamma-hydroxybutyric acid. Trends Pharmacol Sci 2004;25(1):29–34.

86. Nicholson KL, Balster RL. GHB: a new and novel drug of abuse. Drug Alcohol Depend 2001;63(1):1–22.

87. Black J, Houghton WC. Sodium oxybate improves excessive daytime sleepiness in narcolepsy. Sleep 2006;29(7):939–46.

88. Robinson DM, Keating GM. Sodium oxybate: a review of its use in the management of narcolepsy. CNS Drugs 2007;21(4):337–54.

89. Alshaikh MK, Tricco AC, Tashkandi M, et al. Sodium oxybate for narcolepsy with cataplexy: systematic review and meta-analysis. J Clin Sleep Med 2012; 8(4):451–8.

90. Thorpy MJ. Update on therapy for narcolepsy. Curr Treat Options Neurol 2015;17(5):347.

91. Palatini P, Tedeschi L, Frison G, et al. Dose-dependent absorption and elimination of gamma-hydroxybutyric acid in healthy volunteers. Eur J Clin Pharmacol 1993;45(4):353–6.

92. Wang YG, Swick TJ, Carter LP, et al. Safety overview of postmarketing and clinical experience of sodium oxybate (Xyrem): abuse, misuse, dependence, and diversion. J Clin Sleep Med 2009; 5(4):365–71.

93. Administration tUSFaD. Available at: http://www.fda.gov/Drugs/DrugSafety/PostmarketDrugSafetyInformationforPatientsandProviders/ucm332408.htm. Accessed February 9, 2017.

94. Saini P, Rye DB. Hypersomnia: evaluation, treatment, and social and economic aspects. Sleep Med Clin 2017;12(1):47–60.

95. Maitre M, Klein C, Mensah-Nyagan AG. Mechanisms for the specific properties of gamma-hydroxybutyrate in brain. Med Res Rev 2016; 36(3):363–88.

96. Pardi D, Black J. γ-hydroxybutyrate/sodium oxybate. CNS drugs 2006;20(12):993–1018.

97. Andriamampandry C, Taleb O, Viry S, et al. Cloning and characterization of a rat brain receptor that binds the endogenous neuromodulator gamma-hydroxybutyrate (GHB). Faseb J 2003;17(12): 1691–3.

98. Wu MF, Gulyani SA, Yau E, et al. Locus coeruleus neurons: cessation of activity during cataplexy. Neuroscience 1999;91(4):1389–99.

99. Szabadi E. GHB for cataplexy: possible mode of action. J Psychopharmacol 2015;29(6):744–9.

100. Nishino S, Ripley B, Mignot E, et al. CSF hypocretin-1 levels in schizophrenics and controls: relationship to sleep architecture. Psychiatry Res 2002;110(1):1–7.

101. Shiba T. Wake promoting effects of thioperamide, a histamine H3 antagonist in orexin/ataxin-3 narcoleptic mice. Sleep 2004; 27(Suppl):A241–2.

102. Parmentier R, Anaclet C, Guhennec C, et al. The brain H3-receptor as a novel therapeutic target for vigilance and sleep-wake disorders. Biochem Pharmacol 2007;73(8):1157–71.

103. Lin JS, Dauvilliers Y, Arnulf I, et al. An inverse agonist of the histamine H(3) receptor improves wakefulness in narcolepsy: studies in orexin-/- mice and patients. Neurobiol Dis 2008;30(1): 74–83.

104. Dauvilliers Y, Bassetti C, Lammers GJ, et al. Pitolisant versus placebo or modafinil in patients with narcolepsy: a double-blind, randomised trial. Lancet Neurol 2013;12(11):1068–75.

105. Sharif NA, To ZP, Whiting RL. Analogs of thyrotropin-releasing hormone (TRH): receptor affinities in brains, spinal cords, and pituitaries of different species. Neurochem Res 1991;16(2): 95–103.

106. Leu-Semenescu S, Nittur N, Golmard JL, et al. Effects of pitolisant, a histamine H3 inverse agonist, in drug-resistant idiopathic and symptomatic hypersomnia: a chart review. Sleep Med 2014;15(6): 681–7.

107. Swick TJ. Treatment paradigms for cataplexy in narcolepsy: past, present, and future. Nat Sci Sleep 2015;7:159–69.

108. Santarsieri D, Schwartz TL. Antidepressant efficacy and side-effect burden: a quick guide for clinicians. Drugs Context 2015;4:212290.

109. Thase ME. Depression, sleep, and antidepressants. J Clin Psychiatry 1998;59(Suppl 4):55–65.

110. Roth B. Narkolepsie und hypersomnie. Berlin: VEB Verlag Volk und Gesundheit; 1962.

111. Bassetti C, Aldrich MS. Idiopathic hypersomnia. A series of 42 patients. Brain 1997;120(Pt 8): 1423–35.

112. Bassetti C, Gugger M, Bischof M, et al. The narcoleptic borderland: a multimodal diagnostic approach including cerebrospinal fluid levels of hypocretin-1 (orexin A). Sleep Med 2003;4(1):7–12.

113. Vernet C, Leu-Semenescu S, Buzare MA, et al. Subjective symptoms in idiopathic hypersomnia: beyond excessive sleepiness. J Sleep Res 2010; 19(4):525–34.

114. International classification of sleep disorders: diagnostic and coding manual. 3rd edition. Westchester (IL): American Academy of Sleep Medicine; 2014.

115. Mayer G, Benes H, Young P, et al. Modafinil in the treatment of idiopathic hypersomnia without long sleep time–a randomized, double-blind, placebo-controlled study. J Sleep Res 2015;24(1): 74–81.

116. Billiard M, Sonka K. Idiopathic hypersomnia. Sleep Med Rev 2016;29:23–33.

117. Leu-Semenescu S, Louis P, Arnulf I. Benefits and risk of sodium oxybate in idiopathic hypersomnia versus narcolepsy type 1: a chart review. Sleep Med 2016;17:38–44.

118. Nishino S, Kanbayashi T. Symptomatic narcolepsy, cataplexy and hypersomnia, and their implications in the hypothalamic hypocretin/orexin system. Sleep Med Rev 2005;9(4):269–310.

119. Verma A, Anand V, Verma NP. Sleep disorders in chronic traumatic brain injury. J Clin Sleep Med 2007;3(4):357–62.

120. Mathias JL, Alvaro PK. Prevalence of sleep disturbances, disorders, and problems following

traumatic brain injury: a meta-analysis. Sleep Med 2012;13(7):898–905.

121. Baumann CR, Stocker R, Imhof HG, et al. Hypocretin-1 (orexin A) deficiency in acute traumatic brain injury. Neurology 2005;65(1):147–9.

122. Kaiser PR, Valko PO, Werth E, et al. Modafinil ameliorates excessive daytime sleepiness after traumatic brain injury. Neurology 2010;75(20):1780–5.

123. Jha A, Weintraub A, Allshouse A, et al. A randomized trial of modafinil for the treatment of fatigue and excessive daytime sleepiness in individuals with chronic traumatic brain injury. J Head Trauma Rehabil 2008;23(1):52–63.

124. Menn SJ, Yang R, Lankford A. Armodafinil for the treatment of excessive sleepiness associated with mild or moderate closed traumatic brain injury: a 12-week, randomized, double-blind study followed by a 12-month open-label extension. J Clin Sleep Med 2014;10(11):1181–91.

125. Braga-Neto P, da Silva-Junior FP, Sueli Monte F, et al. Snoring and excessive daytime sleepiness in Parkinson's disease. J Neurol Sci 2004;217(1):41–5.

126. Gjerstad MD, Alves G, Wentzel-Larsen T, et al. Excessive daytime sleepiness in Parkinson disease: is it the drugs or the disease? Neurology 2006;67(5):853–8.

127. Verbaan D, van Rooden SM, Visser M, et al. Nighttime sleep problems and daytime sleepiness in Parkinson's disease. Mov Disord 2008;23(1):35–41.

128. Adler CH, Caviness JN, Hentz JG, et al. Randomized trial of modafinil for treating subjective daytime sleepiness in patients with Parkinson's disease. Mov Disord 2003;18(3):287–93.

129. Hogl B, Saletu M, Brandauer E, et al. Modafinil for the treatment of daytime sleepiness in Parkinson's disease: a double-blind, randomized, crossover, placebo-controlled polygraphic trial. Sleep 2002;25(8):905–9.

130. Ondo WG, Fayle R, Atassi F, et al. Modafinil for daytime somnolence in Parkinson's disease: double blind, placebo controlled parallel trial. J Neurol Neurosurg Psychiatr 2005;76(12):1636–9.

131. Ondo WG, Perkins T, Swick T, et al. Sodium oxybate for excessive daytime sleepiness in Parkinson disease: an open-label polysomnographic study. Arch Neurol 2008;65(10):1337–40.

132. Fisone G, Borgkvist A, Usiello A. Caffeine as a psychomotor stimulant: mechanism of action. Cell Mol Life Sci 2004;61(7–8):857–72.

133. Porkka-Heiskanen T, Strecker RE, Thakkar M, et al. Adenosine: a mediator of the sleep-inducing effects of prolonged wakefulness. Science 1997;276(5316):1265–8.

134. Nawrot P, Jordan S, Eastwood J, et al. Effects of caffeine on human health. Food Addit Contam 2003;20(1):1–30.

135. Barone JJ, Roberts HR. Caffeine consumption. Food Chem Toxicol 1996;34(1):119–29.

136. Mieda M, Willie JT, Hara J, et al. Orexin peptides prevent cataplexy and improve wakefulness in an orexin neuron-ablated model of narcolepsy in mice. Proc Natl Acad Sci U S A 2004;101(13):4649–54.

137. Schatzberg SJ, Cutter-Schatzberg K, Nydam D, et al. The effect of hypocretin replacement therapy in a 3-year-old Weimaraner with narcolepsy. J Vet Intern Med 2004;18(4):586–8.

138. Kantor S, Mochizuki T, Janisiewicz AM, et al. Orexin neurons are necessary for the circadian control of REM sleep. Sleep 2009;32(9):1127–34.

139. Deadwyler SA, Porrino L, Siegel JM, et al. Systemic and nasal delivery of orexin-A (Hypocretin-1) reduces the effects of sleep deprivation on cognitive performance in nonhuman primates. J Neurosci 2007;27(52):14239–47.

140. Nagahara T, Saitoh T, Kutsumura N, et al. Design and synthesis of non-peptide, selective orexin receptor 2 agonists. J Med Chem 2015;58(20):7931–7.

141. Baier PC, Hallschmid M, Seeck-Hirschner M, et al. Effects of intranasal hypocretin-1 (orexin A) on sleep in narcolepsy with cataplexy. Sleep Med 2011;12(10):941–6.

142. Mishima K, Fujiki N, Yoshida Y, et al. Hypocretin receptor expression in canine and murine narcolepsy models and in hypocretin-ligand deficient human narcolepsy. Sleep 2008;31(8):1119–26.

143. Kawashima M, Lin L, Tanaka S, et al. Anti-Tribbles homolog 2 (TRIB2) autoantibodies in narcolepsy are associated with recent onset of cataplexy. Sleep 2010;33(7):869–74.

144. Dauvilliers Y, Abril B, Mas E, et al. Normalization of hypocretin-1 in narcolepsy after intravenous immunoglobulin treatment. Neurology 2009;73(16):1333–4.

145. Dauvilliers Y, Carlander B, Rivier F, et al. Successful management of cataplexy with intravenous immunoglobulins at narcolepsy onset. Ann Neurol 2004;56(6):905–8.

146. Ueno R, Honda K, Inoue S, et al. Prostaglandin D2, a cerebral sleep-inducing substance in rats. Proc Natl Acad Sci U S A 1983;80(6):1735–7.

147. Huang ZL, Urade Y, Hayaishi O. Prostaglandins and adenosine in the regulation of sleep and wakefulness. Curr Opin Pharmacol 2007;7(1):33–8.

148. Jordan W, Tumani H, Cohrs S, et al. Narcolepsy increased L-PGDS (beta-trace) levels correlate with excessive daytime sleepiness but not with cataplexy. J Neurol 2005;252:1372–8.

149. Sagawa Y, Sato M, Sakai N, et al. Wake-promoting effects of ONO-4127Na, a prostaglandin DP1 receptor antagonist, in hypocretin/orexin deficient

narcoleptic mice. Neuropharmacology 2016; 110(Part A):268–76.

150. Riehl J, Honda K, Kwan M, et al. Chronic oral administration of CG-3703, a thyrotropin releasing hormone analog, increases wake and decreases cataplexy in canine narcolepsy. Neuropsychopharmacology 2000;23(1):34–45.

151. Nicoll RA. Excitatory action of TRH on spinal motoneurones. Nature 1977;265(5591):242–3.

152. Nishino S, Arrigoni J, Shelton J, et al. Effects of thyrotropin-releasing hormone and its analogs on daytime sleepiness and cataplexy in canine narcolepsy. J Neurosci 1997;17(16):6401–8.

153. Sharp T, Bennett GW, Marsden CA. Thyrotrophin-releasing hormone analogues increase dopamine release from slices of rat brain. J Neurochem 1982;39(6):1763–6.

154. Heuer H, Schafer MK, O'Donnell D, et al. Expression of thyrotropin-releasing hormone receptor 2 (TRH-R2) in the central nervous system of rats. J Comp Neurol 2000;428(2):319–36.

155. Keller HH, Bartholini G, Pletscher A. Enhancement of cerebral noradrenaline turnover by thyrotropin-releasing hormone. Nature 1974;248(448):528–9.

156. Broberger C. Neurotransmitters switching the thalamus between sleep and arousal: functional effects and cellular mechanism. New Frontiers in Neuroscience Research. Showa University International Symposium for Life Science. 1st Annual Meeting Showa University Kamijo Hall. Tokyo, August 31, 2004.

157. Mignot E, Nishino S. Emerging therapies in narcolepsy-cataplexy. Sleep 2005;28(6):754–63.

158. Okura M, Riehl J, Mignot E, et al. Sulpiride, a D2/D3 blocker, reduces cataplexy but not REM sleep in canine narcolepsy. Neuropsychopharmacology 2000;23(5):528–38.

159. Nishino S, Mignot E. Narcolepsy and cataplexy. Handb Clin Neurol 2011;99:783–814.

Nonpharmacologic Management of Excessive Daytime Sleepiness

Matthew R. Ebben, PhD

KEYWORDS

- Excessive daytime sleepiness • Behavioral management • Sleep restriction • Sleep need
- Sleep extension • Sleep debt • Sleep banking • Sleep deprivation

KEY POINTS

- A sleep duration of 7 to 8 hours has been associated with the lowest risk of mortality. At a population level, this information is important; however, for individuals reporting excessive daytime sleepiness, determining personal sleep need is likely to provide the most clinical benefit.
- Excessive daytime sleepiness has been linked to reduced performance, increased work-related accidents, and motor vehicle crashes. Therefore, treating sleepiness is critically important.
- Increasing time in bed before a period of sleep deprivation may help to moderate performance decrements during short periods of reduced sleep.
- Progressively increasing time in bed can help reduce excessive daytime sleepiness in those with chronic partial sleep deprivation. However, care should be taken not to increase time in bed too much at one time because this may result in reduced sleep efficiency.

INTRODUCTION

The focus of this article is to investigate behavioral strategies for improving daytime sleepiness. Other high-quality reviews on this topic have been published in the last several years, including one published in this journal in 2012.[1] In general, previous reviews have focused on sleepiness or hypersomnia secondary to conditions such as sleep apnea, circadian rhythm disorders, narcolepsy, and depression. However, somnolence is so commonly present in these conditions that, often, residual sleepiness is more a function of inadequate treatment of the primary disorder than a separate symptom that needs to be treated independently. Therefore, the goal of this article is to look mainly at sleepiness not stemming from another medical or psychological condition. The only caveat I make to this theme is to briefly discuss behavioral options to address sleepiness associated with narcolepsy because this group of patients develop a unique pattern of somnolence over the course of the day, which makes behavioral management more challenging.

To achieve the goal of understanding behavioral management of sleepiness, it is necessary to first define how nighttime sleep is thought to impact daytime somnolence and performance. Therefore, the literature investigating and discussing optimal sleep in terms of sleep duration, sleep insufficiency, and sleep need is reviewed. This review is followed by prophylactic measures that can be implemented when reduced nighttime sleep is anticipated for short periods of time (banking sleep). As mentioned earlier, behavioral treatment of narcolepsy, including sleep extension and prophylactic naps, is discussed and followed by a description of a technique I have developed in

This article originally appeared in September, 2017 issue of *Sleep Medicine Clinics* (Volume 12, Issue 3).
Disclosure Statement: The author has nothing to disclose.
Department of Neurology, Center for Sleep Medicine, Weill Cornell Medical College of Cornell University, 425 East 61st Street, 5th Floor, New York, NY 10065, USA
E-mail address: mae2001@med.cornell.edu

sleep.theclinics.com

clinical practice to determine sleep need in individuals in order to optimize subjective daytime alertness.

EXCESSIVE DAYTIME SLEEPINESS

Excessive daytime sleepiness (EDS) is a condition characterized by a pressure to sleep during the day, which causes either social or occupational problems for the individual. This condition is different from (idiopathic) hypersomnia, which involves daytime somnolence despite 11 hours or more of sleep.[2] Excessive sleepiness can be defined both objectively with tests, such as the multiple sleep latency test (MSLT)[3] and/or the maintenance for wakefulness test (MWT),[4] or with questionnaires either focused exclusively on sleepiness, such as the Epworth Sleepiness Scale,[5] the Stanford Sleepiness Scale,[6] or the Karolinska Sleepiness Scale,[7] or with questions regarding somnolence imbedded in other surveys. According to the National Sleep Foundation's 2008 Sleep in America poll, 18% of Americans are excessively sleepy.[8]

Daytime sleepiness has been investigated in several studies throughout the world, with prevalence ranging from 9% to 26%.[9] This wide range in prevalence of sleepiness is likely due as much to differences in study design and method used to query sleepiness as it is to true differences in the underlying alertness of populations. However, cultural differences in patterns of sleep, genetic variation, work schedules, and social activities in different countries may also play a role in level of sleepiness. Nonetheless, sleepiness is a major public health concern worldwide and has been found to significantly affect performance when induced experimentally.[10–13] Moreover, sleepiness has been linked to increased motor vehicle and work place accidents.[14–17] A study investigating the optimal duration of sleep to prevent deficits in psychomotor vigilance found that an average of 8.2 hours is needed per night for peak performance.[18] However, the US Department of Health and Human Services estimates that only 65% of Americans get a healthy amount of sleep.[19]

OPTIMAL SLEEP (SLEEP NEED VERSUS SLEEP DURATION VERSUS SLEEP INSUFFICIENCY)

In this section, 3 different but related concepts are examined in relation to optimal sleep. These concepts are sleep duration, sleep insufficiency, and sleep need. Understanding the differences in the terminology used to describe ideal sleep is critical to comprehending the previous research in this area, which can otherwise seem contradictory. Moreover, appreciating these distinctions is necessary to develop a thoughtful treatment approach to behaviorally induced chronic partial sleep deprivation, which is a substantial source of daytime sleepiness.

Sleep duration refers to the total amount of sleep obtained without factoring in whether or not individuals feel rested. More research has been done in this area than in sleep insufficiency or sleep need because questions related to sleep duration are more common than inquiries about whether the current total sleep amount is acceptable in existing large-scale data sets. Sleep duration is also easier to define both objectively and subjectively than other terminology related to optimal sleep.

Several studies have looked at the relationship between sleep length and death. Two relatively recent systematic reviews have shown a U-shaped curve for the association between sleep duration and all-cause mortality.[20,21] The lowest risk of death was found in individuals sleeping 7 to 8 hours per night. Those sleeping more or less than this amount showed an increased risk of mortality. More specifically, coronary heart disease, hypertension, and problems with glucose metabolism have been found to be linked to both short and long sleepers.[22–26] In one study, very short sleep of less than 5 hours per night was associated with increased risk for hypertension, hyperlipidemia, diabetes, and obesity.[27] Interestingly, this study did not find an elevated risk for any of these outcomes for the group self-reporting sleep duration of greater than 9 hours. A study by Altman and colleagues[28] found a significant relationship between sleep duration of less than 5 hours and body mass index, obesity, hypertension, myocardial infarction, and stroke. However, a sleep duration greater than 9 hours was only significantly associated with myocardial infarction and stroke.

A study performed by Van Dongen and colleagues[18] in which subjects were experimentally sleep restricted to 4, 6, or 8 hours in bed found that over the course of 14 days those in the 4- and 6-hour groups had significant decrements in cognitive performance. In fact, the investigators of this study state that 2 weeks of chronic partial sleep deprivation is equivalent to 2 days of total sleep deprivation. This finding is consistent with other studies, which have shown the cumulative effects of sleep restriction on psychomotor performance, mood, and objective measures of daytime sleepiness.[29–31]

In contrast to sleep duration, sleep insufficiency describes when the current amount of sleep is inadequate regardless of total sleep time. For example, someone may sleep 9 hours per night but feel that 10 hours is necessary to feel fully refreshed. Therefore, this person would be considered to have insufficient sleep. On the other hand, another individual may sleep 5 hours per night and feel that their sleep is adequate. As a result, this individual would not be considered to have sleep insufficiency. Sleep need is the most difficult concept out of the 3 to describe. Although not well defined in the literature, within this article it is defined as the amount of sleep a person needs to feel refreshed and alert during the day. In other words, sleep need describes the amount of sleep a person needs to prevent sleep insufficiency. Admittedly, even this straightforward definition leads to ambiguity between whether alertness should be defined subjectively through questionnaires or objectively with tests, such as the MSLT or MWT. Nonetheless, the treatment approach described later in this article is based on determining subjective sleep need in patients complaining of EDS.

The relationship between an individual's optimal sleep requirement and health and cognitive function is more elusive and not as well publicized as the research focused exclusively on duration. From an epidemiologic perspective, the difference between sleep need and duration is simply a function of the population's degree of chronic sleep deprivation. However, from the perspective of an individual, knowing the average sleep duration or need of the population in which they live, although interesting, does not necessarily help them to understand their personal sleep need. Ursin and colleagues[32] calculated a normal distribution of subjective sleep need in middle-aged adults and found a mean for both men and women between 7.0 and 7.5 hours, respectively, with a range of 4 to 10 hours. The standard deviation of sleep need in this study was approximately 1 hour. However, subjective sleepiness has been found to poorly predict objective alertness.[33] Therefore, it is unclear if subjective sleep need is a good indication of biological sleep need.

A few studies have sought to investigate the risks associated with unmet sleep need. In a study by Altman and colleagues,[28] sleep duration alone, sleep insufficiency alone, and the combined effect of sleep duration and insufficiency were examined. The goal of this study was to see if the deleterious effects of sleep duration is moderated by the subjective impression of inadequate sleep. When examined together, sleep insufficiency accounted for an increased risk of hyperlipidemia; duration alone accounted for elevated risk of stroke, myocardial infraction, and obesity.

In a study by Hwangbo and colleagues, daytime sleepiness was investigated based on habitual sleep duration alone and separately controlling for unmet sleep need. The overall prevalence of EDS in their study population was 12%, despite 32% of those studied reporting less than 7 hours of sleep per night. Interestingly, habitual sleep duration was not predictive of EDS when unmet sleep need was taken into account. This study supports the theory that individual sleep need is more important for daytime alertness than overall sleep duration. Unfortunately, overall health status was not explored in this study.

SLEEP DEBT AND BANKING SLEEP

If biological sleep need is not satisfied, sleep pressure will accrue; this process has been termed sleep debt.[34] Several studies have found that when sleep deprivation occurs (and during wakefulness in general), drive to offload slow-wave activity (SWA) and rapid eye movement (REM) sleep amasses such that, once sleep ensues, increased SWA and REM sleep is seen.[34–36] (Usually sleep pressure is thought to relate to SWA, and REM sleep is thought to be regulated by a combination of circadian and sleep-related forces; but REM sleep also shows rebound when deprived.) In fact, the homeostatic process described in Borbely's[37] 2-process model of sleep regulation defines sleep drive as a buildup of homeostatic pressure (process S) during wakefulness, which is measured by the amount of SWA that occurs during the subsequent sleep period. The length of wakefulness is proportional to the amount of SWA discharged.[35] The effects of sleep pressure were initially studied by looking at rebound from periods of either partial or full sleep deprivation.[34–36] More recently, sleep extension protocols have looked at the effects of chronic partial sleep debt.[38–40]

One of the first studies examining extended sleep was performed in the early 1970s by Taub and colleagues.[41] In this study, the sleep of a group of 12 healthy male volunteers was extended from approximately 7 to 9 hours per night. Interestingly, performance on vigilance and pinball tasks decreased after a 1-day recovery period. More recently, Roehrs and colleagues[39] extended the sleep of a group of both sleepy and alert normal subjects, whose group determination was based on MSLT score. The sleepy subjects showed an immediate increase in MSLT sleep latency after sleep extension. However, the alert subjects initially had a decrease in sleep latency; only after 6 days of extended sleep did mean sleep latency on the MSLT increase greater than the baseline level. Although, performance on a divided attention task improved in both groups throughout the extension period.

In 1999, Rupp and colleagues[42] performed a study looking at the effects of extended sleep during a subsequent period of sleep deprivation. On this study, subjects were assigned to either extended time in bed (10 hours) or habitual time in bed (7 hours) for 1 week. This was followed by a week of sleep restricted to 3 hours of time in bed. The extended-sleep group performed significantly better than the habitual-time-in-bed group on psychomotor vigilance tasks and had higher sleep latencies on the MWT. As a result, the term *banking sleep* was coined to describe extending sleep to more than the habitual time in bed in order to improve performance during future episodes of sleep deprivation. Arnal and colleagues[38] performed a follow-up study investigating the benefits of extending sleep before a period of total sleep deprivation. Like Rupp and colleagues,[42] Arnal and colleagues[38] found that sleep extension resulted in enhanced psychomotor vigilance task performance and improved MSLT scores during periods of sleep deprivation. However, some have speculated that sleep extension improves performance and decreases sleepiness during sleep deprivation by decreasing baseline sleep debt instead of truly banking sleep for later use.[43]

Nonetheless, both Rupp and colleagues[42] and Arnal and colleagues[38] show that relieving sleep pressure by extending time in bed to more than habitual time in bed before a period of reduced sleep will result in improved performance during the deprivation period. Therefore, individuals can moderate the discomfort associated with impending reduced sleep by an anticipatory period of extended sleep. Additional studies are required to see if these findings extend to the reduced performance seen with shift workers, who not only have reduced sleep but also battle the effects of being awake during disadvantageous phases of the circadian cycle. Arguably, this group of workers would benefit more from banking sleep than any other group because they can often predict times of reduced sleep based on their work schedule.

BEHAVIORAL TREATMENT OF SLEEPINESS ASSOCIATED WITH NARCOLEPSY

Narcolepsy is a disorder of REM sleep characterized by EDS, hypnogogic and/or hypnopompic hallucinations, sleep paralysis, and cataplexy (in some but not all cases).[2] It is typically diagnosed through a combination of clinical history and objective testing, which includes a polysomnogram followed by a MSLT. A sleep latency of 8 minutes or less with 2 or more REM sleep episodes on the MSLT (or one sleep-onset REM episode on the nighttime study followed by at least one REM episode on the MSLT) is considered diagnostic of narcolepsy.[2] A clinical history of cataplexy is pathognomonic of narcolepsy. However, 15% to 36% of narcoleptic patients do not have cataplexy.[2]

Behavioral treatment of sleepiness associated with narcolepsy has been investigated by a few groups. The most common methods tested for improving daytime sleepiness includes sleep extension and daytime naps (although additional cognitive-behavioral approaches have been investigated to treat other problems associated with narcolepsy). One study extended sleep in narcoleptic patients from 8 to 12 hours and found a significant increase in sleep latency after the extended sleep condition.[11] However, a recent review of studies on sleep satiation in narcoleptic patients found little benefit overall to extending sleep.[44] Narcoleptic patients tend to have fragmented nighttime sleep, but most feel alert upon awakening in the morning. However, as the day progresses, they begin to experience sleepiness at a faster rate than those without narcolepsy,[45] which may explain why sleep extension is not an effective treatment approach.

Studies have generally found daytime napping to improve alertness in narcoleptic patients.[44] A study by Helmus and colleagues[45] prescribed naps of either 15 or 120 minutes and found the longer naps to be more beneficial to daytime alertness. However, regardless of nap length, sleepiness returned when tested 3 hours later, suggesting that multiple brief naps throughout the day are likely to be more helpful than isolated long naps. However, Rogers and colleagues[46] studied the effects of two 15-minute naps on daytime alertness and did not find an overall benefit from the naps alone. Yet, when the scheduled naps were paired with regular bedtimes, daytime alertness was improved. Therefore, a combination of a consistent sleep schedule with multiple daytime naps seems to be the best behavioral strategy to improve alertness in narcoleptic patients.

A NEW BEHAVIORAL APPROACH TO TREAT EXCESSIVE DAYTIME SLEEPINESS (AND DETERMINING SUBJECTIVE SLEEP NEED)

The behavioral approach I describe here stems from my work in sleep restriction therapy (SRT). SRT is one of the elements of cognitive-behavioral therapy for insomnia (CBT-I). This therapy is a collection of nonpharmacologic treatments used to improve nighttime sleep quality in patients complaining of difficulty sleeping. SRT was originally developed by Art Spielman and colleagues[47] in the mid 1980s and involves restricting time in bed in order to increase the likelihood that patients will sleep during the night.

SRT begins by first determining the treatment schedule for patients. This task is done by giving patients sleep logs to fill out for a couple weeks (**Fig. 1**). Once completed, the clinician reviews the logs to determine a new sleep schedule, which is typically done by averaging total sleep time over the period of time tracked by the patients.[48] The patients are then advised to reduce time in bed to approximate their current total sleep time. Therefore, if patients are only sleeping 6.5 hours per night, but they are spending 9 hours in bed, they are advised to reduce the time in bed to 6.5 hours. Ideally, once patients have been on the schedule for 2 to 3 weeks, they have an increase in sleep efficiency and a decrease in sleep latency.

The initial phase of SRT treatment is remarkably successful in improving nighttime sleep quality.[49] However, in many cases, sleepiness remains. When this occurs, patients are advised to increase their time in bed by 15 minutes. They can add this additional time to either their wake time or sleep time. For example, if patients currently have a sleep schedule of 11:00 PM to 5:30 AM, they can extend their time in bed by either going to sleep at 10:45 PM or sleeping in until 5:45 AM (but not both). They are asked to sleep on the new schedule for at least 5 days before making an additional adjustment in the schedule. This allows time for patients to gradually catch up on sleep.

Although a 5-day time period was developed through clinical trial and error, this time period comports with Kitamura and colleagues'[50] recent finding that it takes 4 days of sleep extension to recover from a 1-hour sleep debt. If too much time in bed is given at once, patients may initially be able to generate additional sleep to fill this much larger time in bed but may not be able to sustain the new schedule over the long-term, thus, causing them to develop insomnia once again. The idea that too much time in bed can reduce nighttime sleep quality is evidenced by sleep extension studies. These studies have consistently shown decreased sleep efficiency and increased latency to sleep during periods of extended sleep.[38–40]

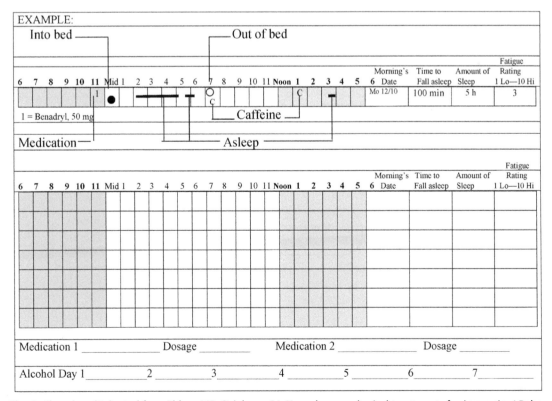

Fig. 1. Sleep log. (*Adapted from* Ebben MR, Spielman AJ. Non-pharmacological treatments for insomnia. J Behav Med 2009;32(3):248; with permission.)

Interestingly, I have found this same technique of extending sleep used in SRT very useful in patients complaining of EDS, who do not report subjective difficulty sleeping at night. Moreover, other elements of CBT-I can also be useful when assessing the likely cause of daytime sleepiness. This subject is described in more detail later.

Behavioral treatment of sleepy patients should begin with a through screening for likely medical and/or psychological causes of the sleepiness (See **Fig. 2** for the treatment decision tree). These causes include (but are not limited to) sleep apnea, narcolepsy, thyroid dysfunction, nutritional/vitamin deficiency, gastroesophageal reflux disease, depression, and/or anxiety. If the clinical history suggests an alternative cause of sleepiness, that condition should be the focus of investigation until it is either ruled out or successfully treated.

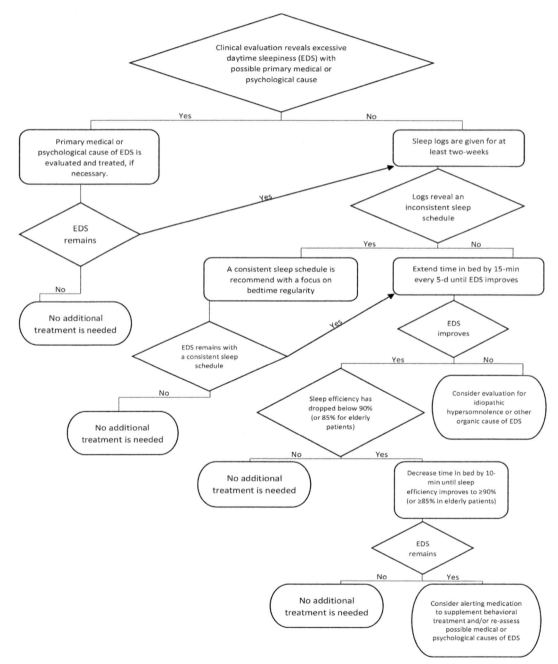

Fig. 2. Algorithm for behavioral management of EDS.

Once cleared for treatment, as with SRT, sleepy patients are asked to fill out sleep logs for at least 2 weeks. When these logs are reviewed, particular attention is paid to sleep efficiency, timing of sleep, sleepiness/fatigue ratings, and weekend versus weekday schedule. Usually behavioral treatment of sleepy patients involves a few phases after the initial sleep logs are reviewed. The first phase of management involves looking at the consistency of the sleep schedule over time. It is known that a variable sleep/wake schedule can cause a misalignment of homeostatic and circadian features of sleep, resulting in increased daytime sleepiness. This theory is informed by the 2-process model of sleep regulation.[37] Therefore, if significant variation in sleep timing is seen on the patients' sleep dairies, this should be addressed. Regularization of the sleep schedule alone without sleep extension has been shown to improve daytime sleepiness.[51] Unlike with SRT, much of the focus on the sleep schedule of sleepy patients is on a consistent bedtime. Wake time, in most of these cases, is determined by work schedule on weekdays, and weekends are often spent catching up on sleep. Once the patient has been on a consistent sleep schedule for at least a couple weeks, if sleepiness remains, the next phase of treatment is begun. If the patient is no longer feeling sleepy during the day on the more consistent sleep schedule, no additional treatment is necessary.

Sleeping longer on weekends versus weekdays, despite a consistent bedtime, is a good indication of chronic sleep deprivation during the week. Therefore, if a patient's sleep log indicates longer bouts of sleep on weekends, the best way to address this issue is to increase total sleep time consistently until the patient feels rested. Using SRT as a model, time in bed is increased by 15 minutes every 5 days until daytime alertness improves. If sleep efficacy is decreased without an increase in alertness, patients are advised to reduce time in bed by 10 minutes. In general, the focus is to increase sleep during the nighttime sleep period because those working during the day may find it difficult to find a place or opportunity to nap. Nonetheless, in those able, additional sleep time can also be added in the form of daytime naps. Adding daytime naps is particularly useful for individuals who have a longer-than-normal sleep need. In some cases, behavioral management alone will not sufficiently treat daytime sleepiness and other treatment approaches to improve alertness may be needed.

The ultimate goal of the sleep extension protocol is to extend total sleep time on a consistent basis until patients feel alert during the day.

Care is also taken to ensure that sleep efficiency is not significantly decreased in this process, as we do not want patients to develop insomnia. Through this process of increasing sleep time without decreasing quality of sleep, we hope to understand the individual sleep need of the patient. Once discovered, the patient now knows how much sleep is needed to feel alert and refreshed during the day. Interestingly, often after determining their sleep need, patients will choose a schedule without sufficient sleep, resulting in mild sleepiness, although at least they know the reason for their somnolence and how to relieve it, if desired.

SUMMARY

The effects of sleep duration on mortality and other important health indicators is well established.[20–26] However, less is known about how the sleep need of the individual moderates the importance of overall sleep duration. Nonetheless, in clinical practice patients are sometimes encountered that cannot generate 7 to 8 hours of sleep or report EDS with the recommended amount of habitual sleep. Assuming, like most other biological systems, that sleep need is normally distributed,[32] it is not surprising that many persons' sleep need will fall outside of the optimal range of sleep duration. Given what is known about the risks associated with long and short sleep duration, there is a natural drive to help patients achieve sleep within this ideal range. However, for those with either long or short biological sleep needs, this task is nearly impossible without the use of hypnotic or alerting medication, which have their own set of risks that likely counteract any benefit obtained by optimizing sleep duration.

Instead of focusing on sleep duration, a more reasonable approach is to attempt to discover the persons' individual sleep need. A recent investigation by Kitamura and colleagues[50] outlines a laboratory-based approach for determining sleep need through a fixed sleep extension protocol. Alternatively, in this article, a clinically based approach to determine sleep need is outlined with an emphasis on increasing daytime alertness without significantly decreasing sleep efficiency and/or increasing sleep latency. However, it is important to note that the method described in this article, although found to be effective clinically in my practice in New York City, has never been empirically evaluated. Although given the limited options available for behavioral interventions in patients with EDS, this approach seems to be a safer alternative to a purely pharmacologic approach.

REFERENCES

1. Conroy DA, Novick DM, Swanson LM. Behavioral management of hypersomnia. Sleep Med Clin 2012;7(2):325–31.
2. American Academy of Sleep Medicine. International classification of sleep disorders. 3rd edition. Darien (IL): American Academy of Sleep Medicine; 2014.
3. Carskadon MA, Dement WC, Mitler MM, et al. Guidelines for the multiple sleep latency test (MSLT): a standard measure of sleepiness. Sleep 1986;9(4):519–24.
4. Mitler MM, Gujavarty KS, Browman CP. Maintenance of wakefulness test: a polysomnographic technique for evaluation treatment efficacy in patients with excessive somnolence. Electroencephalogr Clin Neurophysiol 1982;53(6):658–61.
5. Johns MW. A new method for measuring daytime sleepiness: the Epworth sleepiness scale. Sleep 1991;14(6):540–5.
6. Hoddes E, Dement W, Zarcone V. The development and use of the Stanford sleepiness scale (SSS). Psychophysiology 1972;9:150.
7. Akerstedt T, Gillberg M. Subjective and objective sleepiness in the active individual. Int J Neurosci 1990;52(1–2):29–37.
8. Swanson LM, Arnedt JT, Rosekind MR, et al. Sleep disorders and work performance: findings from the 2008 National Sleep Foundation sleep in America poll. J Sleep Res 2011;20(3):487–94.
9. Ohayon MM. From wakefulness to excessive sleepiness: what we know and still need to know. Sleep Med Rev 2008;12(2):129–41.
10. Banks S, Dinges DF. Behavioral and physiological consequences of sleep restriction. J Clin Sleep Med 2007;3(5):519–28.
11. Cohen DA, Wang W, Wyatt JK, et al. Uncovering residual effects of chronic sleep loss on human performance. Sci Transl Med 2010;2(14):14ra13.
12. Goel N, Rao H, Durmer JS, et al. Neurocognitive consequences of sleep deprivation. Semin Neurol 2009;29(4):320–39.
13. Leproult R, Colecchia EF, Berardi AM, et al. Individual differences in subjective and objective alertness during sleep deprivation are stable and unrelated. Am J Physiol Regul Integr Comp Physiol 2003; 284(2):R280–90.
14. Horne JA, Reyner LA. Driver sleepiness. J Sleep Res 1995;4(S2):23–9.
15. Horne JA, Reyner LA. Sleep related vehicle accidents. BMJ 1995;310(6979):565–7.
16. Ozer C, Etcibasi S, Ozturk L. Daytime sleepiness and sleep habits as risk factors of traffic accidents in a group of Turkish public transport drivers. Int J Clin Exp Med 2014;7(1):268–73.
17. Melamed S, Oksenberg A. Excessive daytime sleepiness and risk of occupational injuries in non-shift daytime workers. Sleep 2002;25(3):315–22.
18. Van Dongen HP, Maislin G, Mullington JM, et al. The cumulative cost of additional wakefulness: dose-response effects on neurobehavioral functions and sleep physiology from chronic sleep restriction and total sleep deprivation. Sleep 2003;26(2):117–26.
19. Liu Y, Wheaton AG, Chapman DP, et al. Prevalence of healthy sleep duration among adults–United States, 2014. MMWR Morb Mortal Wkly Rep 2016; 65(6):137–41.
20. Cappuccio FP, D'Elia L, Strazzullo P, et al. Sleep duration and all-cause mortality: a systematic review and meta-analysis of prospective studies. Sleep 2010;33(5):585–92.
21. Gallicchio L, Kalesan B. Sleep duration and mortality: a systematic review and meta-analysis. J Sleep Res 2009;18(2):148–58.
22. Ayas NT, White DP, Manson JE, et al. A prospective study of sleep duration and coronary heart disease in women. Arch Intern Med 2003;163(2):205–9.
23. Shankar A, Koh WP, Yuan JM, et al. Sleep duration and coronary heart disease mortality among Chinese adults in Singapore: a population-based cohort study. Am J Epidemiol 2008;168(12):1367–73.
24. Nakajima H, Kaneita Y, Yokoyama E, et al. Association between sleep duration and hemoglobin A1c level. Sleep Med 2008;9(7):745–52.
25. Zizi F, Pandey A, Murrray-Bachmann R, et al. Race/ethnicity, sleep duration, and diabetes mellitus: analysis of the National Health interview survey. Am J Med 2012;125(2):162–7.
26. Kachi Y, Ohwaki K, Yano E. Association of sleep duration with untreated diabetes in Japanese men. Sleep Med 2012;13(3):307–9.
27. Grandner MA, Chakravorty S, Perlis ML, et al. Habitual sleep duration associated with self-reported and objectively determined cardiometabolic risk factors. Sleep Med 2014;15(1):42–50.
28. Altman NG, Izci-Balserak B, Schopfer E, et al. Sleep duration versus sleep insufficiency as predictors of cardiometabolic health outcomes. Sleep Med 2012;13(10):1261–70.
29. Carskadon MA, Dement WC. Cumulative effects of sleep restriction on daytime sleepiness. Psychophysiology 1981;18(2):107–13.
30. Dinges DF, Pack F, Williams K, et al. Cumulative sleepiness, mood disturbance, and psychomotor vigilance performance decrements during a week of sleep restricted to 4-5 hours per night. Sleep 1997;20(4):267–77.
31. Belenky G, Wesensten NJ, Thorne DR, et al. Patterns of performance degradation and restoration during sleep restriction and subsequent recovery: a sleep dose-response study. J Sleep Res 2003; 12(1):1–12.
32. Ursin R, Bjorvatn B, Holsten F. Sleep duration, subjective sleep need, and sleep habits of 40- to 45-

year-olds in the Hordaland health study. Sleep 2005; 28(10):1260–9.

33. Richardson GS, Drake CL, Roehrs TA, et al. Habitual sleep time predicts accuracy of self-reported alertness. Sleep 2002;25:A145.

34. Webb WB, Agnew HW. The effects on subsequent sleep of an acute restriction of sleep length. Psychophysiology 1975;12(4):367–70.

35. Dijk DJ, Beersma DG, Daan S. EEG power density during nap sleep: reflection of an hourglass measuring the duration of prior wakefulness. J Biol Rhythms 1987;2(3):207–19.

36. Nakazawa Y, Kotorii M, Ohsima M, et al. Study on the partial differential REM deprivation (PDRD). Folia Psychiatr Neurol Jpn 1977;31(1):1–7.

37. Borbely AA. A two process model of sleep regulation. Hum Neurobiol 1982;1(3):195–204.

38. Arnal PJ, Sauvet F, Leger D, et al. Benefits of sleep extension on sustained attention and sleep pressure before and during total sleep deprivation and recovery. Sleep 2015;38(12):1935–43.

39. Roehrs T, Timms V, Zwyghuizen-Doorenbos A, et al. Sleep extension in sleepy and alert normals. Sleep 1989;12(5):449–57.

40. Wehr TA, Moul DE, Barbato G, et al. Conservation of photoperiod-responsive mechanisms in humans. Am J Physiol 1993;265(4 Pt 2):R846–57.

41. Taub JM, Globus GG, Phoebus E, et al. Extended sleep and performance. Nature 1971;233(5315): 142–3.

42. Rupp TL, Wesensten NJ, Bliese PD, et al. Banking sleep: realization of benefits during subsequent sleep restriction and recovery. Sleep 2009;32(3): 311–21.

43. Axelsson J, Vyazovskiy VV. Banking sleep and biological sleep need. Sleep 2015;38(12):1843–5.

44. Marin Agudelo HA, Jimenez Correa U, Carlos Sierra J, et al. Cognitive behavioral treatment for narcolepsy: can it complement pharmacotherapy? Sleep Sci 2014;7(1):30–42.

45. Helmus T, Rosenthal L, Bishop C, et al. The alerting effects of short and long naps in narcoleptic, sleep deprived, and alert individuals. Sleep 1997;20(4): 251–7.

46. Rogers AE, Aldrich MS, Lin X. A comparison of three different sleep schedules for reducing daytime sleepiness in narcolepsy. Sleep 2001;24(4):385–91.

47. Spielman AJ, Caruso LS, Glovinsky PB. A behavioral perspective on insomnia treatment. Psychiatr Clin North Am 1987;10(4):541–53.

48. Ebben MR, Spielman AJ. Non-pharmacological treatments for insomnia. J Behav Med 2009;32(3): 244–54.

49. Morin CM, Culbert JP, Schwartz SM. Nonpharmacological interventions for insomnia - a meta-analysis of treatment efficacy. Am J Psychiatry 1994;151(8): 1172–80.

50. Kitamura S, Katayose Y, Nakazaki K, et al. Estimating individual optimal sleep duration and potential sleep debt. Sci Rep 2016;6:35812.

51. Manber R, Bootzin RR, Acebo C, et al. The effects of regularizing sleep-wake schedules on daytime sleepiness. Sleep 1996;19(5):432–41.

Treatment of Obstructive Sleep Apnea
Choosing the Best Positive Airway Pressure Device

Neil Freedman, MD

KEYWORDS

- CPAP • Bilevel PAP (BPAP) • AutoPAP (APAP) • AutoBPAP • Expiratory pressure relief
- Humidification • Adherence

KEY POINTS

- Continuous positive airway pressure (CPAP), autotitrating positive airway pressure (APAP), and bilevel positive airway pressure (BPAP) are all reasonable therapies that can be used for patients with uncomplicated obstructive sleep apnea (OSA) across the spectrum of disease severity.
- All of these therapies can be expected to reduce or resolve sleep-disordered breathing and improve symptoms of daytime sleepiness, with the best outcomes being observed in patients with moderate to severe OSA.
- Unattended APAP, either as chronic treatment or as a method to determine a fixed CPAP setting, should be considered first-line therapy for patients with uncomplicated OSA.
- BPAP should be considered for patients who are nonadherent to CPAP or APAP therapy because of pressure intolerance.
- Other factors that should be considered when choosing a PAP device for a given patient include cost, access to online data management software and patient portals, additional technologies such as heated humidification and expiratory pressure relief, and ease of portability for patients who travel frequently.

INTRODUCTION

Treatment with positive airway pressure (PAP) remains the primary therapy for most patients with obstructive sleep apnea (OSA), especially those with moderate to severe OSA. This article focuses on how to determine which type of PAP device may be best for treating a given patient or patient population with OSA. Initially, the author reviews the various forms of PAP therapy for the treatment of OSA, including continuous positive airway pressure (CPAP), autotitrating positive airway pressure (APAP), and bilevel positive airway pressure (BPAP) therapies, focusing on their mechanisms

of action and indications for use in clinical practice. The remainder of the article focuses on how to determine the best PAP device for a given patient or patient population, evaluating factors such as expected outcomes, ease of use and cost of therapy, application of additional technologies, online data management, patient portals and application-based interfaces and compatibility with other manufacturers interfaces and supplies. This review focuses on types of PAP delivery systems and associated technologies and does not make recommendations based on a specific manufacturer because it is not clear from the

This article originally appeared in December 2017 issue of *Sleep Medicine Clinics* (Volume 12, Issue 4).
Disclosure Statement: The author has nothing to disclose.
Pulmonary, Critical Care, Allergy and Immunology, Department of Medicine, North Shore University Health System, 2650 Ridge Avenue, Evanston, IL 60201, USA
E-mail address: Neilfreedman@comcast.net

Sleep Med Clin 15 (2020) 205–218
https://doi.org/10.1016/j.jsmc.2020.02.007

literature that any one manufacturer's devices are consistently superior. Finally, this article only briefly covers interventions that may improve adherence to therapy and various mask interfaces, because these topics will be covered in depth within their own dedicated articles within this issue.

TYPES OF POSITIVE AIRWAY PRESSURE DEVICES

Once the clinician has determined that PAP therapy is the best choice for a given patient with OSA, they initially need to decide which type of PAP technology to use, because there are several modes in which PAP therapy can be delivered. These modes include CPAP, APAP, BPAP, and Auto-BPAP.

Continuous Positive Airway Pressure

CPAP therapy was initially described as a treatment of OSA by Sullivan and colleagues[1] in 1981. Since its initial description, CPAP has become the predominant therapy for the treatment of patients with OSA, because it has been demonstrated to resolve sleep-disordered breathing events and improve several clinical outcomes.[2,3] CPAP delivers a single pressure to the posterior pharynx throughout the night and acts as a pneumatic splint that maintains the patency of the upper airway in a dose-dependent fashion. The best pressure for CPAP treatment is typically determined during an in-laboratory attended sleep study, although a fixed CPAP pressure may also be determined using a short unattended trial of APAP therapy. Treatment with CPAP is typically indicated for patients with moderate to severe OSA (Apnea Hypopnea Index [AHI] ≥15 events per hour) with or without associated symptoms or comorbid diseases, and for patients with mild OSA (AHI ≥5 to ≤14 events per hour) with associated symptoms or comorbid diseases (**Box 1**).

Autotitrating Positive Airway Pressure

APAP (also known as auto-, automated, auto-adjusting, or automatic) incorporates the ability of the PAP device to detect and respond to changes in upper airway flow or resistance in real time.[4] Currently available APAP devices use proprietary algorithms to noninvasively detect and respond to variations in patterns of upper airway inspiratory flow or resistance. Most APAP machines monitor a combination of changes in inspiratory flow patterns, including inspiratory flow limitation, snoring (indirectly measured via mask pressure vibration), reductions of airflow

---

Box 1
Typical indications for positive airway pressure therapies for obstructive sleep apnea

- CPAP
  - ○ Moderate to severe OSA (≥15 events per hour of sleep) with or without associated symptoms or comorbid diseases
  - ○ Mild OSA (≥5 to ≤14 events per hour of sleep) *with* symptoms or associated comorbid diseases:
    - Symptoms:
      - Excessive daytime sleepiness, impaired cognition, mood disorders or insomnia
    - Comorbid diseases:
      - Hypertension, ischemic heart disease, or history of stroke
- APAP
  - ○ Moderate to severe uncomplicated OSA
  - ○ APAP should *not* be used in patients with complicated OSA
    - Complicated OSA is defined as OSA associated with comorbid medical conditions that could potentially affect their respiratory patterns during sleep, including (1) CHF; (2) Lung diseases such as COPD; and (3) Patients expected to have nocturnal arterial oxyhemoglobin desaturation because of conditions other than OSA (eg, obesity hypoventilation syndrome and other hypoventilation syndromes).
  - ○ May be used in an unattended setting for as the exclusive initial and ongoing therapy
  - ○ May also be used as initial therapy to determine a fixed CPAP setting
- Bilevel PAP
  - ○ May be used for the entire spectrum of OSA severity, although is typically considered for patients who have failed CPAP therapy or have pressure intolerance to other initial PAP therapies
- Auto-bilevel PAP
  - ○ Role in OSA therapy and indications not clear

(hypopnea), and absence of flow (apneas), using a pneumotachograph, nasal pressure monitors, or alterations in compressor speed. Another less commonly used technology uses forced oscillation technique (FOT), which is an alternative process that detects changes in patterns of upper airway resistance or impedance.[5–7] Because the FOT method measures changes in upper airway resistance that are independent of patient activity and ventilatory effort, this technology tends to be superior to the flow-based technology at differentiating central apneas from obstructive apneas or mask leak.

Once upper airway flow or impedance changes have been detected, the APAP devices use proprietary algorithms to automatically increase the pressure until the flow or resistance has been normalized. Once a therapeutic pressure has been achieved, the APAP devices typically reduce pressure until flow limitation or increases in airway resistance resume. Most devices have a therapeutic pressure range between 4 cm H_2O and 20 cm H_2O, providing the clinician with the ability to adjust the upper and lower pressure limits based on the clinical conditions and the patient's response to therapy. APAP should be differentiated from BPAP or auto-BPAP (discussed later) in which a separate inspiratory positive airway pressure (IPAP) and expiratory positive airway pressure (EPAP) are set with changes in pressure occurring across each respiratory cycle.

Currently available APAP machines have several potential limitations. Most flow/pressure-based APAP devices are somewhat limited in their ability to distinguish between central and obstructive apneas as well as large mask leaks.[8–11] These flow patterns are "interpreted" by these types of devices as an absence of flow, which, in the cases of central apneas and leaks, may erroneously lead to increases in pressure and worsening of the central events or leaks. Newer APAP algorithms appear to be better at differentiating obstructive from central events as well as compensating for large mask leaks. Also the ability of the APAP devices to respond to sustained hypoventilation in the absence of upper airway obstruction is unclear, because most APAP studies have excluded patients at high risk for hypoventilation, including those patients with obesity hypoventilation syndrome or chronic respiratory diseases.[7,12–21] Given these potential limitations in technology as well as the exclusion of patients with many comorbid diseases from the randomized trials comparing APAP to in-laboratory titrated CPAP therapy, APAP devices are typically recommended for patients with uncomplicated moderate to severe OSA.[13,14,22,23] APAP devices can also be used for patients with mild OSA, although there are less data to support the use of APAP in this patient population.[19] APAP devices typically should *not* be used in patients with comorbid medical conditions that could potentially affect their respiratory patterns (complicated OSA) during sleep, including the following: (1) Congestive heart failure (CHF); (2) Lung diseases such as chronic obstructive pulmonary disease (COPD); and (3) patients expected to have nocturnal arterial oxyhemoglobin desaturation due to conditions other than OSA (eg, obesity hypoventilation syndrome and other hypoventilation syndromes). Patients who do not snore (either due to palatal surgery or naturally) should not be titrated with an APAP device that relies on vibration or sound in the device's algorithm.[13,14,22] Finally, APAP devices are not recommended for split-night titrations given the lack of data to support such a practice (see **Box 1**).

Bilevel Positive Airway Pressure

BPAP therapy's potential benefits in treating patients with OSA were first described in 1990.[24] As opposed to CPAP, which delivers a fixed pressure throughout the respiratory cycle, BPAP therapy allows the independent adjustment of the EPAP and the IPAP. In its initial description, BPAP therapy demonstrated that obstructive events could be eliminated at a lower EPAP compared with conventional CPAP pressures.[24] For patients with uncomplicated OSA, BPAP is typically used in the spontaneous mode (ie, without a back up rate) with an IPAP and EPAP pressure difference of ≥ 4 cm H_2O. To determine the optimal IPAP and EPAP settings, BPAP therapy is typically titrated during an attended in-laboratory sleep study. BPAP may be used for patients with OSA across the spectrum of disease severity, although it is typically recommended as a treatment option for patients with pressure complaints that make it difficult to tolerate CPAP therapy (see **Box 1**). Although intuitively one would predict that BPAP would increase adherence by reducing expiratory pressure–related discomfort and side effects, there are in fact no objective outcomes studies that show that BPAP therapy improves adherence when compared with CPAP therapy for patients with uncomplicated OSA.[25–27] Overall, there have been few studies that objectively evaluate BPAP therapy for the treatment of OSA or compared this mode of PAP therapy to other types of PAP devices for uncomplicated OSA. In addition, there are no short-term or long-term studies evaluating the effects of BPAP on any cardiovascular outcomes in patients with uncomplicated OSA.

Auto-Bilevel Positive Airway Pressure

Auto-BPAP therapy has also been developed, which, using proprietary algorithms, automatically adjusts both the EPAP and the IPAP in response to sleep-disordered breathing events. Limited data indicate that, compared with CPAP, auto-BPAP therapy results in similar compliance and other important outcomes in patients who have had poor initial experiences with CPAP therapy.[28,29] There is currently no peer-reviewed literature evaluating outcomes with auto-BPAP therapy for OSA in PAP-naive patients. Thus, unlike other modes of PAP therapy, there are no specific indications for auto-BPAP use, and no recommendations can be made for auto-BPAP therapy for treating patients with OSA.

CHOOSING THE BEST DEVICE BASED ON EXPECTED OUTCOMES

When determining the best PAP device for a given patient with OSA, the clinician should have a reasonable understanding of which outcomes are most important to the patient and which outcomes are most likely to improve based on the patient's symptoms and comorbid medical problems. Although it is the perception of many non–sleep practitioners and the lay public that PAP treatment consistently resolves or improves several important outcomes including sleep architecture, daytime sleepiness, neurocognitive function, mood, quality of life, and cardiovascular disease in all patients with OSA, this is not the case for many patients.

Resolution of Sleep-Disordered Breathing Events

When titrated appropriately, all types of PAP devices resolve most sleep-disordered breathing across the spectrum of disease severity and have been demonstrated to be superior to placebo, conservative management, and positional therapy with regard to this outcome.[25,26] Randomized controlled trials have also shown CPAP therapy to be superior to placebo at increasing the percent and total time in stages N3 (non–rapid eye movement sleep stage 3) and rapid eye movement (REM) sleep. CPAP's effects on other sleep parameters, including stages N1 and N2 sleep (non–rapid eye movement sleep stages 1 and 2, respectively), total sleep time, and the arousal index, have been inconsistent across studies.[25,26] Compared with standard fixed CPAP therapy, APAP devices as a group are almost always associated with a reduction in mean pressure across a night of therapy in the range of 2 cm H_2O to 2.5 cm H_2O, although peak pressures through the night tend to be higher than fixed CPAP therapy. Despite these differences between CPAP and APAP, there are no clinically significant differences between CPAP and APAP with regards to

important outcomes, such as improvements in daytime sleepiness or adherence to therapy.

Improvement in Daytime Sleepiness

All of the described PAP therapies typically result in significant improvements in subjective symptoms of daytime sleepiness in OSA patients who suffer from this complaint, with the best outcomes being observed in those who suffer from moderate to severe OSA (AHI >15 events per hour).[7,12,15,16,18,19,21,30–51] The minimal and optimal amounts of nocturnal use necessary to improve symptoms of daytime sleepiness are not well defined and appear to be specific to the given individual. Even partial nocturnal use (as little as 2 hours per night) has been associated with significant improvements in daytime symptoms in some patients.[52,53] In general, greater adherence to any of the described PAP therapies on a nightly basis has been associated with greater improvements in symptoms of daytime sleepiness. The data regarding the effects of PAP on more objective measures of daytime sleepiness are more inconsistent across the spectrum of disease severity with results being similar between the different modes of therapy.[21,25,30]

Improvement in Neurocognitive Function, Mood, and Quality of Life

Numerous studies have assessed the effects of sleep-disordered breathing on neurocognitive functioning, mood, and quality of life.[26,37,54–65] Most randomized controlled studies demonstrate inconsistent improvements in several neurobehavioral performance parameters across the spectrum of disease severity.[25,37,39,54–56,66,67] The data regarding the therapeutic effects of PAP treatment on mood and quality of life are also variable and inconsistent, with many randomized trials demonstrating no clear benefits of CPAP therapy compared with placebo or conservative treatments in these parameters.[25,68] Although it is beyond the scope of this article, there are several potential explanations for the inconsistent improvements in neurocognitive function, mood, and quality of life demonstrated with CPAP therapy.[69]

Despite the inconsistent data regarding improvements in neurocognitive function with PAP use, several observational studies support a significant reduction in the incidence of motor vehicle accidents in symptomatic patients with OSA following the initiation of CPAP therapy.[70,71] Although the actual time course to improved driving performance in real-life situations is not clear, driving simulator performance can improve in as little as 2 to 7 nights of therapy. Similar to other aspects of neurobehavioral performance that may be adversely affected by OSA, many patients with OSA may continue to demonstrate impaired driving simulator performance despite several months of high adherence to CPAP therapy.[72] Unfortunately, there is no specific threshold of CPAP use or duration of treatment that can accurately predict a given individual's fitness to safely drive a vehicle. Because the severity of OSA alone is not a reliable predictor of motor vehicle accident risk, the clinician must take into account several factors including improvements in subjective symptoms and adherence with therapy before determining a driver's ability to safely operate a motor vehicle. Although it is likely that all types of PAP therapies for OSA result in a reduction of motor vehicle accidents, all of the literature on this topic is specific to CPAP therapy.

Reductions in Hypertension and Cardiovascular Disease

Although untreated OSA has been associated with an increased risk for hypertension and other cardiovascular diseases in certain populations, the literature and outcomes data supporting the beneficial effects of CPAP on cardiovascular outcomes have been inconsistent.[25,26,73–75] Several randomized clinical trials and meta-analyses have assessed the effects of CPAP on blood pressure.[76–79] Overall, CPAP treatment appears to attenuate the adverse effects of untreated OSA on daytime and nocturnal systolic and diastolic blood pressure, and 24-hour mean blood pressure. These data demonstrate that, compared with placebo, sham CPAP, or supportive therapy alone, CPAP treatment is associated with small (−1.8 to −3.0 mm Hg), but statistically significant, improvements in diurnal mean arterial systolic and diastolic blood pressures. In patients with resistant hypertension and OSA, CPAP tends to improve nighttime blood pressure, although the impact of CPAP on daytime blood pressure has been more unpredictable.[80,81] In general, improvements in blood pressure with CPAP therapy have been associated with greater severity of baseline OSA (higher AHI), the presence of subjective daytime sleepiness, younger age, uncontrolled hypertension at baseline, and greater adherence with CPAP use on a nightly basis.

The most convincing long-term data regarding the potential beneficial effects of CPAP therapy on cardiovascular outcomes comes are based on prospective observational data in a large group of male OSA patients with the spectrum of OSA severity and associated daytime sleepiness.[82]

Results from this study demonstrated that CPAP treatment (>4 hours per night) in patients with severe OSA (AHI ≥30 events per hour) reduced the incidence of adverse cardiovascular outcomes and improved survival, demonstrating outcomes similar to normal controls. Similar improvements in outcomes with CPAP therapy were not observed in OSA patients with mild to moderate obstructive sleep apnea. Aside from these observational data, there are little data that demonstrate that CPAP therapy as typically used reduces mortality or cardiovascular morbidity and no data that demonstrates that CPAP improves cardiovascular outcomes in patients without associated daytime sleepiness.[75,83]

The role of CPAP therapy in resolving or reducing the occurrence or reoccurrence of cardiac arrhythmias is also uncertain. Several observational studies have demonstrated an association between OSA and atrial fibrillation as well as a higher risk of recurrence of atrial fibrillation after electrical cardioversion or catheter ablation therapy. These studies also have shown an association between increased adherence with CPAP therapy and a lower recurrence rate of atrial fibrillation after these procedures.[84–87] Because all of the current data regarding CPAP therapy and atrial fibrillation are based on observational studies, the role of CPAP as an adjunct treatment to improve atrial arrhythmia control remains uncertain. Although there may be an increased risk of ventricular arrhythmias (tachycardia and fibrillation) in some patients with untreated OSA, there are limited data evaluating the effect of PAP therapy for reducing the incidence and prevalence of these events.[88] Thus, the role of PAP therapy for reducing ventricular arrhythmias in patients with OSA is not clear. As is the case with most of the cardiovascular outcomes literature, the data evaluating the effects of PAP therapy on arrhythmia reduction is specific to CPAP therapy because there are no trials looking at the effects of APAP or BPAP on these outcomes.

Given the inconclusive nature of CPAP therapy on cardiovascular outcomes in general, CPAP therapy should be considered adjunctive therapy to lower blood pressure in hypertensive patients with OSA and daytime symptoms.[26] Several authorities and professional societies have recommended that further supporting data are required to better determine the role of CPAP therapy on improving cardiovascular outcomes before making recommendations for its use in various populations.[73,74] Finally, it should be noted that all of the cardiovascular outcomes data are specific to CPAP therapy. There are no short-term or long-term randomized controlled or prospective observational studies specifically focusing on the impact of APAP, BPAP, or auto-BPAP therapies on any cardiovascular outcomes.

POSITIVE AIRWAY PRESSURE USE AND OUTCOMES IN SPECIFIC PATIENT POPULATIONS

Most of the outcomes literature related to PAP therapy has focused predominantly on patients with moderate to severe OSA with associated daytime sleepiness and the absence of comorbid medical problems. As all clinicians know, patients with OSA may present with different phenotypes often exhibiting many different symptoms, with or without the presence of one or more comorbid medical conditions.

Positive Airway Pressure Therapy in Patients with Mild Obstructive Sleep Apnea

As noted previously, most of the literature assessing the effects of PAP on various outcomes has predominantly evaluated OSA patients with moderate to severe disease. Although approximately 28% of patients with mild disease (AHI = 5–14 events per hour) complain of subjective daytime sleepiness,[89] it remains unclear whether treating this group of patients with PAP therapy consistently improves their daytime symptoms. Results from the CPAP Apnea Trial North American Program Trial demonstrated that CPAP therapy significantly improved daytime symptoms as measured by the Functional Outcomes of Sleep Questionnaire (FOSQ) when compared with sham CPAP therapy in symptomatic patients (Mean Epworth Sleepiness Scale score of 15) with mild to moderate OSA over an 8-week period of follow-up.[90] Alternatively, The Apnea Positive Pressure Long Term Efficacy Study showed no significant improvements in objective alertness or subjective sleepiness in patients with mild OSA after 2 and 6 months of CPAP therapy.[39] Limited data evaluating APAP therapy in this patient population have demonstrated some improvement in subjective daytime sleepiness, with results similar to CPAP.[19] Thus, the role of CPAP therapy for this indication in patients with mild disease remains unclear based on the current data.

It appears reasonable to initiate CPAP or APAP therapy in patients with mild OSA and associated daytime sleepiness, but the decision to continue chronic therapy in this patient group should be based on a positive response to therapy. For patients with mild disease without daytime symptoms, it is not clear that treating these patients is beneficial or should be recommended based on the current data.

The Role of Continuous Positive Airway Pressure Therapy in Patients with Rapid Eye Movement–Predominant Obstructive Sleep Apnea

The prevalence of REM sleep–related or REM-predominant OSA is unclear, in part because of the absence of a standard definition for this entity. This OSA variant tends to be more common in women, although it may affect adult patients of both genders across the age spectrum.[91,92] The association of this OSA variant with daytime or nighttime symptoms is not clear, but it appears that a subgroup of patients is affected. Recent studies have also indicated that REM OSA is independently associated with prevalent and incident hypertension, nondipping of nocturnal blood pressure, increased insulin resistance, and impairment of human spatial navigational memory.[93,94]

For those patients who demonstrate this phenotype of OSA and complain of daytime symptoms or nighttime sleep disturbance, it is unclear if treatment with CPAP consistently improves daytime or nighttime symptoms. Limited observational data of CPAP therapy in symptomatic patients with such REM-predominant OSA have demonstrated significant improvements in daytime sleepiness, fatigue, and functional outcomes as assessed by the FOSQ. These improvements with CPAP therapy were similar to patients with OSA not limited to REM sleep.[91] However, it should be noted, there are no randomized controlled data assessing any outcomes in this subgroup of patients, including cardiovascular disease outcomes, and there are no data evaluating the effects of other types of PAP devices in this patient population.

Obstructive Sleep Apnea and Comorbid Diseases: Congestive Heart Failure, Chronic Obstructive Pulmonary Disease, Diabetes Mellitus

CHF is a common disease with an estimated prevalence of concomitant OSA of approximately 33%. Several randomized controlled studies have assessed the effects of CPAP therapy on left ventricular ejection fraction (LVEF) in CHF patients with and without systolic dysfunction.[95] Overall, CPAP therapy has shown statistically significant improvements in LVEF in patients with OSA and concomitant systolic dysfunction, with an average improvement in LVEF across studies of approximately 5%. In patients with diastolic CHF and concomitant OSA, CPAP therapy has not been associated with significant improvements in LVEF (1%). However, it is uncertain if the improvements in LVEF in patients with OSA and concomitant CHF translate into improvements in other important outcomes, such as reductions in hospitalizations and mortality. Most of the studies evaluating this patient population have been limited by small sample sizes and relatively short durations of follow-up (typically 12 weeks or less). These findings are limited to CPAP therapy, because APAP is contraindicated in this group of patients, and there are no data evaluating the use of BPAP in this patient population.

The "overlap syndrome" refers to the coexistence of OSA with COPD. Prospective observational data have shown that CPAP therapy in OSA patients with concomitant COPD has been associated with significant reductions in both acute exacerbations of COPD requiring hospitalizations and death with outcomes similar to COPD patients without OSA.[96] Increased adherence to CPAP therapy has been independently associated with reduced mortality in this patient population, whereas decreased CPAP adherence and increased age have been independently associated with increased mortality.[97] Observational data would suggest that adherence to CPAP therapy for as little as 2 hours per night may be associated with a reduction in mortality in this group of patients. Given the current observational data, it is reasonable to recommend CPAP therapy in patients with the overlap syndrome, although given the absence of randomized controlled data in this patient population, the role of CPAP therapy to reduce exacerbations or improve mortality remains undefined. As is the case with CHF, these recommendations are limited to CPAP therapy because APAP therapy is contraindicated in this patient population.

The role of CPAP therapy for improving important outcomes-associated diabetes mellitus (short-term and long-term glucose control) in patients with coexistent OSA is also unclear, because most of the trials evaluating the use of CPAP in this patient population have yielded inconsistent results.[98,99] The role of CPAP as an adjunct therapy to improve weight loss is also uncertain, and adequate treatment of OSA has not been observed to result in enhanced weight loss in most studies.[100] In fact, some studies have demonstrated a small, but significant weight gain with CPAP use, with greater weight gain being associated with increased adherence to CPAP therapy.[101] The role of APAP or BPAP on weight reduction is not clear.

Positive Airway Pressure in Patients Without Daytime Sleepiness

As noted previously, the presence of subjective daytime sleepiness has generally been associated with a more robust improvement in blood pressure with CPAP therapy. Several large randomized controlled trials have assessed the effect of CPAP therapy in patients with moderate to severe OSA without daytime sleepiness (Epworth Sleepiness Scale score $\leq$10) on various cardiovascular outcomes. In general, CPAP therapy has not been associated with significant improvements in blood pressure, reductions in incident hypertension, or cardiovascular events (nonfatal myocardial infarction or stroke, transient ischemic attack, CHF, or cardiovascular death) or reductions in cardiovascular morbidity or mortality in patients with previously diagnosed cardiovascular diseases.[75,83,102] Thus, the benefit of treating patients with moderate to severe OSA who do not have symptoms of daytime sleepiness with any type of PAP device is unclear and remains to be better defined.

POSITIVE AIRWAY PRESSURE OUTCOMES SUMMARY

CPAP, APAP, and BPAP treatment consistently improve or resolve OSA events across the spectrum of OSA severity and improve symptoms of daytime sleepiness predominantly in patients with moderate to severe OSA. Improvements in other outcomes are less consistent. Treatment with CPAP has been associated with small reductions in blood pressure, with greater reductions being observed in patients with associated daytime sleepiness, poorly controlled or resistant hypertension, and in those who are more adherent to therapy. The role of any type of PAP therapy for reducing long-term cardiovascular risk or mortality in OSA is uncertain based on the current data. Finally, the role of any type of PAP device for patients without daytime symptoms across the spectrum of OSA severity is undefined.

ADDITIONAL QUESTIONS TO ADDRESS WHEN CHOOSING A POSITIVE AIRWAY PRESSURE DEVICE

In addition to the type of PAP delivery system and expected outcomes, there are several other issues to consider when choosing a PAP device for a given patient or patient population. Other factors that should be considered include the following: effect of PAP technology on adherence to therapy, additional options to improve comfort, cost of therapy, including the need for an in-laboratory attended polysomnography (PSG), availability of online data management tools and patient interfaces, portability, and compatibility with other manufacturers masks and supplies.

Effect of Positive Airway Pressure Technology on Adherence to Therapy

Adherence to PAP is typically defined as use ≥4 hours per night on ≥70% of the nights.[103] Using this definition, subjective adherence ranges between 65% and 90%, whereas objective measures of PAP adherence have demonstrated use in the range of 40% to 83% with the average nightly use ranging between 4 and 5 hours per night.[104] Unfortunately, there are few if any consistent predictors of short-term or long-term adherence to PAP therapy.

Given the differences in PAP delivery systems and advancements in technology over time, do any of the PAP platforms consistently result in improved adherence to PAP therapy? The short answer to the question is no. Head-to-head studies comparing APAP and BPAP to CPAP have consistently demonstrated similar adherence and improvements in daytime symptoms among the 3 types of PAP delivery modes.[21,105] Thus, the choice of device for a given individual should be based on other factors, such as symptoms, expected outcomes, cost, underlying comorbid medical problems, and other factors that are outlined in this article.

Additional Options That May Improve Positive Airway Pressure Comfort and Adherence: Heated Humidification and Expiratory Pressure Relief

Given the flow rates generated by most PAP devices, many patients complain of nasal congestion or upper airway dryness without the addition of humidification. Fortunately, most modern-day PAP devices have the capacity to add a humidification system. Although one would assume that heated humidification consistently results in improved adherence with PAP therapy, the data evaluating the effects of heated humidification on adherence to CPAP therapy remain controversial. Although there are some studies that demonstrate that the addition of heated humidification can improve adherence to CPAP therapy, there are several studies demonstrating no improvement in adherence with this intervention.[26,106–110] Patients who tend to benefit the most from the addition of heated humidification are those with symptoms of nasal congestion or rhinitis. Limited data evaluating the role of heated tubing to heated humidification have not consistently shown improvements in adherence in patients with and without nasopharyngeal complaints.[110] With this information in mind, heated humidification should be considered for most patients when initially prescribing a PAP device, given the potential benefits with little

associated risks. Patients can determine the level of heated humidification depending on their symptoms and changes in their local environment.

Another common complaint for many patients with OSA who are treated with PAP therapy is the uncomfortable feeling of exhaling against positive pressure. This consequence has been proposed as one conceivable barrier to the long-term acceptance of PAP therapy. Several PAP manufacturers have developed expiratory pressure relief (EPR) systems in an attempt to remedy this potential problem. EPR device technologies allow pressure relief during exhalation with the goal to make PAP therapy more comfortable. EPR technologies briefly reduce the PAP pressure, between 1 cm H_2O and 3 cm H_2O, during exhalation before returning the pressure to its set PAP setting before the initiation of inspiration. Certain EPR technologies monitor the patient's airflow during exhalation and reduce the expiratory pressure in response to the airflow and patient effort. The amount of pressure relief varies on a breath-by-breath basis, depending on the actual patient's airflow, and is also dictated by the patient's preference setting on the device.

Although several PAP manufacturers have developed EPR technologies for the market place, only the Philips Respironics (Respironics, Inc, Murrysville, PA, USA) technology (CFLEX) has been extensively evaluated in the peer-reviewed literature.[111–113] Several randomized controlled trials have evaluated the role of CFLEX technology compared with standard CPAP therapy in patients with uncomplicated, predominantly moderate to severe OSA. Overall, the use of such CFLEX technology at fixed pressure relief settings between 1 cm H_2O and 3 cm H_2O has not been associated with improved adherence.[113] In addition, improvements in other commonly measured outcomes (subjective sleepiness, objective alertness, vigilance, or residual OSA) were similar to, but not better than, standard CPAP therapy. Similar results have been observed with a similar technology for APAP devices (AFLEX).[20,114] Despite the lack of convincing outcomes data, most of the current PAP devices have EPR or Flex technologies included as standard additions. Thus, patients should be instructed on how to adjust these technologies and may self-titrate the amount of pressure relief based on comfort.

Cost of Therapy Including the Need for an In-Laboratory Attended Polysomnography

Current general trends in US health care economics have payers focusing on reducing costs, while improving quality and value. Although the

Affordable Care Act has increased the availability of health insurance, one unfortunate result has been increased out-of-pocket costs for patients in the forms of higher deductibles and increased annual health insurance costs. Finally, as payment systems move away from fee-for-service payment models, management approaches that reduce costs while maintaining or improving quality will become more important. Thus, the clinician needs to be aware of the patient's and health system's (where appropriate) costs, when prescribing PAP therapy for the patient with OSA.

In general, CPAP devices are less expensive than APAP and BPAP devices for patients and payers. The main advantage of APAP therapy is that it can be prescribed and used in an unattended setting obviating the need and costs associated with an in-laboratory titration study. As noted previously, APAP used in the proper patient population results in similar outcomes as CPAP. Thus, when reductions in cost are considered in the management strategy for a given patient or population, APAP should be considered the initial PAP treatment either as a primary therapy or as a method to determine a fixed CPAP setting for ongoing treatment in patients with moderate to severe uncomplicated OSA.[115,116]

Availability of Online Data Management Tools and Patient Interfaces

Unfortunately, as noted previously, most studies have not been able to identify factors that consistently predict short- or long-term adherence with CPAP therapy.[32,103,117–120] Because adherence with PAP therapy tends to be suboptimal, subjective adherence tends to overestimate objective PAP use, and there are no consistent early predictors of PAP adherence, professional societies currently recommend and many payer policies require, objective adherence data assessment to document adherence with therapy and potentially identify problems that can be addressed.[3] Although most randomized controlled trials have used objective adherence data to monitor outcomes related to PAP therapy, the overall impact of assessing objective compliance data either in person or remotely via a telemedicine approach for all patients on PAP therapy is uncertain.[121,122]

Most of the PAP manufacturers have developed sophisticated online software programs for monitoring several parameters of PAP therapy, including nightly adherence, efficacy of therapy (residual AHI), and problems with mask fit (primarily amount of air leak). Many of the same manufacturers have also developed computer-based patient portals or phone-based applications that allow the patient to monitor their progress with therapy. Despite the absence of outcomes data demonstrating consistent benefits of using this information to improve adherence to therapy, the author's group finds this information invaluable for managing patients on a day-to-day basis. Factors to consider when choosing a specific manufacturer's software should include ease of use for the clinician and the patient, compatibility with a given electronic medical record system, and the ability to monitor progress and make adjustments remotely. In reality, most clinicians will need to get comfortable using more than one data-management system given the array of PAP manufacturers currently on the market.

Portability and Compatibility with Other Manufacturers Masks and Supplies

Practical issues to consider when prescribing a PAP device include the patient's occupation and travel plans as it relates to the ease of portability. Most modern-day PAP devices, regardless of delivery technology, are approximately similar in size and weight when considering the PAP device and supplies. More recently, several companies market much smaller CPAP and APAP devices that may be more suitable for patients who frequently travel for their job or leisure. It is not clear if these smaller portable PAP devices will be durable enough for everyday use. Finally, because it is common for patients to use masks made by different manufacturers, it is good to know that most current PAP devices are compatible with masks made by several manufacturers.

SUMMARY

CPAP, APAP, and BPAP all are reasonable therapies that can be used for patients with uncomplicated OSA across the spectrum of disease severity. All of these therapies can be expected to reduce or resolve sleep-disordered breathing and improve symptoms of daytime sleepiness, with the best outcomes to be expected in patients with moderate to severe OSA. Unattended APAP, either as chronic treatment or as a method to determine a fixed CPAP setting, should be considered first-line therapy for patients with uncomplicated OSA when the cost of treatment is a priority for the patient. BPAP should be considered for patients who are nonadherent to CPAP or APAP therapy because of pressure intolerance. When choosing the best PAP device for a given patient, the clinician should consider several other factors including cost of the device and management strategy, access to online data management software and patient portals, additional technologies such as heated humidification and EPR, ease of portability for patients who travel frequently, and compatibility with other manufacturers' supplies.

REFERENCES

1. Sullivan C, Issa F, Berthon-Jones M, et al. Reversal of obstructive sleep apnea by continuous positive airway pressure applied through the nares. Lancet 1981;1:862–5.
2. Loube DI, Gay PC, Strohl KP, et al. Indications for positive airway pressure treatment of adult obstructive sleep apnea patients: a consensus statement. Chest 1999;115(3):863–6.
3. Epstein LJ, Kristo D, Strollo PJ Jr, et al. Clinical guideline for the evaluation, management and long-term care of obstructive sleep apnea in adults. J Clin Sleep Med 2009;5(3):263–76.
4. Roux F, Hilbert J. Continuous positive airway pressure: new generations. In: Lee-Chiong T, Mohsenin V, editors. Clinics in chest medicine, vol. 24. Philadelphia: W.B. Saunders Company; 2003. p. 315–42.
5. Randerath WJ, Parys K, Feldmeyer F, et al. Self-adjusting nasal continuous positive airway pressure therapy based on measurement of impedance: a comparison of two different maximum pressure levels. Chest 1999;116(4):991–9.
6. Randerath WJ, Schraeder O, Galetke W, et al. Autoadjusting CPAP therapy based on impedance efficacy, compliance and acceptance. Am J Respir Crit Care Med 2001;163(3):652–7.
7. Randerath W, Galetke W, David M, et al. Prospective randomized comparison of impedance-controlled auto-continuous positive airway pressure (APAP(FOT)) with constant CPAP. Sleep Med 2001;2:115–24.
8. Abdenbi F, Chambille B, Escourrou P. Bench testing of auto-adjusting positive airway pressure devices. Eur Respir J 2004;24(4):649–58.
9. Rigau J, Montserrat JM, Wohrle H, et al. Bench model to simulate upper airway obstruction for analyzing automatic continuous positive airway pressure devices. Chest 2006;130(2):350–61.
10. Farre R, Montserrat JM, Rigau J, et al. Response of automatic continuous positive airway pressure devices to different sleep breathing patterns: a bench study. Am J Respir Crit Care Med 2002;166(4):469–73.
11. Lofaso F, Desmarais G, Leroux K, et al. Bench evaluation of flow limitation detection by automated continuous positive airway pressure devices. Chest 2006;130(2):343–9.
12. Hudgel DW, Fung C. A long-term randomized cross-over comparison of auto-titrating and standard nasal continuous positive airway pressure. Sleep 2000;23:1–4.
13. Berry R, Parish J, Hartse K. The use of auto-titrating continuous positive airway pressure for the treatment of adult obstructive sleep apnea. Sleep 2002;25(2):148–73.
14. Littner M, Hirshkowitz M, Davilla D, et al. Practice parameters for the use of autotitrating continuous positive airway pressure devices for titrating pressures and treating adult patients with obstructive sleep apnea syndrome. Sleep 2002; 25(2):143–7.
15. Ayas N, Patel S, Malhotra A, et al. Auto-titrating vs standard continuous positive airway pressure for the treatment of obstructive sleep apnea: results of a meta-analysis. Sleep 2004;27(2):249–53.
16. Hukins CA. Comparative study of autotitrating and fixed-pressure CPAP in the home: a randomized, single-blind crossover trial. Sleep 2004;27(8): 1512–7.
17. Stammnitz A, Jerrentrup A, Penzel T, et al. Automatic CPAP titration with different self-setting devices in patients with obstructive sleep apnoea. Eur Respir J 2004;24(2):273–8.
18. Nussbaumer Y, Bloch KE, Genser T, et al. Equivalence of autoadjusted and constant continuous positive airway pressure in home treatment of sleep apnea. Chest 2006;129(3):638–43.
19. Nolan G, Doherty L, McNicholas W. Auto-adjusting versus fixed positive pressure therapy in mild to moderate obstructive sleep apnoea. Sleep 2007; 30(2):189–94.
20. Kushida CA, Berry RB, Blau A, et al. Positive airway pressure initiation: a randomized controlled trial to assess the impact of therapy mode and titration process on efficacy, adherence, and outcomes. Sleep 2011;34(8):1083–92.
21. Ip S, D'Ambrosio C, Patel K, et al. Auto-titrating versus fixed continuous positive airway pressure for the treatment of obstructive sleep apnea: a systematic review with meta-analyses. Syst Rev 2012; 1:20.
22. Morgenthaler T, Aurora R, Brown T, et al. Practice parameters for the use of autotitrating continuous positive airway pressure devices for titrating pressures and treating adult patients with obstructive sleep apnea syndrome: an update for 2007. An American Academy of Sleep Medicine report. Sleep 2008;31:141–7.
23. Freedman N. Positive airway pressure therapy for obstructive sleep apnea. In: Kyrger MRT, Dement W, editors. The principles and practice of sleep medicine. 6th edition. New York: Elsevier Saunders Press; 2016. p. 1125–37.
24. Sanders M, Kern N. Obstructive sleep apnea treated by independently adjusted inspiratory and expiratory positive airway pressures via nasal

mask. Physiologic and clinical implications. Chest 1990;98(2):317–24.

25. Gay P, Weaver T, Loube D, et al. Evaluation of positive airway pressure treatment for sleep related breathing disorders in adults. Sleep 2006;29(3): 381–401.

26. Kushida C, Littner M, Hirshkowitz M, et al. Practice parameters for the use of continuous and bilevel positive airway pressure devices to treat adult patients with sleep-related breathing disorders. Sleep 2006;29(3):375–80.

27. Reeves-Hoche M, Hudgel D, Meck R, et al. Continuous versus bilevel positive airway pressure for obstructive sleep apnea. Am J Respir Crit Care Med 1995;151(2):443–9.

28. Carlucci A, Ceriana P, Mancini M, et al. Efficacy of bilevel-auto treatment in patients with obstructive sleep apnea not responsive to or intolerant of continuous positive airway pressure ventilation. J Clin Sleep Med 2015;11(9):981–5.

29. Powell ED, Gay PC, Ojile JM, et al. A pilot study assessing adherence to auto-bilevel following a poor initial encounter with CPAP. J Clin Sleep Med 2012; 8(1):43–7.

30. Patel SR, White DP, Malhotra A, et al. Continuous positive airway pressure therapy for treating sleepiness in a diverse population with obstructive sleep apnea: results of a meta-analysis. Arch Intern Med 2003;163(5):565–71.

31. Engleman HM, Douglas NJ. Sleep 4: sleepiness, cognitive function, and quality of life in obstructive sleep apnoea/hypopnoea syndrome. Thorax 2004; 59(7):618–22.

32. Douglas NJ, Engleman HM. CPAP therapy: outcomes and patient use. Thorax 1998;53(90003): 47S–8S.

33. Douglas NJ. Systematic review of the efficacy of nasal CPAP. Thorax 1998;53(5):414–5.

34. Jenkinson C, Davies R, Mullins R, et al. Comparison of therapeutic and subtherapeutic nasal continuous airway pressure for obstructive sleep apnea: a randomized prospective parallel trial. Lancet 1999;353:2100–5.

35. Ballester E, Badia JR, Hernandez L, et al. Evidence of the effectiveness of continuous positive airway pressure in the treatment of sleep apnea/hypopnea syndrome. Am J Respir Crit Care Med 1999;159(2): 495–501.

36. Masa JF, Jimenez A, Duran J, et al. Alternative methods of titrating continuous positive airway pressure: a large multicenter study. Am J Respir Crit Care Med 2004;170(11):1218–24.

37. Engleman H, Martin S, Kingshott R, et al. Randomised, placebo-controlled trial of daytime function after continuous positive airway pressure therapy for the sleep apnoea/hypopnoea syndrome. Thorax 1998;53:341–5.

38. Berry R, Hill G, Thompson L, et al. Portable monitoring and autotitration versus polysomnography for the diagnosis and treatment of sleep apnea. Sleep 2008;31(10):1423–31.

39. Kushida CA, Nichols DA, Holmes TH, et al. Effects of continuous positive airway pressure on neurocognitive function in obstructive sleep apnea patients: the apnea positive pressure long-term efficacy study (APPLES). Sleep 2012;35(12): 1593–602.

40. Schwartz SW, Rosas J, Iannacone MR, et al. Correlates of a prescription for bilevel positive airway pressure for treatment of obstructive sleep apnea among veterans. J Clin Sleep Med 2013;9(4): 327–35.

41. Massie CA, McArdle N, Hart RW, et al. Comparison between automatic and fixed positive airway pressure therapy in the home. Am J Respir Crit Care Med 2003;167(1):20–3.

42. Teschler H, Wessendorf T, Farhat A, et al. Two months auto-adjusting versus conventional nCPAP for obstructive sleep apnoea syndrome. Eur Respir J 2000;15(6):990–5.

43. Meurice J, Marc I, Series F. Efficacy of auto-CPAP in the treatment of obstructive sleep apnea/hypopnea syndrome. Am J Respir Crit Care Med 1996;153(2):794–8.

44. Series F, Marc I. Efficacy of automatic continuous positive airway pressure therapy that uses an estimated required pressure in the treatment of the obstructive sleep apnea syndrome. Ann Intern Med 1997;127(8 Pt 1):588–95.

45. d'Ortho M-P, Grillier-Lanoir V, Levy P, et al. Constant vs automatic continuous positive airway pressure therapy: home evaluation. Chest 2000;118(4): 1010–7.

46. Konermann M, Sanner B, Vyleta M, et al. Use of conventional and self-adjusting nasal continuous positive airway pressure for treatment of severe obstructive sleep apnea syndrome: a comparative study. Chest 1998;113(3):714–8.

47. Planes C, d'Ortho M, Foucher A, et al. Efficacy and cost of home-initiated auto-nCPAP versus conventional nCPAP. Sleep 2003;26(2):156–60.

48. Noseda A, Kempenaers C, Kerkhofs M, et al. Constant vs auto-continuous positive airway pressure in patients with sleep apnea hypopnea syndrome and a high variability in pressure requirement. Chest 2004;126(1):31–7.

49. Pevernagie DA, Proot PM, Hertegonne KB, et al. Efficacy of flow- vs impedance-guided autoadjustable continuous positive airway pressure: a randomized cross-over trial. Chest 2004;126(1): 25–30.

50. Smith I, Lasserson T. Pressure modification for improving usage of systematic age of continuous positive airway pressure machines in adults with

obstructive sleep apnoea. Cochrane Database Rev 2009;(4):CD003531.

51. Vennelle M, White S, Riha RL, et al. Randomized controlled trial of variable-pressure versus fixed-pressure continuous positive airway pressure (CPAP) treatment for patients with obstructive sleep apnea/hypopnea syndrome (OSAHS). Sleep 2010;33(2):267–71.

52. Weaver T, Maislin G, Dinges D, et al. Relationship between hours of CPAP use and achieving normal levels of sleepiness and daily functioning. Sleep 2007;30:711–9.

53. Antic NA, Catcheside P, Buchan C, et al. The effect of CPAP in normalizing daytime sleepiness, quality of life, and neurocognitive function in patients with moderate to severe OSA. Sleep 2011; 34(1):111–9.

54. Engleman H, Martin S, Deary I, et al. The effect of continuous positive airway pressure therapy on daytime function in the sleep apnoea/hyponoea syndrome. Lancet 1994;343:572–5.

55. Engleman H, Martin S, Deary I, et al. Effect of CPAP therapy on daytime function in patients with mild sleep apnoea/hypopnoea syndrome. Thorax 1997;52:114–9.

56. Engleman H, Kingshott R, Wraith P, et al. Randomized placebo-controlled crossover trial of CPAP for mild sleep apnea/hypopnea syndrome. Am J Respir Crit Care Med 1999;159:461–7.

57. Engleman H, Kingshott R, Martin S, et al. Cognitive function in the sleep apnea/hyponea syndrome (SAHS). Sleep 2000;23(Suppl 4):S102–8.

58. Greenberg G, Watson R, Deptula D. Neuropsychological dysfunction in sleep apnea. Sleep 1987;10: 254–62.

59. Redline S, Strauss M, Adams N, et al. Neuropsychological function in mild sleep-disordered breathing. Sleep 1997;20:160–7.

60. Kim H, Young T, Matthews C, et al. Sleep-disordered breathing and neuropsychological deficits: a population based study. Am J Respir Crit Care Med 1997;156:1813–9.

61. Bedard M, Montplaisir J, Richer F, et al. Obstructive sleep apnea syndrome: pathogenesis of neuropsychological deficits. J Clin Exp Neuropsychol 1991; 13:950–64.

62. Borak J, Cieslicki J, Koziej M, et al. Effects of CPAP treatment on psychological status in patients with severe obstructive sleep apnea. J Sleep Res 1996;5(2):123–7.

63. Naegele B, Thouvard V, Pepin J, et al. Deficits of cognitive executive functions in patients with sleep apnea syndrome. Sleep 1995;18:43–52.

64. Ramos Platon M, Espinar Sierra J. Changes in psychopathological symptoms in sleep apnea patients after treatment with nasal continuous airway pressure. Int J Neurosci 1992;62(3–4):173–95.

65. Munoz A, Mayoralas L, Barbe F, et al. Long-term effects of CPAP on daytime functioning in patients with sleep apnoea syndrome. Eur Respir J 2000; 15(4):676–81.

66. Zimmerman ME, Arnedt JT, Stanchina M, et al. Normalization of memory performance and positive airway pressure adherence in memory-impaired patients with obstructive sleep apnea. Chest 2006;130(6):1772–8.

67. Olaithe M, Bucks RS. Executive dysfunction in OSA before and after treatment: a meta-analysis. Sleep 2013;36(9):1297–305.

68. Batool-Anwar S, Goodwin JL, Kushida CA, et al. Impact of continuous positive airway pressure (CPAP) on quality of life in patients with obstructive sleep apnea (OSA). J Sleep Res 2016;25(6):731–8.

69. Quan SF, Chan CS, Dement WC, et al. The association between obstructive sleep apnea and neurocognitive performance–the Apnea Positive Pressure Long-term Efficacy Study (APPLES). Sleep 2011;34(3):303–314b.

70. Tregear S, Reston J, Schoelles K, et al. Continuous positive airway pressure reduces risk of motor vehicle crash among drivers with obstructive sleep apnea: systematic review and meta-analysis. Sleep 2010;33(10):1373–80.

71. Ayas N, Skomro R, Blackman A, et al. Obstructive sleep apnea and driving: a Canadian Thoracic Society and Canadian Sleep Society position paper. Can Respir J 2014;21(2):114–23.

72. Vakulin A, Baulk SD, Catcheside PG, et al. Driving simulator performance remains impaired in patients with severe OSA after CPAP treatment. J Clin Sleep Med 2011;7(3):246–53.

73. Gottlieb DJ, Craig SE, Lorenzi-Filho G, et al. Sleep apnea cardiovascular clinical trials-current status and steps forward: the International collaboration of sleep apnea cardiovascular trialists. Sleep 2013;36(7):975–80.

74. Parati G, Lombardi C, Hedner J, et al. Position paper on the management of patients with obstructive sleep apnea and hypertension: joint recommendations by the European Society of Hypertension, by the European Respiratory Society and by the members of European COST (COoperation in Scientific and Technological research) ACTION B26 on obstructive sleep apnea. J Hypertens 2012;30(4): 633–46.

75. McEvoy RD, Antic NA, Heeley E, et al. CPAP for prevention of cardiovascular events in obstructive sleep apnea. N Engl J Med 2016;375(10):919–31.

76. Fava C, Dorigoni S, Dalle Vedove F, et al. Effect of CPAP on blood pressure in patients with OSA/hypopnea a systematic review and meta-analysis. Chest 2014;145(4):762–71.

77. Montesi SB, Edwards BA, Malhotra A, et al. The effect of continuous positive airway pressure

treatment on blood pressure: a systematic review and meta-analysis of randomized controlled trials. J Clin Sleep Med 2012;8(5):587–96.

78. Haentjens P, Van Meerhaeghe A, Moscariello A, et al. The impact of continuous positive airway pressure on blood pressure in patients with obstructive sleep apnea syndrome: evidence from a meta-analysis of placebo-controlled randomized trials. Arch Intern Med 2007;167(8):757–64.

79. Bakker JP, Edwards BA, Gautam SP, et al. Blood pressure improvement with continuous positive airway pressure is independent of obstructive sleep apnea severity. J Clin Sleep Med 2014;10(4):365–9.

80. Pepin JL, Tamisier R, Barone-Rochette G, et al. Comparison of continuous positive airway pressure and valsartan in hypertensive patients with sleep apnea. Am J Respir Crit Care Med 2010;182(7):954–60.

81. Muxfeldt ES, Margallo V, Costa LM, et al. Effects of continuous positive airway pressure treatment on clinic and ambulatory blood pressures in patients with obstructive sleep apnea and resistant hypertension: a randomized controlled trial. Hypertension 2015;65(4):736–42.

82. Marin J, Carrizo S, Vincente E, et al. Long-term cardiovascular outcomes in men with obstructive sleep apnoea-hypopnea with or without treatment with continuous positive airway pressure: an observational study. Lancet 2005;365(9464):1046–53.

83. Barbe F, Duran-Cantolla J, Sanchez-de-la-Torre M, et al. Effect of continuous positive airway pressure on the incidence of hypertension and cardiovascular events in nonsleepy patients with obstructive sleep apnea: a randomized controlled trial. JAMA 2012;307(20):2161–8.

84. Holmqvist F, Guan N, Zhu Z, et al. Impact of obstructive sleep apnea and continuous positive airway pressure therapy on outcomes in patients with atrial fibrillation-results from the outcomes registry for better informed treatment of atrial fibrillation (ORBIT-AF). Am Heart J 2015;169(5):647–54. e2.

85. Fein AS, Shvilkin A, Shah D, et al. Treatment of obstructive sleep apnea reduces the risk of atrial fibrillation recurrence after catheter ablation. J Am Coll Cardiol 2013;62(4):300–5.

86. Kanagala R, Murali NS, Friedman PA, et al. Obstructive sleep apnea and the recurrence of atrial fibrillation. Circulation 2003;107(20):2589–94.

87. Ng CY, Liu T, Shehata M, et al. Meta-analysis of obstructive sleep apnea as predictor of atrial fibrillation recurrence after catheter ablation. Am J Cardiol 2011;108(1):47–51.

88. Raghuram A, Clay R, Kumbam A, et al. A systematic review of the association between obstructive sleep apnea and ventricular arrhythmias. J Clin Sleep Med 2014;10(10):1155–60.

89. Kapur VK, Baldwin CM, Resnick HE, et al. Sleepiness in patients with moderate to severe sleep-disordered breathing. Sleep 2005;28(4):472–7.

90. Weaver TE, Mancini C, Maislin G, et al. Continuous positive airway pressure treatment of sleepy patients with milder obstructive sleep apnea: results of the CPAP Apnea Trial North American Program (CATNAP) randomized clinical trial. Am J Respir Crit Care Med 2012;186(7):677–83.

91. Su CS, Liu KT, Panjapornpon K, et al. Functional outcomes in patients with REM-related obstructive sleep apnea treated with positive airway pressure therapy. J Clin Sleep Med 2012;8(3):243–7.

92. Khan A, Harrison SL, Kezirian EJ, et al. Obstructive sleep apnea during rapid eye movement sleep, daytime sleepiness, and quality of life in older men in Osteoporotic Fractures in Men (MrOS) Sleep Study. J Clin Sleep Med 2013;9(3):191–8.

93. Mokhlesi B, Hagen EW, Finn LA, et al. Obstructive sleep apnoea during REM sleep and incident non-dipping of nocturnal blood pressure: a longitudinal analysis of the Wisconsin sleep cohort. Thorax 2015;70(11):1062–9.

94. Alzoubaidi M, Mokhlesi B. Obstructive sleep apnea during rapid eye movement sleep: clinical relevance and therapeutic implications. Curr Opin Pulm Med 2016;22(6):545–54.

95. Sun H, Shi J, Li M, et al. Impact of continuous positive airway pressure treatment on left ventricular ejection fraction in patients with obstructive sleep apnea: a meta-analysis of randomized controlled trials. PLoS One 2013;8(5):e62298.

96. Marin JM, Soriano JB, Carrizo SJ, et al. Outcomes in patients with chronic obstructive pulmonary disease and obstructive sleep apnea: the overlap syndrome. Am J Respir Crit Care Med 2010;182(3):325–31.

97. Stanchina ML, Welicky LM, Donat W, et al. Impact of CPAP use and age on mortality in patients with combined COPD and obstructive sleep apnea: the overlap syndrome. J Clin Sleep Med 2013;9(8):767–72.

98. Iftikhar IH, Hoyos CM, Phillips CL, et al. Meta-analyses of the association of sleep apnea with insulin resistance, and the effects of CPAP on HOMA-IR, adiponectin, and visceral adipose fat. J Clin Sleep Med 2015;11(4):475–85.

99. Pamidi S, Wroblewski K, Stepien M, et al. Eight hours of nightly CPAP treatment of obstructive sleep apnea improves glucose metabolism in prediabetes: a randomized controlled trial. Am J Respir Crit Care Med 2015;192(1):96–105.

100. Redenius R, Murphy C, O'Neill E, et al. Does CPAP lead to change in BMI? J Clin Sleep Med 2008;4(3):205–9.

101. Quan SF, Budhiraja R, Clarke DP, et al. Impact of treatment with continuous positive airway pressure (CPAP) on weight in obstructive sleep apnea. J Clin Sleep Med 2013;9(10):989–93.

102. Martinez-Garcia MA, Capote F, Campos-Rodriguez F, et al. Effect of CPAP on blood pressure in patients with obstructive sleep apnea and resistant hypertension: the HIPARCO randomized clinical trial. JAMA 2013;310(22):2407–15.

103. Kribbs N, Pack A, Kline L, et al. Objective measurement of patterns of nasal CPAP use by patients with obstructive sleep apnea. Am Rev Respir Dis 1993; 147:887–95.

104. Parthasarathy S, Subramanian S, Quan SF. A multicenter prospective comparative effectiveness study of the effect of physician certification and center accreditation on patient-centered outcomes in obstructive sleep apnea. J Clin Sleep Med 2014;10(3):243–9.

105. Mansukhani MP, Kolla BP, Olson EJ, et al. Bilevel positive airway pressure for obstructive sleep apnea. Expert Rev Med Devices 2014;11(3):283–94.

106. Massie CA, Hart RW, Peralez K, et al. Effects of humidification on nasal symptoms and compliance in sleep apnea patients using continuous positive airway pressure. Chest 1999;116(2):403–8.

107. Martins de Araujo MT, Vieira SB, Vasquez EC, et al. Heated humidification or face mask to prevent upper airway dryness during continuous positive airway pressure therapy. Chest 2000;117(1):142–7.

108. Rakotonanahary D, Pelletier-Fleury N, Gagnadoux F, et al. Predictive factors for the need for additional humidification during nasal continuous positive airway pressure therapy. Chest 2001;119(2):460–5.

109. Ryan S, Doherty LS, Nolan GM, et al. Effects of heated humidification and topical steroids on compliance, nasal symptoms, and quality of life in patients with obstructive sleep apnea syndrome using nasal continuous positive airway pressure. J Clin Sleep Med 2009;5(5):422–7.

110. Nilius G, Franke KJ, Domanski U, et al. Effect of APAP and heated humidification with a heated breathing tube on adherence, quality of life, and nasopharyngeal complaints. Sleep Breath 2016; 20(1):43–9.

111. Aloia MS, Stanchina M, Arnedt JT, et al. Treatment adherence and outcomes in flexible vs standard continuous positive airway pressure therapy. Chest 2005;127(6):2085–93.

112. Nilius G, Happel A, Domanski U, et al. Pressure-relief continuous positive airway pressure vs constant continuous positive airway pressure: a comparison of efficacy and compliance. Chest 2006;130(4): 1018–24.

113. Bakker JP, Marshall NS. Flexible pressure delivery modification of continuous positive airway pressure for obstructive sleep apnea does not improve compliance with therapy: systematic review and meta-analysis. Chest 2011;139(6):1322–30.

114. Dungan GC 2nd, Marshall NS, Hoyos CM, et al. A randomized crossover trial of the effect of a novel method of pressure control (SensAwake) in automatic continuous positive airway pressure therapy to treat sleep disordered breathing. J Clin Sleep Med 2011;7(3):261–7.

115. Parish JM, Freedman NS, Manaker S. Evolution in reimbursement for sleep studies and sleep centers. Chest 2015;147(3):600–6.

116. Freedman N. COUNTERPOINT: does laboratory polysomnography yield better outcomes than home sleep testing? No. Chest 2015;148(2): 308–10.

117. Reeves-Hoche M, Meck R, Zwillich C. Nasal CPAP: an objective evaluation of patient compliance. Am J Respir Crit Care Med 1994;149(1):149–54.

118. Rauscher H, Formanek D, Popp W, et al. Self-reported vs measured compliance with nasal CPAP for obstructive sleep apnea. Chest 1993;103(6): 1675–80.

119. Engleman H, Martin S, Douglas N. Compliance with CPAP therapy in patients with the sleep apnoea/hypopnoea syndrome. Thorax 1994;49(3): 263–6.

120. Rosen CL, Auckley D, Benca R, et al. A multisite randomized trial of portable sleep studies and positive airway pressure autotitration versus laboratory-based polysomnography for the diagnosis and treatment of obstructive sleep apnea: the HomePAP study. Sleep 2012;35(6):757–67.

121. Sparrow D, Aloia M, Demolles DA, et al. A telemedicine intervention to improve adherence to continuous positive airway pressure: a randomised controlled trial. Thorax 2010;65(12):1061–6.

122. Fox N, Hirsch-Allen AJ, Goodfellow E, et al. The impact of a telemedicine monitoring system on positive airway pressure adherence in patients with obstructive sleep apnea: a randomized controlled trial. Sleep 2012;35(4):477–81.

Treatment of Obstructive Sleep Apnea
Choosing the Best Interface

Marie Nguyen Dibra, MD[a],*, Richard Barnett Berry, MD[b],
Mary H. Wagner, MD[c]

KEYWORDS

- OSA • CPAP interface • Nasal mask • Mask fitting • PAP initiation • PAP compliance • Mask leak

KEY POINTS

- Difficulty with the mask interface is common and no one type of mask is clearly superior. Changing mask type or improving fit to can dramatically improve adherence and satisfaction.
- Trying several mask types and sizes may improve mask seal and comfort; fitting a mask under pressure is suggested (ideally with the patient reclining).
- An oronasal mask may be useful in patients with mouth leak or severe nasal congestion; however, a higher pressure may be needed when switching from a nasal mask to an oronasal mask.
- Hybrid masks may be helpful in patients who could benefit from an oronasal mask but in whom claustrophobia or obtaining a good seal around the upper nose is difficult.
- Proper adjustment, cleaning, and replacement are important for maintaining a good seal. When a mask worked initially but begins to leak over time, the cushion may have deteriorated.

OVERVIEW

There is a range of interface or mask options available for delivering positive pressure therapy in obstructive sleep apnea (OSA). These include masks that fit into the nostrils (nasal pillows) or that cover the nose (nasal mask), are inserted into the mouth, cover both the nose and the mouth (oronasal mask or full face mask), or even the entire face (total face mask or helmet).[1–3] Adherence to continuous positive airway pressure (CPAP) is a crucial aspect of therapy and the benefits of positive airway pressure (PAP) are most evident in patients who comply with treatment and have longer durations of CPAP use.

Nevertheless, an estimated 46% to 83% of patients are nonadherent with CPAP when compliance is defined as usage for 4 or more hours a night.[2] Predictors of adherence to CPAP therapy include the severity of OSA, the degree of daytime sleepiness, the socioeconomic status, the level of patient understanding of the therapy, and the type of mask used.[3]

It can be challenging to find a mask that fits well and is, at the same time, comfortable to wear. Patients receiving nasal CPAP often complain about side effects related to mask fit such as eye irritation owing to air leak into the eyes, skin reactions to the cushion material, pain or abrasion to the bridge of the nose, residual imprints on the face

This article originally appeared in December 2017 issue of *Sleep Medicine Clinics* (Volume 12, Issue 4).

Disclosures: The authors listed above have identified no professional or financial affiliations for themselves or their spouse/partner.

[a] Division of Pulmonary, Critical Care, and Sleep Medicine, Department of Sleep Medicine, UF Health Sleep Center, University of Florida, 4740 Northwest 39th Place, Gainesville, FL 32606, USA; [b] Department of Sleep Medicine, UF Health Sleep Center, University of Florida, 4740 Northwest 39th Place, Gainesville, FL 32606, USA; [c] Department of Sleep Medicine, UF Health Sleep Disorders Center, UF Health Sleep Center, 4740 Northwest 39th Place, Gainesville, FL 32606, USA

* Corresponding author.

E-mail address: Marie.Nguyen@medicine.ufl.edu

in the morning owing to pressure from mask or straps, or pressure sores and noisy air leaks, all of which reduce the tolerability of treatment. A change in mask type or size may be a required to intervene for these problems. Changes in interface may also be needed if the patient develops chronic skin irritation at the point of contact with the mask, if changes in the patient's weight that compromise the mask's fit, or if increases in pressure lead to increased leak issues.[1] For patients who experience symptomatic mouth leak while wearing a nasal mask, the addition of a chin strap or change to an oral nasal interface may be helpful.

MASK TYPE

A nasal mask is usually the first interface tried for PAP titration and treatment (**Fig. 1**). The biggest challenge with a nasal mask is providing a comfortable seal around the nasal bridge. Given the large variability in the shape and size of noses and the associated nasal bridge, it is not surprising that several masks must often be tried before a satisfactory seal can be obtained. Air leak into the eyes is poorly tolerated by patients. For a nasal mask to work well, the patient must be able to breathe nasally with the mouth closed. If more than a mild degree of expiratory venting through the mouth occurs during sleep, this may result in dryness or arouse the patient frequently. Oronasal masks are an alternative interface that can be used for patients with significant nasal congestion and predominant oral breathing or those with a large mouth leak during sleep.[4] However, an oronasal interface must seal over a large area, which can make finding a good fit very difficult in some

patients. In edentulous patients, there is a lack of structural support under the lower face for oronasal masks. In these patients, oronasal masks may compress soft tissues and create an air leak. Several studies have found that oronasal masks generally require a higher treatment pressure than nasal masks and are associated with higher leak or a higher residual apnea–hypopnea index. In an occasional patient, a substantially lower pressure may be effective with a nasal mask compared with a full face mask.[5] It has been hypothesized that use of an oronasal mask may cause the jaw or tongue to move posteriorly, narrowing the upper airway. In addition, some patients may not tolerate an oronasal mask owing to claustrophobia or difficulty obtaining a mask seal. Hybrid masks, which use nasal pillows or a nasal cradle combined with a portion of the mask covering the mouth may be a solution in some patients. Only the lower part of the nose fits down into the cradle, the bottom of which contains an opening hole, allowing air to enter and leave the nares. This type of mask also avoids the need to maintain a seal in the nasal bridge area. For example, the Amara View (Philips Respironics, Murrysville, PA; **Fig. 2**) uses a nasal cradle cushion on top of a portion of the mask that covers the mouth.

Nasal pillows consist of 2 nasal inserts and have emerged as an alternative to nasal masks because they are smaller and have less contact with the face.[3] CPAP applied through nasal pillows and a nasal mask are equally effective in treating mild, moderate, and severe sleep apnea.[6] A variety of nasal pillows are

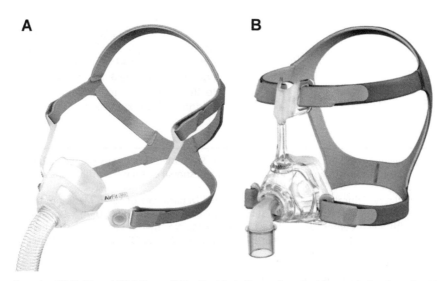

Fig. 1. Nasal masks. (*A*) N-10 and (*B*) Mirage FX by ResMed. (Reproduced with permission from ResMed. ResMed, Air10, Swift, Mirage are trademarks and/or registered trademarks of the ResMed family of companies.)

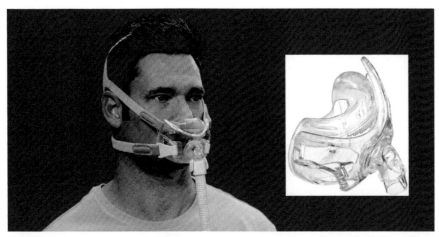

Fig. 2. Amara View. This interface uses a nasal cradle on top of a portion of the mask that covers the mouth. (*Courtesy of* Philips Respironics, Murrysville, PA.)

available; one major issue is finding the correct sized pillow (**Figs. 3** and **4**). Finding a mask with the proper pillow shape may require trying several brands of masks. Some models of nasal pillows are lighter, such as the Airfit P10 (ResMed, San Diego, CA), whereas others more stable, like the Swift LT (ResMed). Using too small a pillow size causes leak unless the mask is overtightened, which may cause nasal pain with prolonged use. In clinical practice, it has been found that, when patients are switched from a nasal mask to nasal pillows, they sometimes complain that the pressure feels much higher. This is due to the fact that the pressure drop across the nasal inlet is eliminated.

Therefore, a slightly lower pressure may be needed when changing to nasal pillows.[7]

Nasal pillows may benefit patients by minimizing side effects such as claustrophobia, pressure sores, and air leak into the eyes.[8] They may also be useful in patients with mustaches or edentulous patients who have no dental support for the upper lip. A study by Zhu and colleagues[8] found that nasal pillows are as efficacious and subjectively as acceptable as nasal masks when treating OSA with high CPAP pressures. Therefore, one should not assume that nasal pillows will not work in patients on higher pressure. Nasal pillows are lighter and their initial acceptance might be higher; however, they can cause more nasal

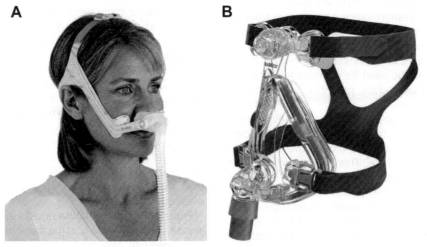

Fig. 3. (*A*) Nasal pillows mask (Swift LT) and (*B*) full face mask (Mirage Quattro) by ResMed. (Reproduced with permission from ResMed. ResMed, Air10, Swift, Mirage are trademarks and/or registered trademarks of the ResMed family of companies.)

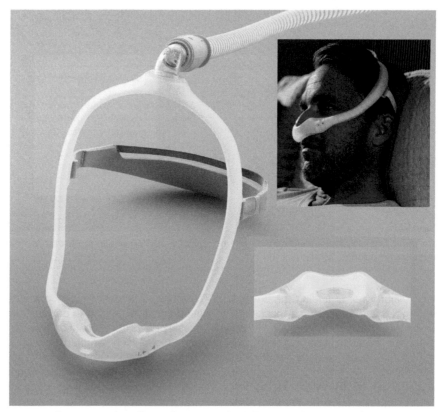

Fig. 4. DreamWear. This is a nasal cradle mask optimized to allow side sleeping. Airflow can enter from either side of the mask. (*Courtesy of* Philips Respironics, Murrysville, PA.)

problems, particularly when a CPAP greater than 12 cm H_2O is used.[3] Ryan and colleagues studied 21 patients with severe OSA using nasal masks and nasal pillows for 4 weeks each. The authors found no differences between the 2 types of CPAP masks in terms of their impact on treatment adherence. However, the participants complained of nasal congestion, nasal dryness, nosebleeds, and headaches more frequently when they used nasal pillows than when they used nasal masks.[3] Use of adequate humidification, proper pillow size (avoiding the need for overtightening), and a saline gel may reduce potential problems with nasal pillows masks.

There are also specialty masks such as the total face mask, which covers the entire face including the eyes. The seal wraps around the outer most perimeter of the face. This moves the pressure off the cheeks and nose and may be an option for patients who have great difficulty obtaining an adequate seal with a nasal or oronasal mask. Oral interfaces (Oracle, Fisher Paykel, Auckland, New Zealand) are an option for patients with severe nasal congestion. However, dryness is a problem and the acceptance of oral interfaces is generally low (**Table 1**).

GENERAL CONSIDERATIONS

Frequently, a trial of several masks is needed to find one that a patient can tolerate. Patients should try different mask types in the sleep center before the start of a split or titration sleep study. Proper sizing and mask adjustment are crucial and should be checked at every clinic visit. It is important to ensure that mask fittings are performed properly because they are often done incorrectly. The mask is initially put on with the patient sitting upright; however, the straps should be adjusted while the patient is reclined because head position can affect mask tension. Some newer PAP devices have a check mask fit feature that gives the patient an estimate of mask fit before starting therapy. The machine attempts to do this by measuring the amount of leak. When trying on a new mask, it is essential to test the mask fit with the patient's treatment pressure to determine if the seal is adequate.

Patients tend to overtighten masks and this may actually impair the ability of the mask to seal properly. Adequate care and regular replacement of masks are paramount to maintain proper mask seal. Proper cleaning of the cushion with a gentle

Table 1
Different types of CPAP masks: advantages/disadvantages

	Advantages/Indications	Disadvantages
Nasal pillows masks	Patients with claustrophobia Intractable air leak into eyes with a nasal mask Difficult obtaining a seal over upper nasal bridge with a nasal mask No upper teeth or mustache makes obtaining a seal with a nasal mask difficult	Sensation of higher pressure in some patients Nasal irritation (saline gel may help) May not be tolerated in patients requiring high pressure
Oronasal masks	Patients with mouth leak or nasal congestion	Large area to obtain a seal (often associated with higher leak) May be challenging in edentulous patients or those with facial creases May worsen claustrophobia May require higher treatment pressure than a nasal mask in some patients
Nasal masks	Smaller area to obtain a seal In some patients, a lower pressure than needed with a full face mask may be effective	May require intervention for mouth leak (chin strap) or nasal congestion (medications and adequate humidification) Air leak into eyes a potential problem

soap and water to remove facial oils may increase the lifespan of the membrane. Wiping the cushion with a damp cloth after each night may also be effective. With sleep onset, facial muscles relax (resulting in mouth opening or "jaw drop") and this slackening may change the ability of an oronasal mask to provide a good seal. In the case of intractable mouth leak owing to jaw drop, it may be necessary to use a larger size mask or wear a chin strap along with using an oronasal mask (under the mask).

INTERVENTIONS FOR SIDE EFFECTS

Air leakage is a significant problem during CPAP therapy. It is experienced by up to 50% of nasal CPAP users and can cause a drop in mask pressure leading to suboptimal treatment, severe dryness, or repeated arousal from noise or eye irritation and these problems may result in poor compliance.[2] Oronasal masks are frequently used because of presumptive excessive mouth leak in some patients while using nasal masks.[9] Unintentional leaks may be caused by mouth opening or a poorly fitting mask. A disturbing leak may stem from air blowing toward the eyes and can also cause a disturbing noise (waking the patient or bed partner). Some leaks may occur only when PAP pressures are high. Some patients experience air leak when sleeping in the lateral position. The pillow under the head may push against the mask. "CPAP pillows" are available that have a recess on the side to prevent pressure against the mask.

Patients who breathe through their mouth either by habit or because of nasal obstruction.[3] In the presence of mouth leak, an early switch from a nasal mask to an oronasal mask is a reasonable decision.[2] In 1 study of obese patients with OSA changing from a nasal to an oronasal mask, there was increased leak and residual apnea–hypopnea index; however, this did not affect the therapeutic pressure requirement.[10] Other studies suggest that a higher treatment pressure is required with oronasal compared with nasal masks.[5,11] A history of mouth breathing is not a clear contraindication to the use of nasal masks. There is evidence that the use of nasal CPAP leads to a change of habit, reducing mouth opening and the number of oral breaths. Some patients breathing through the nose and mouth while awake may switch to a nasal breathing route during sleep.[4] Use of a chin strap may be an effective intervention for mouth leak. In some individuals, intensive medical treatment of nasal congestion may allow a nasal interface to be used in a patient with difficulty breathing through the nose. Adequate humidification may also help to maintain nasal patency during the night. Drying of the nasal mucosa can increase nasal resistance.[12] Despite the potential problems with oronasal masks, many patients adapt well to them and exhibit good adherence and treatment efficacy.[3] Sometimes a mask leak with any interface will respond to a slight lowering of pressure. Also, switching from CPAP to an auto-PAP device may result in a lower mean nightly pressure and reduce leak.[7]

Claustrophobia is an important influential factor in CPAP adherence and an important clinical problem. Anxiety disorders are common among adults with OSA. Evidence suggests that anxiety disorders and the fear of choking may be more prevalent in severe OSA and in those adults with a higher body mass index.[13] Nasal pillow masks are often better tolerated compared with traditional nasal masks by patients with claustrophobia. Mask desensitization may also be an effective approach to reducing or eliminating claustrophobia in OSA treated with CPAP.[13] For patients with intractable mouth leak or mouth dryness who cannot tolerate an oronasal mask, they may prefer using a nasal mask with a chin strap (or a hybrid mask).

Facial pain related to CPAP, which may be described as dental or periodontal pain, is mainly caused by direct pressure of the device on the gums. This can occur in 15% to 20% of CPAP users.[14] In this case, nasal pillows may be better tolerated than nasal or oronasal masks. For skin irritation or a rash that develops from use of a PAP mask, there are CPAP mask liners that provide a soft layer between the face and CPAP mask cushion. The liner can help to prevent leaks and irritation while absorbing facial oils and moisture. Cloth PAP masks are also available and are made from a soft cloth, which can prevent pressure points from developing on the face during use. Gel nasal pads are available that can be placed across the nasal bridge and can help to reduce facial sores, minimize air leak into the eyes, and improve mask comfort.

Nasal congestion is a common symptom among PAP users. To manage nasal stuffiness, the cause should be treated and a mask change should be considered.[1] For dry or irritated nasal passages, which can be caused by the use of nasal pillows, the use of a saline nasal gel is recommended. If nasal congestion worsens over the night on PAP treatment, this is a clue that the patient may benefit from more humidification.

ADJUNCTS TO MASKS

For patients who report entanglement of the CPAP hose during use of their machine, a hose caddy is a device that is used to lift the hose above the user while they are asleep. As mentioned, mask barriers such as CPAP mask liners act as a soft barrier between the silicone mask cushion and face. The liner can be used to prevent leaks and irritation around the cushion seal and protect skin from excessive moisture or residual red marks. To prevent skin irritation owing to the CPAP mask headstraps, there are pads that slide over the lower strap of the CPAP mask headgear. As mentioned, patients who are side sleepers may find it difficult to keep the mask in place when they sleep in the lateral position. CPAP pillows are designed with contoured cutouts to prevent that mask from shifting toward 1 side of the face.

REFERENCES

1. Bachour A, Vitikainen P, Maasilta P. Rates of initial acceptance of PAP masks and outcomes of mask switching. Sleep Breath 2016;20:733–8.
2. Neuzeret PC, Morin L. Impact of different nasal masks on CPAP therapy for obstructive sleep apnea: a randomized comparative trial. Clin Respir J 2016. [Epub ahead of print].
3. Andrade R, Piccin V, Nascimento J, et al. Impact of the type of mask on the effectiveness of and adherence to continuous positive airway pressure treatment for obstructive sleep apnea. J Bras Pneumol 2014;40:658–68.
4. Prosise GL, Berry RB. Oral-nasal continuous positive airway pressure as a treatment for obstructive sleep apnea. Chest 1994;106:180–6.
5. Ng JR, Aiyappan V, Mercer J, et al. Choosing an oronasal mask to deliver continuous positive airway pressure may cause more upper airway obstruction or lead to higher continuous positive airway pressure requirements than a nasal mask in some patients: a case series. J Clin Sleep Med 2016;12(9): 1227–32.
6. Ebben MR, Oyegbile T, Pollak CP. The efficacy of three different mask styles on a PAP titration night. Sleep Med 2012;13:645–9.
7. Berry RB, Wagner MH. Sleep medicine pearls. 3rd edition. Philadelphia: Saunders; 2014.
8. Zhu X, Wimms AJ, Benjafield AV. Assessment of the performance of nasal pillows at high CPAP pressures. J Clin Sleep Med 2013;9:873.
9. Bettinzoli M, Taranto-Montemurro L, Messineo L, et al. Oronasal masks require higher levels of positive airway pressure than nasal masks to treat obstructive sleep apnea. Sleep Breath 2014;18: 845–9.
10. Bakker JP, Neill AM, Campbell AJ. Nasal versus oronasal continuous positive airway pressure masks for obstructive sleep apnea: a pilot investigation of pressure requirement, residual disease, and leak. Sleep Breath 2012;16:709–16.
11. Deshpande S, Joosten S, Turton A, et al. Oronasal masks require a higher pressure than nasal and

nasal pillow masks for the treatment of obstructive sleep apnea. J Clin Sleep Med 2016;12(9): 1263–8.

12. Richard GL, Cistulli PA, Ugar G, et al. Mouth leak with nasal continuous positive airway pressure increases nasal airway resistance. Am J Respir Crit Care Med 1996;154:182–6.

13. Edmonds JC, Yang H, King TS, et al. Claustrophobic tendencies and continuous positive airway pressure therapy non-adherence in adults with obstructive sleep apnea. Heart Lung 2015;44:100–6.

14. Mermod M, Broome M, Hoarau R, et al. Facial pain associated with CPAP use: intra-sinusal third molar. Case Rep Otolaryngol 2014;2014:837252.

Treatment of Obstructive Sleep Apnea
Achieving Adherence to Positive Airway Pressure Treatment and Dealing with Complications

Christopher J. Lettieri, MD[a],*, Scott G. Williams, MD[a], Jacob F. Collen, MD[a], Emerson M. Wickwire, PhD[b,c]

KEYWORDS

- Obstructive sleep apnea • Positive airway pressure • Patient adherence
- Motivational enhancement therapy

KEY POINTS

- Patient education and proactive support throughout the evaluation and treatment processes are the basis for maximal adherence.
- Pharmacologic and behavioral treatment of comorbid conditions, such as sinus congestion and insomnia, should be incorporated early in the treatment course or before initiating PAP.
- Multidisciplinary care teams are instrumental for achieving optimal patient care; members should include sleep medicine physicians, midlevel providers, behavioral specialists, and durable medical equipment support.
- Technical features of PAP platforms, including variable pressure delivery, expiratory pressure reductions, integrated humidification, and more advanced settings can improve patient comfort and enhance treatment effectiveness.
- Leveraging technology and implementing frequent follow-up assessments can help analyze patterns of PAP use and identify patients needing more intensive support or targeted adherence interventions.

INTRODUCTION

Obstructive sleep apnea (OSA) is a common condition that is associated with multiple adverse consequences, including worsened health outcomes, diminished quality of life, and increased health care-related costs (**Box 1**).[1–3] The standard treatment for OSA is positive airway pressure (PAP), which has been in use since the early 1980s.[4,5] When used consistently, PAP therapy has been shown to reduce the negative health impact of many comorbid medical and psychiatric disorders.[6–8] Unfortunately, PAP adherence remains suboptimal.[9] Despite advances in both mask and PAP platform technology, which have incorporated multiple features to improve both comfort

This article originally appeared in December, 2017 issue of *Sleep Medicine Clinics* (Volume 12, Issue 4).

Disclaimer: The views expressed in this review reflect those of the authors, and do not constitute official policy of the United States Army or Department of Defense.

[a] Department of Pulmonary, Critical Care, and Sleep Medicine, Walter Reed National Military Medical Center, 8901 Wisconsin Avenue, Bethesda, MD 20889, USA; [b] Department of Psychiatry, University of Maryland School of Medicine, 100 North Greene Street, 2nd Floor, Baltimore, MD 21201, USA; [c] Sleep Disorders Center, Division of Pulmonary and Critical Care Medicine, Department of Medicine, University of Maryland School of Medicine, 100 North Greene Street, 2nd Floor, Baltimore, MD 21201, USA

* Corresponding author.

E-mail address: christopher.j.lettieri.mil@mail.mil

Sleep Med Clin 15 (2020) 227–240

https://doi.org/10.1016/j.jsmc.2020.02.009

1556-407X/20/Published by Elsevier Inc.

sleep.theclinics.com

Box 1
Complications of positive airway pressure

Mask interface problems

  Skin irritation

  Skin breakdown

  Change in dentitions

  Mask discomfort

Claustrophobia

Vasomotor rhinitis

Transient insomnia

Dry mouth

Aerophagia

Central or complex sleep apnea

---

and the effective delivery of pressure, adherence has not improved substantially.

By any measure, the optimal treatment of OSA requires long-term behavior changes, which include sleep habits, diet and exercise, and adherence with therapeutic interventions. Poor adoption is evident throughout the continuum of care. This is particularly true of PAP. Whether this lack of adherence is unique to PAP, or reflects multiple overlapping confounders and merely highlighted because this therapy includes integrated objective measures of use, remains a source on ongoing debate. Regardless, both acceptance of and adherence to PAP therapy remains problematic. For example, up to 30% of patients fail to initiate therapy after diagnosis.[10] Of those starting therapy, approximately 25% stop within the first year, and fewer than 50% remain adherent in the long term.[11–14] Even among those who use CPAP regularly, average nighttime use is only 3.5 to 5.3 hours.[15–17]

Despite these challenges, several interventions have been shown to improve PAP use and, subsequently, improve patient outcomes. The purpose of this review is to define PAP adherence, identify and discuss current challenges faced by clinicians as they provide PAP therapy to their patients, and provide an overview of the various strategies to increase PAP use, with an emphasis on understanding, recognizing, and overcoming common barriers to care and using high-yield interventions early in the treatment course.

QUANTIFYING ADHERENCE WITH POSITIVE AIRWAY PRESSURE TREATMENT

Currently accepted insurance criteria in the United States contend that "adherent" equates to the use of PAP greater than 4 hours per night for at least 70% of nights.[15,18] Therefore, an individual only has to use PAP 86 hours per month, or 35% of the total recommended sleep time, to be considered adherent. Although many argue that this definition of adherence is grossly insufficient and most likely contributes to the limited ability of PAP to resolve both symptoms and consequences associated with OSA, the fact remains that despite using a low threshold for adherence, most patients do not achieve it. PAP use is commonly measured objectively. Although objective measures are intuitively superior to subjective reports, they do not always reflect the entire history. For PAP, adherence reports reveal the amount of time the PAP device was in use. They do not include time spent awake, nor do they record sleep without PAP. As such, they can both overestimate and underestimate sleep. In addition, these reports do not differentiate between patients who only intermittently use PAP, those who use it every night but only for part of the night, or those who use PAP during every sleep period but are grossly sleep restricted. As a result, commonly reported objective measures represent an upperbound estimate of how long PAP was worn during sleep, which is frequently an inaccurate reflection of both total sleep time and true adherence. All of these possibilities can be attributed to the persistence of symptoms, with significant variability regarding the effectiveness of PAP between each of these three scenarios. In other words, the persistence of symptoms may reflect insufficient sleep, insufficient use of PAP, limitations in the efficacy of PAP, or some combination of each. And, despite their objective nature, PAP use reports do not answer this question. Clinical assessment and results of PAP outcomes research should be interpreted with this limitation in mind.

Regardless of the limitations related to the accuracy of how PAP use is measured, there is sufficient evidence regarding the efficacy of PAP. And, it is clear that increased use leads to greater improvements in outcomes. In short, this therapy is efficacious, but its effectiveness is limited by insufficient use. Multiple studies have reported a dose–response relationship between hours of PAP use and improvements in OSA severity,[19] neurocognitive performance,[20] symptoms, and mortality.[21] Some outcomes have been shown to improve with even limited PAP use, and some seem to have a ceiling effect, where additional use may not lead to further improvements. This circumstance has contributed to the low threshold defining PAP adherence. However, improvements in other outcomes are not observed unless PAP is used for more than 6 or 7 hours per night. For example, a 2007 study by Weaver and colleagues[22] showed that, depending on the outcome, different durations of nightly PAP use were required to show improvement. Subjective alertness improved after 4 hours of use, whereas objective improvements in mean sleep latency required at least 6 hours, and functional outcomes required at least 7 hours of PAP use per night for optimization. Similarly, Antic and colleagues[23] reported a variable dose response for changes in subjective and objective somnolence, as well as improvements in neurobehavioral assessments.

Unfortunately, many studies do not report the dose response to PAP therapy, so it is challenging to define the beneficial impact of "optimal" use. As an example, a recent study considered the effect of PAP therapy on resistant hypertension and found that PAP resulted in a significant decrease in systolic blood pressure (3.08 mm Hg; 95% CI, 1.79–4.37), diastolic blood pressure (2.28 mm Hg; 95% CI, 1.56–3.00), and mean arterial pressure (2.54 mm Hg; 95% CI, 1.73–3.36) within the first year of treatment.[24] This effect size is less than a typical antihypertensive.[25] However, this study did not stratify PAP users by hours of therapy per night, or regular use. Thus, it was impossible to discern the optimal duration of PAP use in this sample. Nonetheless, in a clinical context, we recommend that patients are advised to wear PAP during all sleep periods.

WHAT FACTORS AFFECT ADHERENCE TO POSITIVE AIRWAY PRESSURE TREATMENT?

A number of factors have been identified that influence both acceptance of and adherence to PAP therapy. More easily measured factors relate to demographic, physiologic, and disease-specific variables. Perhaps more important, the influence of a patient's understanding of the underlying disorder and therapeutic strategy, their perceived benefit of treatment, their initial experiences with an intervention, and their overall health behaviors are becoming increasingly recognized as impactful determinants of both therapeutic adherence and outcomes.

Several variables regarding patient demographics, such as age, gender, ethnicity, socioeconomic status, and education level, have been shown to influence PAP adherence, although with variable results.[13,26–32] The impact of disease-specific features, such as OSA severity, degree of symptoms, and presence of medical comorbidities, are similarly inconsistent.[13,26–28,33] Although more well-defined markers of OSA severity have not always been shown to influence adherence, certain physiologic factors, such as

increased nasal resistance and claustrophobia, are clearly associated with increased difficulty in adapting to PAP and represent modifiable risk factors for adherence.[34,35]

Both the perceived benefit of, and subjective response to, therapy represent the most robust determinants of PAP adherence. Adherence requires that a patient perceive the treatment as being beneficial, be motivated to initiate therapy, and have a sense of self-efficacy regarding the use of PAP.[36] Self-efficacy, or a patient's belief that they can use PAP successfully, is a modifiable psychological variable that is consistently related to PAP adherence.[37] Patients who lack a sense of motivation or perceived benefit, or those who endorse negative perceptions regarding inconvenience or discomfort with PAP, are not likely to use therapy. The patient's understanding of the underlying condition, the consequences of remaining untreated, and the available therapies and their benefits substantially influence these perceptions. These understandings can be enhanced through education and an individualized approach to therapeutic decisions.

A patient's understanding of OSA and benefits of PAP will not improve adherence in isolation. Although their perception of how PAP will benefit them can greatly influence acceptance of PAP, their response to therapy greatly influences their continued use of PAP. Although baseline symptoms have been shown to predict subsequent PAP use, adherence is significantly higher among those who experience greater reductions of these symptoms. Those who are more symptomatic have the potential of perceiving more symptomatic improvements. Equally important, those who have more comfort and a better initial experience with PAP are more likely to continue use, and early experiences with PAP predict long-term use.[27,38,39] This can be achieved by addressing 2 fundamental aspects in initiating PAP therapy. First, clinicians must identify and overcome common conditions, as explained elsewhere in this article, that can reduce the initial comfort and tolerance of PAP. Second, the initial PAP settings must optimize both comfort and the ablation of obstructive events. The quality of the PAP titration can impact subsequent compliance and persistent sleep apnea will quickly lead to a poor perception regarding the benefits of therapy.[40] Thus, it is imperative that clinicians adopt a proactive approach toward PAP adherence and seek to identify facilitators and barriers to PAP use as early as possible. Early impressions are critical, and a patient's attitude toward treatment and initial experiences can predict subsequent use.[41] Indeed, psychological instruments assessing subjective well-being and health status were able to correctly predict 85.7% of nonadherent patients in 1 study.[42]

In our clinical experience, PAP adherence and other health-related behaviors are frequently correlated. Medication nonadherence, inconsistent bedtimes,[43] smoking, alcohol use, and other unhealthy behaviors may be markers for both poor adherence and a reduced therapeutic response.[44,45] We found that PAP use paralleled medications adherence.[46] Although it is well-shown that PAP use remains problematic, it may not be unique to this specific treatment, but rather reflect an overall poor adherence with medical therapies and healthy behaviors, which is only recognized and highlighted because PAP includes objective measures of use. Regardless, these behaviors reflect, and can help to identify patients at an increased risk for PAP nonadherence.

As presented, there are numerous factors that can negatively impact PAP adherence. However, these also represent both a means to identify high-risk patients and potential targets for intervention. Although a multitude of interventions aimed to improve PAP use have been studied, they each require additional costs and resources. Given the increasing prevalence of OSA, it would be prohibitive to apply all interventions to all patients. Recognizing those at an increased risk for poor adherence or discontinuation of PAP can help to focus the correct intervention toward the correct patient to individualize care and maximize the benefits of therapy.

COMMON BARRIERS TO ADHERENCE TO POSITIVE AIRWAY PRESSURE TREATMENT AND HOW TO OVERCOME THEM

Initial experience with PAP predicts long-term use, so potential barriers to adherence should be addressed early and readdressed on an ongoing basis.[19,27,40] A proactive clinical approach is particularly important, because many new PAP users report side effects during the acclimatization phase of therapy.[47] Common complaints impacting adherence are sinus congestion, mask discomfort, insomnia, and claustrophobia. Early assessment and intervention may improve adherence and long-term patient outcomes.

Intolerance of the mask interface is the most common complaint leading to PAP discontinuation or exploration of other, non-PAP treatments for OSA. Several studies have evaluated the impact of mask type on PAP adherence. Although the type of mask interface is often considered interchangeable, the available literature suggests that nasal masks may provide better patient

acceptance and comfort, lower required pressure and residual apnea–hypopnea index (AHI), and fewer side effects compared with other mask types.[48–53] Oronasal masks may induce anatomic obstruction by pushing the tongue posteriorly[54] and studies have noted that these masks are associated with increased pressure requirements, higher residual AHIs, and lower rates of adherence compared with nasal masks.[48,55–59] The importance of proper mask selection and sizing cannot be overemphasized and can frequently mitigate this common barrier to PAP use. When PAP therapy is initiated, patients should have a formal custom mask fitting and assistance with mask selection by a specially trained respiratory therapist. Patients should be educated about proper fit, donning, and care of their mask. Many patients are unaware that masks should be periodically replaced. Over time, the mask liner deteriorates, resulting in skin irritation and leak, and potentially promoting patient discomfort and poor adherence.

Nasal congestion is both a frequent complaint among patients with OSA and is a common barrier to PAP use. Up to 14% of the US population has chronic sinus disease, with an even higher proportion experiencing acute allergic flares.[60] This prevalence is significantly higher among patients with OSA, with 40% reporting chronic rhinitis. Sinus congestion is a common cause of PAP discomfort and decreases its efficacy. As such, it is important to recognize and treat before initiating PAP. Not only is preexisting nasal congestion common among those with OSA, it can also occur as a result of PAP therapy, typically early in the course of treatment. As many as 30% of patients report developing nasal congestion during the initial weeks of therapy, with 10% having persistent symptoms for several months.[61] PAP-induced vasomotor rhinitis occurs as a dose–response phenomenon, with higher pressures causing more significant symptoms.[62] Heated, humidified air can reduce congestion,[63] and this consequence of PAP use has greatly decreased with wide adaptation of integrated humidifiers in most PAP platforms. However, nasal steroids or nasal antimuscarinics may be required for those who develop nasal congestion despite the use of a humidifier.

Comorbid insomnia occurs in up to 55% of patients with OSA and a bidirectional relationship between insomnia and OSA has been postulated.[64] Clinical experience suggests that, when insomnia is caused by sleep fragmentation arising from intermittent airway obstruction, symptoms frequently resolve with PAP therapy.[65–67] However, the existence of both sleep initiation and maintenance insomnia pose significant barriers to PAP use, and adapting to therapy can often prove challenging and cause further difficulties with sleep onset and continuity.[68] Similarly, insomnia-related posttraumatic stress disorder has been shown to both worsen OSA-related symptoms and quality of life measures, but also significantly reduces the use of and response to PAP.[69–71] A brief course of sedative-hypnotics may assist with the initial adaptation of PAP for those with preexisting insomnia.[72] However, nonpharmacologic therapy is the preferred treatment for insomnia, including for those with comorbid OSA, and the National Institutes of Health, American Academy of Sleep Medicine, and American College of Physicians all recommend cognitive-behavioral treatment for insomnia as first-line treatment for chronic insomnia, including insomnia occurring in the context of other medical, psychiatric, or sleep disorders.[73–75] In patients with OSA, CBT for insomnia has been shown to improve tolerance, effectiveness, and patient satisfaction with PAP.[76]

PAP-induced anxiety and claustrophobia can also present substantial barriers to therapy.[77] Even after proper mask selection and fitting, a subset of patients continues to describe difficulty sleeping with the mask interface. Although sometimes confused with insomnia, claustrophobia is a very different barrier and can be treated with simple desensitization in most cases. For persistent symptoms, referral to a behavioral sleep medicine specialist is often very helpful in these instances.[78] Use of an abbreviated daytime polysomnogram (ie, "PAP NAP") may also facilitate accommodation to PAP therapy and improve adherence.[79]

ADDITIONAL NONPHARMACOLOGIC INTERVENTIONS TO IMPROVE ADHERENCE TO POSITIVE AIRWAY PRESSURE TREATMENT
Education

Successful treatment with PAP starts with a comprehensive patient education plan. The decision to use PAP, like any medical treatment, involves both a commitment and associated lifestyle changes. It is important to realize that the treating clinician is asking the patient to change the way they sleep every single night. This means that one-third of their lives will be directly altered by this decision. And, the transition to PAP therapy may initially worsen their sleep. Education must be an ongoing process, starting from the initial assessment and continuing at every patient encounter. And, it must extend beyond OSA and PAP and include information regarding sleep health, proper sleep habits, and the benefits of

resolving sleep disorders. Although this might seem like common sense and can significantly improve outcomes, thorough patient education is, unfortunately, not common practice. A recent trial randomizing patients to either simply reviewing the results of their polysomnogram with a clinician or not found, not surprisingly, that those who spoke with sleep medicine staff and understood the importance of treating sleep-disordered breathing had significantly greater PAP use.[80]

Numerous studies have evaluated a range of programs, including video-education protocols,[81,82] patient education literature,[83] small group problem-based learning,[84] and CBT. Although improvements in adherence for some programs have been inconsistent,[36,83,85,86] programs using CBT (including desensitization, CBT for insomnia, and motivational enhancement [ME]) have been largely effective.[87–92] Unfortunately, these programs require a significant amount of time and expertise, and may not feasible in all practices.

The importance of spousal involvement for optimizing patient outcomes cannot be overstated. However, there is little high-quality objective evidence to discern the exact contribution of bed partner involvement in care. In a recent review, Ye and colleagues[93] considered the qualitative nature of the bed partner dynamic. Of 30 studies included in the most recent Cochrane review of behavioral interventions to improve PAP adherence, only 2 included the spouses of patients with OSA.[94] Given that the most common impetus for referral to a sleep facility is bed partner complaint, and considering patients frequently report potential PAP-induced spousal sleep disturbances as a primary excuses not to use therapy,[95] it is critical to include them in the education and treatment plan.[96] Clinical experience suggests that inclusion of bed partners and family members in routine clinical care can produce dramatic results. One study comparing those who slept alone with those with a consistent bed partner found PAP use increased 1.3 hours per night if a bed partner was present.[39] In another study, PAP was used more often during nights when married couples slept in the same bed.[97] It is essential, therefore, to educate patients that PAP tends to improve sleep quality for both patients and spouses.[98–100]

Group appointments can offer additional benefits related to PAP adherence. Not only do they reduce per-patient resources, they also provide less tangible benefits such as a shared sense of purpose and bonding over a common experience. Brostrom and colleagues[84] used a problem-based learning small group tutorial to improve PAP adherence in 25 subjects. After this educational program, 72% were adherent with PAP, with persistent benefits noted 6 months later.[84] In contrast, Basoglu and colleagues[81] failed to find a benefit from the addition of an educational video compared with standard physician instructions alone. We previously published the benefits of a comprehensive group educational program during PAP initiation.[101] Compared with individual counseling, group education led to both improved adherence and a 3-to 4-fold increase in access to care. The benefits of patient education and improved outcomes are well-established, and group education strategies may be a useful option for clinics that lack the resources to provide intensive education on an individual basis.

Motivational Enhancement

Motivational interviewing and ME are patient-centered psychological approaches that have demonstrated effectiveness for improving patient adherence in conditions ranging from cardiovascular disease and diabetes to nutrition and substance use disorders.[102] Multiple authors have found positive results from ME-based interventions among patients with OSA.[87,91,103–105] Although most of the ME research in the OSA population has been conducted by the same group, there is a consistent trend toward positive results.[87] In 2007, Aloia and colleagues[103] compared standard education, ME, and a control group. The probability of PAP discontinuation in the control group was 51%, compared with 30% in the education group and 26% in the ME group. Although the probability of reaching adherence was not significant different (61% control group, 68% education group, 67% ME group). Although ME might not significantly improve adherence, it may help to identify those who will discontinue therapy and allow clinics to manage these patients differently. This study was followed by a recent paper in which individual at greater risk did demonstrate a 97-minute per night increase after ME compared with controls.[104] Although behavioral treatments are often considered a "fix" for poor adherence, we believe that patient motivation is an essential aspect of OSA care. One of the key features of ME is that it is useful only if the patient desires to make a change. Therefore, identifying motivated patients before PAP initiation is critical to maximizing the success of ME and help to prioritize and appropriately allocate other resources intended to promote adherence.

Telehealth and Technology

As a result of technological advancements, PAP automated tracking technologies offer the opportunity to improve medical care for patients with OSA that is unlike the monitoring capabilities we have for most other chronic diseases. Historically, these technologies have provided clinicians with data on how much the patient is using PAP, how effective it is (based on indirect measurements of airflow limitation, which are interpreted as a residual AHI), and mask leak (which may indicate mask fit and comfort). The 2013 American Thoracic Society guidance for interpreting PAP compliance reports recommends a cutoff value for the residual AHI of fewer than 10 events per hour as indicative of satisfactory control of OSA.[106] It should be noted that a high residual AHI may lead to persistence of symptoms, poor sleep quality, and a loss of confidence in the value of PAP, and subsequently lead to its discontinuation by patients. As such, this threshold may be too high for most patients and it is recommended to optimize the ablation of obstructive events to promote better outcomes and adherence.

Heated humidification is a comfort feature that is felt to improve adherence, potentially by reducing symptoms of dry mouth and nasal congestion. The available literature suggests that there is little evidence that heated humidification provides substantial or clinically significant benefits for PAP adherence and a systematic Cochrane review found little impact on compliance.[107,108] However, humidification can mitigate some discomfort with PAP therapy, particularly oronasal dryness. Further, 1 study demonstrated that heated humidification could increase PAP use by 36 minutes per night.[95] Nonetheless, we provide heated humidification to all our patients. Our clinical experience is that most patients derive benefit from the heated humidification, either from comfort, or from having a sense of control in adjusting the setting on their appliance.

Transient and synchronized flexible alterations in the delivered pressure during both the inspiratory and expiratory portions of the respiratory phase has become a common feature in most PAP platforms, and is intended to improve comfort and tolerability to improve adherence. Although similar in design, each manufacturer uses its own patented technology: for example, ResMed (ResMed Corp, San Diego, CA) uses EPR and Philips-Respironics (Koninklijke Philips Electronics, NV, Eindhoven, the Netherlands) use A-Flex or C-Flex. There are few data in the published literature regarding the impact that these technologies have on PAP adherence.[36] Aloia and colleagues[109] found that C-Flex improved adherence compared with standard CPAP. However, there were no differences noted in symptomatic improvement. Chihara and colleagues[110] compared the impact on adherence between standard APAP, APAP plus C-Flex, and APAP plus A-Flex. The investigators demonstrated that C-Flex was superior to both standard APAP and APAP plus A-Flex. Although these features can improve comfort, they largely have not shown benefit in significantly improving PAP use or adherence. In addition, the changes in pressure can lead to sleep fragmentation and the reduced pressure during exhalation may result in instability of the airways and a persistence of apneic events. Ultimately, more studies are needed to evaluate the impact of these technologies on adherence.

PHARMACOLOGIC INTERVENTIONS TO IMPROVE ADHERENCE TO POSITIVE AIRWAY PRESSURE TREATMENT

Sedative hypnotics, in particular nonbenzodiazepine receptor agonists (NBRAs), offer an attractive option for improving adherence, particularly when used during the initial experiences with PAP. NBRAs do not adversely impact the AHI, oxygen saturation (SpO_2), sleep architecture, or response to PAP therapy.[111–113] The use of a sedative hypnotic during initial polysomnography has been shown to improve adherence, likely by facilitating a more accurate pressure determination and by improving the initial experience with PAP.[114–117] Similarly, the transient use of these agents should improve the transition to PAP therapy. However, studies assessing the usefulness of NBRAs for improving the transition to PAP therapy have had mixed results. In a study by Bradshaw and colleagues,[112] zolpidem failed to demonstrate a benefit on improving PAP compliance. In contrast, we found that 2 weeks of eszopiclone during PAP initiation led to more PAP use, less PAP discontinuation, and a greater likelihood of achieving adherence compared with placebo.[72] Eszopiclone has a longer duration of action than zolpidem, facilitating increased sleep continuity, which may explain the differences noted in these studies. Although most studies have evaluated nonselected patients with OSA, it is likely that the greatest benefit of NBRAs is for patients with comorbid insomnia.[36,118] Given that insomnia is a substantial barrier to PAP acceptance, means to facilitate the transition to therapy are needed to prevent abandonment of treatment.

Not only do sedatives have a role in aiding in the initial transition of PAP therapy, they may be beneficial in the management of sleep-disordered breathing. There is increasing recognition regarding the arousal threshold in sleep apnea, and patients with a low arousal threshold may represent a unique phenotype of OSA. In these individuals, airflow limitations may lead to sleep fragmentation in the absence of significant gas exchange abnormalities, possibly owing to sensitivity to the degree of stimuli required to cause an arousal or awakening.[119,120] Both trazodone and eszopiclone have been shown to improve the AHI and sleep continuity in patients with the low arousal threshold phenotype, and may provide a mechanism for improving adherence and outcomes.[119] However, these potential benefits need to be weighed against the effects of long-term use of sedatives.

COMPLICATIONS OF POSITIVE AIRWAY PRESSURE THERAPY AND HOW TO PREVENT OR OVERCOME THEM

Although safe and typically well-tolerated, there are several potential complications of PAP therapy, in addition to vasomotor rhinitis already discussed, that may have a negative impact on adherence. Proper patient education may mitigate the development of many of these complications. In addition, patients should be queried regarding their occurrence during each follow-up visit to promptly recognize and treat them to minimize their effect on PAP tolerance.

Aerophagia may result from positive pressure therapy. Patients may experience reflux, belching, distension, cramping, flatulence, and generalized gastrointestinal discomfort. Aerophagia is a challenging topic for clinicians, with limited evidence to guide management. Two physiologic mechanisms may contribute to this phenomenon. Air that enters the oropharynx under positive pressure may be swallowed and misdirected to the esophagus. Swallowed air can contribute to lower esophageal relaxation and cause or worsen reflux and nocturnal symptoms of gastroesophageal reflux disease.[121–123] Swallowed air can also trigger a reflexive closure of the upper esophageal sphincter, preventing escape of air, which can lead to abdominal distention and flatulence. Aerophagia is more common in patients with gastroesophageal reflux disease and those on antireflux medication. It also occurs more commonly in those with chronic sinus congestion, likely owing to an increase in upper airway resistance. In addition, hyperflexion of the neck from pillows can lead to partial closure of the upper airways, facilitating air to enter the esophagus instead of the trachea. By routine and unless otherwise contraindicated, we advise all patients with OSA to elevate the head of their beds 4 to 6 inches and use only a single, flat pillow to minimize this occurrence. In addition, we recommend treatment of sinus congestion before initiation of PAP to both reduce

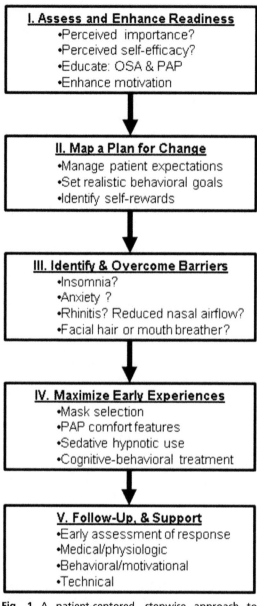

I. Assess and Enhance Readiness
- Perceived importance?
- Perceived self-efficacy?
- Educate: OSA & PAP
- Enhance motivation

II. Map a Plan for Change
- Manage patient expectations
- Set realistic behavioral goals
- Identify self-rewards

III. Identify & Overcome Barriers
- Insomnia?
- Anxiety ?
- Rhinitis? Reduced nasal airflow?
- Facial hair or mouth breather?

IV. Maximize Early Experiences
- Mask selection
- PAP comfort features
- Sedative hypnotic use
- Cognitive-behavioral treatment

V. Follow-Up, & Support
- Early assessment of response
- Medical/physiologic
- Behavioral/motivational
- Technical

Fig. 1. A patient-centered, stepwise approach to maximizing adherence to positive airway pressure (PAP) treatment. From a motivational perspective, patients must be ready to attempt PAP. Clinicians and care teams should provide comprehensive disease education including not only personalized consequences of obstructive sleep apnea (OSA) and potential health benefits of treatment, but also patient-centered and patient-defined improvements in quality of life that might result from treatment. Next, patient expectations should be managed, and a detailed care plan with deadline and rewards for adherence should be established. Potential barriers to PAP adherence such as insomnia or rhinitis should be identified and addressed as early in the treatment plan as possible. Early experiences are essential to long-term PAP success, and clinicians and care teams should strive to

the development of aerophagia and to address this common barrier to PAP tolerability, as discussed. For patients using an oronasal mask interface who develop aerophagia, switching to a nasal mask may resolve this. Compared with full-face masks, nasal masks produce a relatively greater negative pressure gradient in the posterior oropharynx that, in theory, should result in less air swallowing. When these techniques are unsuccessful, clinicians may elect to reduce the prescribed PAP pressure. Although there is no literature supporting pressure change as an avenue to improve aerophagia, anecdotal experiences have fund this to be beneficial in some patients. However, this should be balanced with the potential for inadequately treated OSA. Ultimately, patients with ongoing complaints should be referred to a gastroenterologist to assess for hiatal hernia or other conditions outside the scope of a sleep physician that may be causing these symptoms.

Central apneas and periodic breathing may occur in patients with OSA following the initiation of PAP therapy. "Treatment-emergent" or "complex" sleep apnea develops in up to 19% of patients. In the majority of cases, these central events resolve with continued PAP use, likely owing to normalization of P_{CO_2} and the hypercarbic threshold. However, 5% to 26% of patients will have persistent (>3 months) complex sleep apnea.[124] This condition highlights the multitude of physiologic underpinnings of sleep-disordered breathing, with upper airway collapsibility promoting obstructive events, and correction of airway tone with PAP promoting central apneas and an unstable respiratory pattern owing to increased chemosensitivity, low arousal threshold, and increased loop gain. Conservative measures, including optimization of heart failure therapies when indicated, weight loss, improved sleep hygiene, and reducing use of opioid medications, may alleviate the condition, to a degree. Non-PAP medical therapies, such as sedatives to increase the arousal threshold (decrease the number of arousals), respiratory stimulants such as acetazolamide, inhaled CO_2, addition of deadspace ventilation, and supplemental oxygen, are often less feasible owing to cost, difficult

"front-load" support to patients and family members. Finally, ongoing follow-up with attention to medical, physiologic, behavioral, motivational, and technical factors is essential. (*From* Wickwire EM, Lettieri CJ, Cairns AA, et al. Maximizing positive airway pressure adherence in adults: a common-sense approach. Chest 2013;144(2):689; with permission.)

implementation, lack of availability or expertise, and limited empiric evidence.[125] When identified, the continued use of CPAP with close observation is the first option for most practitioners and, as stated, resolution of central events occurs in most patients after several weeks on PAP therapy.[125] Patients with persistent complex sleep apnea can be treated with biphasic PAP or adaptive servo-ventilation (ASV). ASV is well-tolerated by most patients and will resolve central apneas and periodic breathing faster and more effectively than CPAP, especially in the short term.[124,126] Deciding whether to use a watchful waiting approach with continued CPAP, or adopting ASV early in the course of treatment depends on many considerations, including cost and how quickly a treatment response is needed.[125] Because PAP adherence is determined early, a more conservative strategy with CPAP may lead some patients to abandon therapy. Our practice is to provide close clinical follow-up and consider ASV in those whose central events do not resolve with CPAP. Given the recent results of SERVE-HF, we avoid the use of ASV in patients with a left ventricular ejection fraction of less than or equal to 45%.[127]

Local complications resulting from mask interfaces include skin irritation, visible indentations that are cosmetically unappealing, and skin ulceration in regions of maximal contact (ie, nasal bridge).[128] Eye irritation and keratitis from mask leak have also been reported. Often, these events can be resolved or even prevented with proper mask selection and educating patients on the proper way to don and adjust the mask. Patients often overtighten masks to resolve air leaks. This overtightening is not only counterproductive in most cases, it can also cause or contribute to skin ulcerations. Proper mask selection and sizing that is both compatible with the patient's facial features and pressure requirements and minimized air leak is crucial because this measure will enhance comfort and efficacy while also reducing complications. Several lotions and barriers intended to reduce mask-induced skin irritation and ulceration are commercially available; however, no clinical data are available to assess their usefulness.

Craniofacial changes and alterations in bite occlusion may occur with PAP, particularly among those using nasal masks. In a prospective study assessing craniofacial changes after 2 years of PAP use, Tsuda and coworkers[129] found that nasal CPAP led to significant retrusion of the anterior maxilla, a setback of the chin positions, a subluxation of the maxillary incisors, and bite malocclusion.

SUMMARY

PAP remains the most efficacious treatment for OSA and is the first choice of treatment for most patients. However, challenges with adherence remain problematic. Numerous trials show improved subjective and objective outcomes from successfully treating OSA. In contrast, several studies have failed to observe that PAP significantly improves symptoms or end-organ dysfunction. However, these studies are largely limited by insufficient use of therapy. The fact remains that PAP only works if it is being used. And, despite the barriers to PAP use, the majority of motivated patients can become adherent. If clinicians adopt a comprehensive strategy to systematically assess and remedy barriers to care, the likelihood of optimal treatment dramatically increases. We recommend a patient-centered, stepwise approach to maximizing PAP adherence (**Fig. 1**). We also recommend that patients failing to achieve adherence with PAP should receive a retrial of therapy using these strategies. For patients who continue to refuse or are intolerant of therapy, alternatives to PAP, particularly oral appliances, should be used as the primary objective is to ensure their OA is sufficiently treated.

REFERENCES

1. Punjabi NM, Shahar E, Redline S, et al. Sleep-disordered breathing, glucose intolerance, and insulin resistance: the Sleep Heart Health Study. Am J Epidemiol 2004;160(6):521–30.
2. Shahar E, Whitney CW, Redline S, et al. Sleep-disordered breathing and cardiovascular disease: cross-sectional results of the Sleep Heart Health Study. Am J Respir Crit Care Med 2001;163(1):19–25.
3. Shepard JW Jr. Hypertension, cardiac arrhythmias, myocardial infarction, and stroke in relation to obstructive sleep apnea. Clin Chest Med 1992; 13(3):437–58.
4. Kushida CA, Littner MR, Hirshkowitz M, et al. Practice parameters for the use of continuous and bilevel positive airway pressure devices to treat adult patients with sleep-related breathing disorders. Sleep 2006;29(3):375–80.
5. Sullivan CE, Issa FG, Berthon-Jones M, et al. Reversal of obstructive sleep apnoea by continuous positive airway pressure applied through the nares. Lancet 1981;1(8225):862–5.
6. Guo J, Sun Y, Xue LJ, et al. Effect of CPAP therapy on cardiovascular events and mortality in patients with obstructive sleep apnea: a meta-analysis. Sleep Breath 2016;20(3):965–74.
7. Montserrat JM, Ferrer M, Hernandez L, et al. Effectiveness of CPAP treatment in daytime function in

sleep apnea syndrome: a randomized controlled study with an optimized placebo. Am J Respir Crit Care Med 2001;164(4):608–13.

8. Sanchez AI, Buela-Casal G, Bermudez MP, et al. The effects of continuous positive air pressure treatment on anxiety and depression levels in apnea patients. Psychiatry Clin Neurosci 2001;55(6): 641–6.

9. Weaver TE, Grunstein RR. Adherence to continuous positive airway pressure therapy: the challenge to effective treatment. Proc Am Thorac Soc 2008;5(2):173–8.

10. Collard P, Pieters T, Aubert G, et al. Compliance with nasal CPAP in obstructive sleep apnea patients. Sleep Med Rev 1997;1(1):33–44.

11. Edinger JD, Carwile S, Miller P, et al. Psychological status, syndromatic measures, and compliance with nasal CPAP therapy for sleep apnea. Percept Mot Skills 1994;78(3 Pt 2):1116–8.

12. Marquez-Baez C, Paniagua-Soto J, Castilla-Garrido JM. Treatment of sleep apnea syndrome with CPAP: compliance with treatment, its efficacy and secondary effects. Rev Neurol 1998;26(151): 375–80 [in Spanish].

13. McArdle N, Devereux G, Heidarnejad H, et al. Long-term use of CPAP therapy for sleep apnea/hypopnea syndrome. Am J Respir Crit Care Med 1999;159(4 Pt 1):1108–14.

14. Pepin JL, Krieger J, Rodenstein D, et al. Effective compliance during the first 3 months of continuous positive airway pressure. A European prospective study of 121 patients. Am J Respir Crit Care Med 1999;160(4):1124–9.

15. Kribbs NB, Pack AI, Kline LR, et al. Objective measurement of patterns of nasal CPAP use by patients with obstructive sleep apnea. Am Rev Respir Dis 1993;147(4):887–95.

16. Loube DI, Gay PC, Strohl KP, et al. Indications for positive airway pressure treatment of adult obstructive sleep apnea patients: a consensus statement. Chest 1999;115(3):863–6.

17. Reeves-Hoche MK, Meck R, Zwillich CW. Nasal CPAP: an objective evaluation of patient compliance. Am J Respir Crit Care Med 1994;149(1): 149–54.

18. Brown LK. Use it or lose it: Medicare's new paradigm for durable medical equipment coverage? Chest 2010;138(4):785–9.

19. Stepnowsky CJ, Dimsdale JE. Dose-response relationship between CPAP compliance and measures of sleep apnea severity. Sleep Med 2002;3(4): 329–34.

20. Zimmerman ME, Arnedt JT, Stanchina M, et al. Normalization of memory performance and positive airway pressure adherence in memory-impaired patients with obstructive sleep apnea. Chest 2006;130(6):1772–8.

21. Campos-Rodriguez F, Pena-Grinan N, Reyes-Nunez N, et al. Mortality in obstructive sleep apnea-hypopnea patients treated with positive airway pressure. Chest 2005;128(2):624–33.

22. Weaver TE, Maislin G, Dinges DF, et al. Relationship between hours of CPAP use and achieving normal levels of sleepiness and daily functioning. Sleep 2007;30(6):711–9.

23. Antic NA, Catcheside P, Buchan C, et al. The effect of CPAP in normalizing daytime sleepiness, quality of life, and neurocognitive function in patients with moderate to severe OSA. Sleep 2011;34(1):111–9.

24. Walia HK, Griffith SD, Foldvary-Schaefer N, et al. Longitudinal effect of CPAP on BP in resistant and nonresistant hypertension in a large clinic-based Cohort. Chest 2016;149(3):747–55.

25. Law MR, Morris JK, Wald NJ. Use of blood pressure lowering drugs in the prevention of cardiovascular disease: meta-analysis of 147 randomised trials in the context of expectations from prospective epidemiological studies. BMJ 2009;338:b1665.

26. Sin DD, Mayers I, Man GC, et al. Long-term compliance rates to continuous positive airway pressure in obstructive sleep apnea: a population-based study. Chest 2002;121(2):430–5.

27. Budhiraja R, Parthasarathy S, Drake CL, et al. Early CPAP use identifies subsequent adherence to CPAP therapy. Sleep 2007;30(3):320–4.

28. Pieters T, Collard P, Aubert G, et al. Acceptance and long-term compliance with nCPAP in patients with obstructive sleep apnoea syndrome. Eur Respir J 1996;9(5):939–44.

29. Billings ME, Auckley D, Benca R, et al. Race and residential socioeconomics as predictors of CPAP adherence. Sleep 2011;34(12):1653–8.

30. Campbell A, Neill A, Lory R. Ethnicity and socioeconomic status predict initial continuous positive airway pressure compliance in New Zealand adults with obstructive sleep apnoea. Intern Med J 2012; 42(6):e95–101.

31. Platt AB, Field SH, Asch DA, et al. Neighborhood of residence is associated with daily adherence to CPAP therapy. Sleep 2009;32(6):799–806.

32. Scharf SM, Seiden L, DeMore J, et al. Racial differences in clinical presentation of patients with sleep-disordered breathing. Sleep Breath 2004; 8(4):173–83.

33. Loube DI, Gay PC, Strohl KP, et al. Indications for positive airway pressure treatment of adult obstructive sleep apnea patients: a consensus statement. Chest 1999;115(3):863–6.

34. Li HY, Engleman H, Hsu CY, et al. Acoustic reflection for nasal airway measurement in patients with obstructive sleep apnea-hypopnea syndrome. Sleep 2005;28(12):1554–9.

35. Morris LG, Setlur J, Burschtin OE, et al. Acoustic rhinometry predicts tolerance of nasal continuous

positive airway pressure: a pilot study. Am J Rhinol 2006;20(2):133–7.

36. Wickwire EM, Lettieri CJ, Cairns AA, et al. Maximizing positive airway pressure adherence in adults: a common-sense approach. Chest 2013; 144(2):680–93.

37. Dzierzewski JM, Wallace DM, Wohlgemuth WK. Adherence to continuous positive airway pressure in existing users: self-efficacy enhances the association between continuous positive airway pressure and adherence. J Clin Sleep Med 2016; 12(2):169–76.

38. Aloia MS, Arnedt JT, Stanchina M, et al. How early in treatment is PAP adherence established? Revisiting night-to-night variability. Behav Sleep Med 2007;5(3):229–40.

39. Lewis KE, Seale L, Bartle IE, et al. Early predictors of CPAP use for the treatment of obstructive sleep apnea. Sleep 2004;27(1):134–8.

40. Drake CL, Day R, Hudgel D, et al. Sleep during titration predicts continuous positive airway pressure compliance. Sleep 2003;26(3):308–11.

41. Balachandran JS, Yu X, Wroblewski K, et al. A brief survey of patients' first impression after CPAP titration predicts future CPAP adherence: a pilot study. J Clin Sleep Med 2013;9(3):199–205.

42. Poulet C, Veale D, Arnol N, et al. Psychological variables as predictors of adherence to treatment by continuous positive airway pressure. Sleep Med 2009;10(9):993–9.

43. Sawyer AM, King TS, Sawyer DA, et al. Is inconsistent pre-treatment bedtime related to CPAP nonadherence? Res Nurs Health 2014;37(6):504–11.

44. Russo-Magno P, O'Brien A, Panciera T, et al. Compliance with CPAP therapy in older men with obstructive sleep apnea. J Am Geriatr Soc 2001; 49(9):1205–11.

45. Woehrle H, Graml A, Weinreich G. Age- and gender-dependent adherence with continuous positive airway pressure therapy. Sleep Med 2011;12(10):1034–6.

46. Walter RJ, Lettieri CJ, Sheikh K, et al. Does medication adherence predict cpap compliance? Sleep 2015;36:A200.

47. Engleman HM, Wild MR. Improving CPAP use by patients with the sleep apnoea/hypopnoea syndrome (SAHS). Sleep Med Rev 2003;7(1):81–99.

48. Borel JC, Tamisier R, Dias-Domingos S, et al. Type of mask may impact on continuous positive airway pressure adherence in apneic patients. PLoS One 2013;8(5):e64382.

49. Anderson FE, Kingshott RN, Taylor DR, et al. A randomized crossover efficacy trial of oral CPAP (Oracle) compared with nasal CPAP in the management of obstructive sleep apnea. Sleep 2003;26(6):721–6.

50. Beecroft J, Zanon S, Lukic D, et al. Oral continuous positive airway pressure for sleep apnea: effectiveness, patient preference, and adherence. Chest 2003;124(6):2200–8.

51. Khanna R, Kline LR. A prospective 8 week trial of nasal interfaces vs. a novel oral interface (Oracle) for treatment of obstructive sleep apnea hypopnea syndrome. Sleep Med 2003;4(4):333–8.

52. Mortimore IL, Whittle AT, Douglas NJ. Comparison of nose and face mask CPAP therapy for sleep apnoea. Thorax 1998;53(4):290–2.

53. Ryan S, Garvey JF, Swan V, et al. Nasal pillows as an alternative interface in patients with obstructive sleep apnoea syndrome initiating continuous positive airway pressure therapy. J Sleep Res 2011; 20(2):367–73.

54. Schorr F, Genta PR, Gregorio MG, et al. Continuous positive airway pressure delivered by oronasal mask may not be effective for obstructive sleep apnoea. Eur Respir J 2012;40(2):503–5.

55. Bachour A, Vitikainen P, Maasilta P. Rates of initial acceptance of PAP masks and outcomes of mask switching. Sleep Breath 2016;20(2):733–8.

56. Bachour A, Vitikainen P, Virkkula P, et al. CPAP interface: satisfaction and side effects. Sleep Breath 2013;17(2):667–72.

57. Deshpande S, Joosten S, Turton A, et al. Oronasal masks require a higher pressure than nasal and nasal pillow masks for the treatment of obstructive sleep apnea. J Clin Sleep Med 2016;12(9):1263–8.

58. Ebben MR, Narizhnaya M, Segal AZ, et al. A randomised controlled trial on the effect of mask choice on residual respiratory events with continuous positive airway pressure treatment. Sleep Med 2014;15(6):619–24.

59. Ng JR, Aiyappan V, Mercer J, et al. Choosing an oronasal mask to deliver continuous positive airway pressure may cause more upper airway obstruction or lead to higher continuous positive airway pressure requirements than a nasal mask in some patients: a case series. J Clin Sleep Med 2016; 12(9):1227–32.

60. Kaliner MA, Osguthorpe JD, Fireman P, et al. Sinusitis: bench to bedside. Current findings, future directions. J Allergy Clin Immunol 1997;99(6 Pt 3):S829–48.

61. Ulander M, Johansson MS, Ewaldh AE, et al. Side effects to continuous positive airway pressure treatment for obstructive sleep apnoea: changes over time and association to adherence. Sleep Breath 2014;18(4):799–807.

62. Alahmari MD, Sapsford RJ, Wedzicha JA, et al. Dose response of continuous positive airway pressure on nasal symptoms, obstruction and inflammation in vivo and in vitro. Eur Respir J 2012;40(5):1180–90.

63. Koutsourelakis I, Vagiakis E, Perraki E, et al. Nasal inflammation in sleep apnoea patients using CPAP

and effect of heated humidification. Eur Respir J 2011;37(3):587–94.

64. Beneto A, Gomez-Siurana E, Rubio-Sanchez P. Comorbidity between sleep apnea and insomnia. Sleep Med Rev 2009;13(4):287–93.

65. Krakow B, Melendrez D, Ferreira E, et al. Prevalence of insomnia symptoms in patients with sleep-disordered breathing. Chest 2001;120(6): 1923–9.

66. Krakow B, Melendrez D, Lee SA, et al. Refractory insomnia and sleep-disordered breathing: a pilot study. Sleep Breath 2004;8(1):15–29.

67. Krakow B, Melendrez D, Warner TD, et al. To breathe, perchance to sleep: sleep-disordered breathing and chronic insomnia among trauma survivors. Sleep Breath 2002;6(4):189–202.

68. Wickwire EM, Smith MT, Birnbaum S, et al. Sleep maintenance insomnia complaints predict poor CPAP adherence: a clinical case series. Sleep Med 2010;11(8):772–6.

69. Collen JF, Lettieri CJ, Hoffman M. The impact of posttraumatic stress disorder on CPAP adherence in patients with obstructive sleep apnea. J Clin Sleep Med 2012;8(6):667–72.

70. El-Solh AA, Ayyar L, Akinnusi M, et al. Positive airway pressure adherence in veterans with posttraumatic stress disorder. Sleep 2010;33(11): 1495–500.

71. Lettieri CJ, Williams SG, Collen JF. OSA syndrome and posttraumatic stress disorder: clinical outcomes and impact of positive airway pressure therapy. Chest 2016;149(2):483–90.

72. Lettieri CJ, Shah AA, Holley AB, et al. Effects of a short course of eszopiclone on continuous positive airway pressure adherence: a randomized trial. Ann Intern Med 2009;151(10):696–702.

73. National Institute of Health, et al. NIH Consens State Sci Statements 2005;22:1.

74. Qaseem A, Kansagara D, Forciea MA, et al, Clinical Guidelines Committee of the American College of Physicians. Management of chronic insomnia disorder in adults: a clinical practice guideline from the American College of Physicians. Ann Intern Med 2016;165(2):125–33.

75. Schutte-Rodin S, Broch L, Buysse D, et al. Clinical guideline for the evaluation and management of chronic insomnia in adults. J Clin Sleep Med 2008;4(5):487–504.

76. Luyster FS, Buysse DJ, Strollo PJ Jr. Comorbid insomnia and obstructive sleep apnea: challenges for clinical practice and research. J Clin Sleep Med 2010;6(2):196–204.

77. Chasens ER, Pack AI, Maislin G, et al. Claustrophobia and adherence to CPAP treatment. West J Nurs Res 2005;27(3):307–21.

78. Haynes PL. The role of behavioral sleep medicine in the assessment and treatment of sleep disordered breathing. Clin Psychol Rev 2005; 25(5):673–705.

79. Krakow B, Ulibarri V, Melendrez D, et al. A daytime, abbreviated cardio-respiratory sleep study (CPT 95807-52) to acclimate insomnia patients with sleep disordered breathing to positive airway pressure (PAP-NAP). J Clin Sleep Med 2008;4(3):212–22.

80. Jurado-Gamez B, Bardwell WA, Cordova-Pacheco LJ, et al. A basic intervention improves CPAP adherence in sleep apnoea patients: a controlled trial. Sleep Breath 2015;19(2):509–14.

81. Basoglu OK, Midilli M, Midilli R, et al. Adherence to continuous positive airway pressure therapy in obstructive sleep apnea syndrome: effect of visual education. Sleep Breath 2012;16(4):1193–200.

82. Jean Wiese H, Boethel C, Phillips B, et al. CPAP compliance: video education may help! Sleep Med 2005;6(2):171–4.

83. Chervin RD, Theut S, Bassetti C, et al. Compliance with nasal CPAP can be improved by simple interventions. Sleep 1997;20(4):284–9.

84. Brostrom A, Fridlund B, Ulander M, et al. A mixed method evaluation of a group-based educational programme for CPAP use in patients with obstructive sleep apnea. J Eval Clin Pract 2013;19(1): 173–84.

85. Aloia MS, Di Dio L, Ilniczky N, et al. Improving compliance with nasal CPAP and vigilance in older adults with OAHS. Sleep Breath 2001;5(1):13–21.

86. Sedkaoui K, Leseux L, Pontier S, et al. Efficiency of a phone coaching program on adherence to continuous positive airway pressure in sleep apnea hypopnea syndrome: a randomized trial. BMC Pulm Med 2015;15:102.

87. Aloia MS, Arnedt JT, Riggs RL, et al. Clinical management of poor adherence to CPAP: motivational enhancement. Behav Sleep Med 2004;2(4): 205–22.

88. Bartlett D, Wong K, Richards D, et al. Increasing adherence to obstructive sleep apnea treatment with a group social cognitive therapy treatment intervention: a randomized trial. Sleep 2013; 36(11):1647–54.

89. Edinger JD, Radtke RA. Use of in vivo desensitization to treat a patient's claustrophobic response to nasal CPAP. Sleep 1993;16(7):678–80.

90. Lai AY, Fong DY, Lam JC, et al. The efficacy of a brief motivational enhancement education program on CPAP adherence in OSA: a randomized controlled trial. Chest 2014;146(3):600–10.

91. Olsen S, Smith SS, Oei TP, et al. Motivational interviewing (MINT) improves continuous positive airway pressure (CPAP) acceptance and adherence: a randomized controlled trial. J Consult Clin Psychol 2012;80(1):151–63.

92. Richards D, Bartlett DJ, Wong K, et al. Increased adherence to CPAP with a group cognitive

behavioral treatment intervention: a randomized trial. Sleep 2007;30(5):635–40.

93. Ye L, Malhotra A, Kayser K, et al. Spousal involvement and CPAP adherence: a dyadic perspective. Sleep Med Rev 2015;19:67–74.

94. Wozniak DR, Lasserson TJ, Smith I. Educational, supportive and behavioural interventions to improve usage of continuous positive airway pressure machines in adults with obstructive sleep apnoea. Cochrane Database Syst Rev 2014;(1): CD007736.

95. Weaver TE, Maislin G, Dinges DF, et al. Self-efficacy in sleep apnea: instrument development and patient perceptions of obstructive sleep apnea risk, treatment benefit, and volition to use continuous positive airway pressure. Sleep 2003;26(6):727–32.

96. McArdle N, Kingshott R, Engleman HM, et al. Partners of patients with sleep apnoea/hypopnoea syndrome: effect of CPAP treatment on sleep quality and quality of life. Thorax 2001;56(7):513–8.

97. Cartwright R. Sleeping together: a pilot study of the effects of shared sleeping on adherence to CPAP treatment in obstructive sleep apnea. J Clin Sleep Med 2008;4(2):123–7.

98. Doherty LS, Kiely JL, Lawless G, et al. Impact of nasal continuous positive airway pressure therapy on the quality of life of bed partners of patients with obstructive sleep apnea syndrome. Chest 2003;124(6):2209–14.

99. McFadyen TA, Espie CA, McArdle N, et al. Controlled, prospective trial of psychosocial function before and after continuous positive airway pressure therapy. Eur Respir J 2001;18(6): 996–1002.

100. Parish JM, Lyng PJ. Quality of life in bed partners of patients with obstructive sleep apnea or hypopnea after treatment with continuous positive airway pressure. Chest 2003;124(3):942–7.

101. Lettieri CJ, Walter RJ. Impact of group education on continuous positive airway pressure adherence. J Clin Sleep Med 2013;9(6):537–41.

102. Miller WR, Rollnick S. Motivational interviewing: helping people change. 3rd edition. New York: Guilford Press; 2013.

103. Aloia MS, Smith K, Arnedt JT, et al. Brief behavioral therapies reduce early positive airway pressure discontinuation rates in sleep apnea syndrome: preliminary findings. Behav Sleep Med 2007;5(2): 89–104.

104. Bakker JP, Wang R, Weng J, et al. Motivational enhancement for increasing adherence to CPAP: a randomized controlled trial. Chest 2016;150(2): 337–45.

105. Dantas AP, Winck JC, Figueiredo-Braga M. Adherence to APAP in obstructive sleep apnea syndrome: effectiveness of a motivational intervention. Sleep Breath 2015;19(1):327–34.

106. Schwab RJ, Badr SM, Epstein LJ, et al. An official American Thoracic Society statement: continuous positive airway pressure adherence tracking systems. The optimal monitoring strategies and outcome measures in adults. Am J Respir Crit Care Med 2013;188(5):613–20.

107. Haniffa M, Lasserson TJ, Smith I. Interventions to improve compliance with continuous positive airway pressure for obstructive sleep apnoea. Cochrane Database Syst Rev 2004;(4):CD003531.

108. Massie CA, Hart RW, Peralez K, et al. Effects of humidification on nasal symptoms and compliance in sleep apnea patients using continuous positive airway pressure. Chest 1999;116(2):403–8.

109. Aloia MS, Stanchina M, Arnedt JT, et al. Treatment adherence and outcomes in flexible vs standard continuous positive airway pressure therapy. Chest 2005;127(6):2085–93.

110. Chihara Y, Tsuboi T, Hitomi T, et al. Flexible positive airway pressure improves treatment adherence compared with auto-adjusting PAP. Sleep 2013; 36(2):229–36.

111. Berry RB, Patel PB. Effect of zolpidem on the efficacy of continuous positive airway pressure as treatment for obstructive sleep apnea. Sleep 2006;29(8):1052–6.

112. Bradshaw DA, Ruff GA, Murphy DP. An oral hypnotic medication does not improve continuous positive airway pressure compliance in men with obstructive sleep apnea. Chest 2006;130(5): 1369–76.

113. Coyle MA, Mendelson WB, Derchak PA, et al. Ventilatory safety of zaleplon during sleep in patients with obstructive sleep apnea on continuous positive airway pressure. J Clin Sleep Med 2005;1(1): 97.

114. Collen J, Lettieri C, Kelly W, et al. Clinical and polysomnographic predictors of short-term continuous positive airway pressure compliance. Chest 2009; 135(3):704–9.

115. Lettieri CJ, Collen JF, Eliasson AH, et al. Sedative use during continuous positive airway pressure titration improves subsequent compliance: a randomized, double-blind, placebo-controlled trial. Chest 2009;136(5):1263–8.

116. Lettieri CJ, Eliasson AH, Andrada T, et al. Does zolpidem enhance the yield of polysomnography? J Clin Sleep Med 2005;1(2):129–31.

117. Lettieri CJ, Quast TN, Eliasson AH, et al. Eszopiclone improves overnight polysomnography and continuous positive airway pressure titration: a prospective, randomized, placebo-controlled trial. Sleep 2008;31(9):1310–6.

118. Zhang XJ, Li QY, Wang Y, et al. The effect of nonbenzodiazepine hypnotics on sleep quality and severity in patients with OSA: a meta-analysis. Sleep Breath 2014;18(4):781–9.

119. Eckert DJ, Owens RL, Kehlmann GB, et al. Eszopi-clone increases the respiratory arousal threshold and lowers the apnoea/hypopnoea index in obstructive sleep apnoea patients with a low arousal threshold. Clin Sci (Lond) 2011;120(12): 505–14.

120. Edwards BA, Eckert DJ, McSharry DG, et al. Clinical predictors of the respiratory arousal threshold in patients with obstructive sleep apnea. Am J Respir Crit Care Med 2014;190(11):1293–300.

121. Shepherd K, Hillman D, Eastwood P. CPAP-induced aerophagia may precipitate gastroesophageal reflux. J Clin Sleep Med 2013;9(6):633–4.

122. Shepherd K, Hillman D, Eastwood P. Symptoms of aerophagia are common in patients on continuous positive airway pressure therapy and are related to the presence of nighttime gastroesophageal reflux. J Clin Sleep Med 2013;9(1):13–7.

123. Watson NF, Mystkowski SK. Aerophagia and gastroesophageal reflux disease in patients using continuous positive airway pressure: a preliminary observation. J Clin Sleep Med 2008;4(5):434–8.

124. Morgenthaler TI, Kuzniar TJ, Wolfe LF, et al. The complex sleep apnea resolution study: a prospective randomized controlled trial of continuous positive airway pressure versus adaptive servoventilation therapy. Sleep 2014;37(5):927–34.

125. Kuzniar TJ, Morgenthaler TI. Treatment of complex sleep apnea syndrome. Chest 2012;142(4): 1049–57.

126. Dellweg D, Kerl J, Hoehn E, et al. Randomized controlled trial of noninvasive positive pressure ventilation (NPPV) versus servoventilation in patients with CPAP-induced central sleep apnea (complex sleep apnea). Sleep 2013;36(8): 1163–71.

127. Cowie MR, Woehrle H, Wegscheider K, et al. Adaptive servo-ventilation for central sleep apnea in systolic heart failure. N Engl J Med 2015;373(12): 1095–105.

128. Yamaguti WP, Moderno EV, Yamashita SY, et al. Treatment-related risk factors for development of skin breakdown in subjects with acute respiratory failure undergoing noninvasive ventilation or CPAP. Respir Care 2014;59(10):1530–6.

129. Tsuda H, Almeida FR, Tsuda T, et al. Craniofacial changes after 2 years of nasal continuous positive airway pressure use in patients with obstructive sleep apnea. Chest 2010;138:870–4.

Oral Appliances in the Management of Obstructive Sleep Apnea

Jing Hao Ng, BDS (Singapore), MDS Orthodontics (Singapore),
MOrth RCS (Edinburgh, UK)*, Mimi Yow, BDS (Singapore), FDS RCS (Edinburgh),
MSc (London) (Orthodontics), FAMS (Craniofacial Orthodontics)

KEYWORDS

- OSA • Oral appliance • Mandibular advancement • Tongue stabilizer

KEY POINTS

- The concept in oral appliances for obstructive sleep apnea (OSA) management is protrusion of the mandible and/or tongue for structural effects on the upper airway.
- The upper airway is a muscular tube and its dimensions are enlarged with mandibular and tongue advancement.
- Protrusion of the mandible and tongue stretches the muscles, thereby reducing upper airway collapsibility with airway shape change and increase in muscle tone.
- Oral appliances are effective and evidence-based options in managing OSA.

TYPES OF ORAL APPLIANCES

The primary oral appliance (OA) used in obstructive sleep apnea (OSA) treatment is the mandibular advancement device (MAD). MADs may be either an over-the-counter stock device or customized for individual patients. MADs come in various designs and materials, but most comprise upper and lower splints mounted over the dentition as either a 1-piece monoblock (**Fig. 1**) or a 2-piece biblock (**Fig. 2**). Connectors or blocks relate the upper and lower splints in a biblock to protrude the mandible in a forward position during sleep.[1]

Tongue-retaining devices, or tongue-stabilizing devices (TSDs) (**Fig. 3**), are a second type of OA, which displace the tongue anteriorly and may be customized or come in different stock sizes. TSDs use negative pressure and salivary adhesion to hold onto the tongue and anterior lip shields to elongate and reposition the tongue in a more forward position independent of the mandible during sleep, thereby opening the oropharyngeal airway.[1,2]

TSDs have similar efficacy as MADs but poorer compliance. More than 90% of patients preferred MADs over TSDs for OA therapy.[3] The evidence base is stronger for MADs and considerably lower for TSDs.[2,4,5]

ORAL APPLIANCE EFFECTS ON AIRWAY
Cross-Sectional Area

Airway imaging with cone-beam computed tomography, magnetic resonance imaging and nasal endoscopy showed anteroposterior (AP) mandibular protrusion predominantly increases the caliber of the airway at the retropalatal area via lateral expansion and displacement of parapharyngeal fat pads[2,6–13] while the tongue and tongue-base muscles shift forward.[2,9,13]

The lateral widening from AP movement is attributed to stretching of soft tissue connections

This article originally appeared in March, 2019 issue of *Sleep Medicine Clinics* (Volume 14, Issue 1).
Disclosure Statement: The authors declare no conflicts of interest and no funding was received in the preparation of this article.
Department of Orthodontics, National Dental Centre Singapore, 5 Second Hospital Avenue, Singapore 168938, Singapore
* Corresponding author.
E-mail address: ng.jing.hao@singhealth.com.sg

Sleep Med Clin 15 (2020) 241–250
https://doi.org/10.1016/j.jsmc.2020.02.010

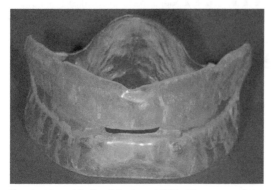

Fig. 1. Monoblock of 1-piece MAD. (*Courtesy of* the Orthodontic Laboratory in the National Dental Centre of Singapore, Singapore.)

between the tongue, soft palate, and lateral pharyngeal walls.[11,14,15] Dynamic MRI suggests a direct connection between lateral pharyngeal walls and the ramus, postulated to be the pterygomandibular raphe.[13]

TSDs increase airway AP diameter to a greater degree than MADs, and traction on intrapharyngeal connections through the tongue base additionally increases the lateral dimension of the airway. Compared with MADs, TSDs produce greater increases in retropalatal and retroglossal cross-sectional area (CSA). This is attributed to greater anterior tongue movement with TSDs.[2]

Other Effects

Lateral expansion with both MADs and TSDs promotes an elliptical cross-sectional shape with a transverse long axis.[2] A small but significant decrease in upper airway length has been found with MAD use,[2] which may counteract the airway length increase from lying supine demonstrated in OSA patients.[16]

Electromyography shows that MADs increase activation of masseter, lateral pterygoid, genioglossus, and geniohyoid muscles. It is postulated that on top of the purely structural anatomic effects of MADs, increased neuromuscular activation contributes to upper airway patency.[17–19]

Collapsibility

Morphologic increase in CSA, change in cross-sectional shape, decrease in airway length, and neuromuscular activation with MAD may contribute to reduced collapsibility.[2,12,20] Empirically, a significant reduction in upper airway collapsibility in stage 2 and stage 3 sleep was observed with MAD use. Improvement in collapsibility was significantly greater in complete responders than in partial responders or nonresponders.[21] Airway collapsibility may have a dose-dependent relationship with mandibular advancement.[10]

ORAL APPLIANCE EFFECTS ON OBSTRUCTIVE SLEEP APNEA COMPARED WITH CONTINUOUS POSITIVE AIRWAY PRESSURE

Continuous positive airway pressure (CPAP) and MADs are chronic, noninvasive, symptomatic treatments for OSA that do not treat the underlying

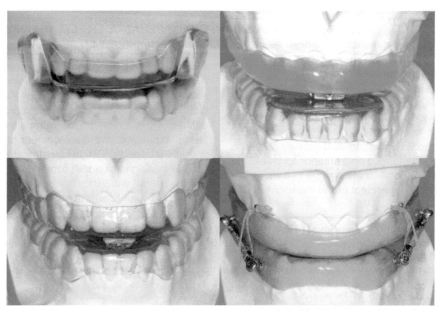

Fig. 2. Biblock or 2-piece MADs with different connectors. (*Courtesy of* [*upper left*] SomnoMed, Sydney, Australia; and [*upper right, lower left,* and *lower right*] Orthodontic Master, Singapore.)

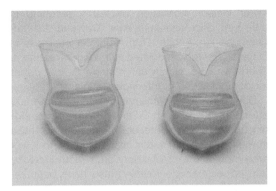

Fig. 3. TSD. (*Courtesy of* Innovative Health Technologies Ltd, Dunedin, New Zealand.)

anatomic basis of the condition. Pneumatic splinting of the airway with CPAP is acknowledged as the gold standard for treatment of OSA, although MAD has been progressively recommended with each iteration of the American Academy of Sleep Medicine (AASM) guidelines.[4,22,23] The latest AASM guidelines do not specify a particular disease severity for MAD use due to lack of evidence relating MAD efficacy to disease severity.[4]

Apnea-Hypopnea Index

MADs are efficacious in reducing apnea-hypopnea index (AHI) although there is individual variability.[24] A nonlinear dose-dependent relationship with degree of advancement is reported.[25–30]

The efficacy of CPAP over MAD in reducing AHI is well established and has been consistently reported by meta-analyses comparing the 2,[4,31–34] even with increasing numbers of primary studies. According to the AASM/American Academy of Dental Sleep Medicine (AADSM) task force, CPAP is significantly better than MAD at reducing AHI scores (difference of 6.24 events per hour).[4] A recent meta-analysis of 14 randomized controlled trials reported that CPAP reduced AHI by an additional 8.43 events per hour over MAD.[34]

Oxygenation

MADs are efficacious in improving minimum arterial oxygen saturation (Sao_2), and the improvement has been reported to have a nonlinear dose-dependent relationship with degree of advancement.[10]

Similar to AHI, the finding of better improvement in Sao_2 with CPAP over MAD has been consistently reported.[4,31,32,34] The AASM/AADSM task force reported that CPAP is slightly better at improving oxygenation (Sao_2 difference of 3.11%) compared with MADs.[4] More recently, a significant effect on Sao_2 in favor of CPAP was reported.[34]

Compliance

Comparing subjective self-reported MAD compliance with objective recorded CPAP compliance, MAD compliance is better. The AASM/AADSM task force reported that MADs were used 0.70 more hours per night than CPAP.[4] Objective measurements of OA usage after 3 months of OA treatment ranged from a mean of 6.4 hours to 6.6 hours per night.[35,36] A meta-analysis of 6 studies encompassing both subjective and objective MAD compliance measures reported an additional 1.1 hours per night use of MAD over CPAP.[33]

A majority of crossover trials report that MADs are preferred to CPAP, which may imply better patient compliance with MADs.[4,37,38] Depending on OSA severity and total sleep time, less than ideal compliance with CPAP can substantially decrease its effectiveness. Better MAD compliance over CPAP could be why health outcomes of the 2 treatment modalities are similar despite better CPAP efficacy at reducing AHI and increasing oxygenation.[37]

Subjective Sleepiness

MADs improve subjective daytime sleepiness measured by Epworth Sleepiness Scale (ESS) scores significantly.[39]

Despite better efficacy with CPAP than MADs in reducing AHI and improving Sao_2, differences in ESS scores are more ambiguous. A network meta-analysis of 67 studies found that CPAP and MADs are both effective in reducing excessive daytime sleepiness as assessed by the ESS, but CPAP is likely to be more effective than MADs, with a greater reduction in ESS by an average of 0.8 points.[40] Other reviews have reported either similar outcomes[4,32] or slightly better outcomes with CPAP.[33,34]

Function and Quality of Life

Aside from long-term health effects, untreated OSA also affects health-related quality of life, with hypersomnolence impacting ability to function.[41] Function and quality of life are commonly measured using both the sleep-specific Functional Outcomes of Sleep Questionnaire (FOSQ) and generic Medical Outcomes Study 36-Item Short Form Health Survey (SF-36). MADs are associated with improvements in FOSQ subscale and total scores as well as SF-36 scores.[4,42,43]

Minimal difference was found between CPAP and MAD with respect to improvements in daytime functional outcomes measured by SF-36 and FOSQ scores.[4] This finding was corroborated in a meta-analysis,[44] with direct comparisons as well as network meta-analysis showing no significant difference in treatment outcomes between

CPAP and MAD in the mental and physical components of SF-36. Other meta-analyses have also reported no difference in FOSQ or SF-36 scores.[31–34]

Cardiovascular Effects

Meta-analyses by multiple groups have found MADs to be the equivalent of CPAP at reducing blood pressure in adults with OSA.[4,34,45–47] A network meta-analysis reported that CPAP was associated with a reduction in systolic blood pressure of 2.5 mm Hg and diastolic blood pressure reduction of 2.0 mm Hg. MADs were associated with reduction in systolic blood pressure of 2.1 mm Hg and diastolic blood pressure of 1.9 mm Hg. There was no significant difference between CPAP and MADs.[40]

Studies on other cardiovascular markers (heart rate variability, circulating cardiovascular biomarkers, endothelial function, and arterial stiffness) were deemed heterogeneous and inconclusive.[46]

Mortality

A prospective cohort study on long-term cardiovascular mortality in 208 subjects found CPAP and MAD equally effective in reducing the risk of fatal cardiovascular events in patients with severe OSA, despite higher residual AHI for MAD compared with CPAP users (16.3 vs 4.5 events per hour). There was no difference in the cumulative cardiovascular mortality between OSA patients treated with CPAP or MAD and that of the nonapneic controls, suggesting effective symptomatic treatment with either modality despite differences in residual AHI.[48] This outcome, however, is from a single observational study. More longitudinal studies with better methodology are needed to answer key questions on cardiovascular morbidity and mortality outcomes.[46,48]

ORAL APPLIANCE ADVERSE EFFECTS

Similar to efficacy, adverse side effects have a dose-dependent relationship with protrusion.[29] A balance must be struck between efficacy and side effects because more adverse effects reduce long-term compliance,[35,49] resulting in patients terminating MAD therapy.[50,51] Most adverse effects caused by MADs are mild and transient, occur during the initial phase of therapy, and tend to resolve with time.[51,52]

Dental Effects

Long-term use of OAs leads to occlusal changes. A meta-analysis reported a significant increase in lower incisor inclination by 2.07°, resulting in 0.99-mm decrease in overjet (OJ) and 1.0-mm decrease in overbite (OB). A greater decrease in OJ and OB was associated with longer treatment. There was no significant change in the upper incisor inclination or interincisal angle.[53]

Due to the lower incisor inclination change and attendant decrease in OJ and OB, there was significant increase in anterior crossbites,[54] increase in mandibular arch width, and reduction in lower arch crowding.[54,55] Maxillary arch width increase and upper arch decrowding also have been reported.[55] A decrease in posterior occlusal contacts[54,56–58] may result in a transient difficulty with chewing.[51] Although the magnitude of dental changes are small, they may be significant to patient perception of developing dental malocclusion.[59]

Craniofacial Changes

A meta-analysis of skeletal changes from MAD use reported no significant skeletal changes.[53] Other investigators, however, report significant increase in lower and total anterior facial height from long-term MAD use of more than 2 years.[60,61]

Temporomandibular Joint Disorders

Transient muscle soreness and temporomandibular joint (TMJ) discomfort have been reported after MAD use, especially during the initial titration period.[3,51] A 5-year follow-up study of MAD patients found mild, temporary subjective side effects, such as muscular or TMJ discomfort, but no changes in temporomandibular disorder prevalence using the Research Diagnostic Criteria for Temporomandibular Disorders.[57]

Other Effects

Other MAD side effects include increased salivation, more frequent and excessive dry mouth, tongue discomfort, and a sense of suffocation.[3,35,51] TSD side effects include excess salivation, drooling, dry mouth, and soft tissue irritation.[3]

PREDICTING AND IMPROVING ORAL APPLIANCE TREATMENT RESPONSE

Although most patients show an increased airway CSA with mandibular advancement, a minority of patients show no change or even a decreased CSA.[9,12] MAD is a primarily structural treatment[9] for a heterogeneous condition with nonanatomic etiology in up to 56% of patients.[62,63] Consequently, MAD treatment completely resolves AHI to fewer than 5 events per hour in only 36% to 70% of OSA patients.[24,38] Patients of female gender, younger age, smaller neck circumference, lower body mass index, lower AHI, and supine-dependent OSA are predicted to have better treatment success with MADs.[38,50,64,65] For TSDs, the best predictor of success is believed to be the presence of a single-site airway obstruction in supine-dependent OSA.[1]

There is currently no validated clinical method to reliably differentiate responders from nonresponders.[24] Uncertainty of MAD treatment response is exacerbated by cost of treatment.[66] The literature lacks consensus in successful treatment outcome, with a majority of success criteria used in research not meshing with clinical definitions of OSA severity. Discordant success criteria makes comparing results of different studies difficult.[67] Prospective trials are under way to determine predictive potential of wakeful nasoendoscopy with Müller maneuver, drug-induced sleep endoscopy (DISE), and computational fluid dynamics.[68,69] In the meantime, careful diagnosis and patient selection can increase the chances of success.

Cephalometry

Classically, shorter soft palate length, larger retropalatal airway space, lower hyoid bone position, and a smaller mandible are associated with favorable MAD treatment response.[1,65] Two recent systematic reviews,[70,71] however, exploring cephalometric predictors for MAD response found a majority of observational studies on cephalometric predictors had flawed designs and failed to control for known confounding factors such as age, gender, body mass index, and baseline AHI. Definitions of treatment success were inconsistent, and heterogeneity in design prevented data synthesis and meta-analysis. Cephalometric parameters warranting further study included mandibular plane angle, hyoid to mandibular plane distance, and soft palate length.

Mandibular Advancement Device Design

Customized versus noncustomized

Both customized and noncustomized MADs reduce AHI in adult patients with OSA, but meta-analysis by the AASM/AADSM task force shows the improvements to be far greater in customized than noncustomized, with an AHI reduction of 13.89 events compared with 6.28 events per hour.[4] Noncustomized MADs do not improve minimum Sao_2, whereas customized MADs increase Sao_2 by 3.22%.[4] They also do not reduce ESS scores to any significant level,[72] whereas modest improvements in ESS scores can be expected from customized MADs.[4]

Titratable versus nontitratable

Both custom titratable and custom nontitratable MADs reduce AHI, improve Sao_2 and reduce ESS scores, with meta-analyses by the AASM/AADSM task force showing the improvements to be approximately equivalent. Titratable MADs are recommended, however, over nontitratable MADs because the confidence interval for the effect of custom, titratable MADs is considerably smaller than for custom, nontitratable MADs.[4]

Due to dose-dependent effects, a clinical titration can improve MAD response and increase the amount of achievable protrusion. This is only possible with titratable MADs.[27]

Therapeutic Diagnosis

Visualizing airway response

Treatment response to MAD can be estimated by visualizing airway response to mandibular protrusion or tongue thrust with nasoendoscopy or MRI in awake supine patients, or in patients using DISE. An increase in velopharyngeal CSA with mandibular advancement was significantly associated with greater AHI reduction with MADs.[8,9,73,74] This was not fully predictive, however, with some patients without velopharyngeal widening showing high AHI reductions and vice versa.[2,73]

Müller maneuver during nasoendoscopy induced significantly greater collapse in velopharyngeal and oropharyngeal CSA in MAD nonresponders than responders. With mandibular advancement, Müller maneuver induced a significantly greater collapse at all airway levels in nonresponders.[8]

On MRI, TSD responders showed a greater increase with TSD in AP diameter, minimum and mean CSA, and volume compared with nonresponders.[2]

Mandibular advancement device titration using polysomnography

Due to the dose-dependent relationship between efficacy and protrusion, increasing protrusion can increase treatment response in OSA patients. Conventional titration protocols use subjective symptoms to adjust mandibular advancement over several months and an outcome polysomnography (PSG) to confirm efficacy. There is no consensus, however, on an optimal titration protocol.[67]

Manually increasing MAD advancement during overnight PSG can increase therapeutic efficacy of mandibular protrusion while reducing the number of titration visits required by most therapeutic protocols. After a clinical titration period, overnight MAD titration with PSG using the final MAD increased treatment response by an additional

9.9% to 30.4% of study subjects.[28,75] Disappointing outcomes were reported, however, using an interim MAD without a period of clinical titration because efficacy of the interim MAD was not translated to the final MAD.[76]

Overnight MAD titration with PSG may require large single-night mandibular advancements to relieve respiratory events, in contrast to slow titration with conventional protocols. Significant jaw discomfort was noted with PSG titration without prior MAD use[76] but was not reported by patients who had an adaptation period with conventional clinical MAD titration.[28]

Remote-controlled mandibular positioners

Using remote-controlled mandibular positioners (RCMPs) for single-night titration of MADs is similar to overnight MAD titration with PSG, with the advantage of adjustment done remotely without waking the patient or removing the appliance. Sleep architecture is maintained while protruding the mandible progressively until respiratory events are eliminated.[26,77–80]

RCMPs can determine an effective target protrusion that is correlated with successful MAD treatment, may be able to identify nonresponders early, and reduce the number of titration reviews needed compared with conventional titration protocols.[81] RCMP titration, however, necessitates large single-night mandibular advancements, which can cause significant jaw discomfort.[26]

Combination Therapy

Mandibular advancement device and tongue-stabilizing devices

Because TSDs have somewhat different anatomic effects on the airway compared with MADs,[2] combining the therapies using a novel hybrid appliance resulted in augmentative treatment effects. Tongue suction with 6 mm mandibular protrusion produced better treatment response than 8 mm mandibular protrusion alone.[30] Combination therapy might improve OA treatment response and prove useful in patients with limited mandibular protrusion.

Mandibular advancement device and continuous positive airway pressure

Combining MAD and CPAP lowered the therapeutic CPAP pressure.[82–85] An augmentative treatment effect on reducing AHI was found in patients not responding to CPAP or MAD use alone.[82–84]

PRACTICE RECOMMENDATIONS
Indications

OAs in the form of MADs can be used as an alternative for patients of all OSA severities who are intolerant of CPAP or prefer an alternative therapy.[4]

Contraindications

Patients who are generally unsuitable for MAD treatment include edentulous patients and patients with inadequate number of sound teeth, severe periodontitis, and/or history of TMJ disease. There are exceptions, and MADs can sometimes be worn successfully by edentulous patients with good dentoalveolar ridges.[1] TSDs are not dependent on the dentition for retention and can be prescribed for edentulous or insufficiently dentate patients.

Appliance Selection

A plethora of designs is currently in use.[86] Based on current evidence, customized, titratable MADs are the preferred form of OAs.[4] TSDs can be used in MAD nonresponders who want OA therapy.

Clinical Follow-up

Trained dentists in sleep practice should follow-up patients using MADs to reduce dental side effects and occlusal changes.[4] Initial side effects are transient and reversible.[51,52] Close monitoring and coaching through the initial period may improve compliance.[35,50,51]

For initial comfort, mandibular advancement is 75% of maximum protrusion.[1] Clinical titration with an adaptation period increases the achievable protrusion and improves treatment response.[27]

Clinical titration should be followed by overnight PSG. Subjective feedback is not sufficient to determine the optimal setting of MAD. Post-PSG titration has been shown to improve MAD efficacy significantly.[4,28,75]

REFERENCES

1. Yow M, Lye EKW. Obstructive sleep apnea: orthodontic startegies to establish and maintain a patent airway. In: Krishnan V, Davidovitch Z, editors. Integrated clinical orthodontics. 1st edition. New Jersey (USA): Wiley-Blackwell Publishing Ltd; 2012. p. 214–39.
2. Sutherland K, Deane SA, Chan AS, et al. Comparative effects of two oral appliances on upper airway structure in obstructive sleep apnea. Sleep 2011; 34(4):469–77.
3. Deane SA, Cistulli PA, Ng AT, et al. Comparison of mandibular advancement splint and tongue stabilizing device in obstructive sleep apnea: a randomized controlled trial. Sleep 2009;32(5):648–53.

4. Ramar K, Dort LC, Katz SG, et al. Clinical practice guideline for the treatment of obstructive sleep apnea and snoring with oral appliance therapy: an update for 2015. J Clin Sleep Med 2015;11(7): 773–827.

5. Chang ET, Fernandez-Salvador C, Giambo J, et al. Tongue retaining devices for obstructive sleep apnea: a systematic review and meta-analysis. Am J Otolaryngol 2017;38(3):272–8.

6. Ishida M, Inoue Y, Suto Y, et al. Mechanism of action and therapeutic indication of prosthetic mandibular advancement in obstructive sleep apnea syndrome. Psychiatry Clin Neurosci 1998;52(2):227–9.

7. Ryan CF, Love LL, Peat D, et al. Mandibular advancement oral appliance therapy for obstructive sleep apnoea: effect on awake calibre of the velopharynx. Thorax 1999;54(11):972–7.

8. Chan AS, Lee RW, Srinivasan VK, et al. Nasopharyngoscopic evaluation of oral appliance therapy for obstructive sleep apnoea. Eur Respir J 2010; 35(4):836–42.

9. Chan AS, Sutherland K, Schwab RJ, et al. The effect of mandibular advancement on upper airway structure in obstructive sleep apnoea. Thorax 2010; 65(8):726–32.

10. Kato J, Isono S, Tanaka A, et al. Dose-dependent effects of mandibular advancement on pharyngeal mechanics and nocturnal oxygenation in patients with sleep-disordered breathing. Chest 2000; 117(4):1065–72.

11. Kuna ST, Woodson LC, Solanki DR, et al. Effect of progressive mandibular advancement on pharyngeal airway size in anesthetized adults. Anesthesiology 2008;109(4):605–12.

12. Choi JK, Hur YK, Lee JM, et al. Effects of mandibular advancement on upper airway dimension and collapsibility in patients with obstructive sleep apnea using dynamic upper airway imaging during sleep. Oral Surg Oral Med Oral Pathol Oral Radiol Endod 2010;109(5):712–9.

13. Brown EC, Cheng S, McKenzie DK, et al. Tongue and lateral upper airway movement with mandibular advancement. Sleep 2013;36(3):397–404.

14. Isono S, Tanaka A, Sho Y, et al. Advancement of the mandible improves velopharyngeal airway patency. J Appl Physiol (1985) 1995;79(6):2132–8.

15. Isono S, Tanaka A, Tagaito Y, et al. Pharyngeal patency in response to advancement of the mandible in obese anesthetized persons. Anesthesiology 1997;87(5):1055–62.

16. Pae EK, Lowe AA, Fleetham JA. A role of pharyngeal length in obstructive sleep apnea patients. Am J Orthod Dentofacial Orthop 1997;111(1):12–7.

17. Yoshida K. Effect of a prosthetic appliance for treatment of sleep apnea syndrome on masticatory and tongue muscle activity. J Prosthet Dent 1998;79(5): 537–44.

18. Johal A, Gill G, Ferman A, et al. The effect of mandibular advancement appliances on awake upper airway and masticatory muscle activity in patients with obstructive sleep apnoea. Clin Physiol Funct Imaging 2007;27(1):47–53.

19. Kurtulmus H, Cotert S, Bilgen C, et al. The effect of a mandibular advancement splint on electromyographic activity of the submental and masseter muscles in patients with obstructive sleep apnea. Int J Prosthodont 2009;22(6):586–93.

20. Malhotra A, Huang Y, Fogel RB, et al. The male predisposition to pharyngeal collapse: importance of airway length. Am J Respir Crit Care Med 2002; 166(10):1388–95.

21. Ng AT, Gotsopoulos H, Qian J, et al. Effect of oral appliance therapy on upper airway collapsibility in obstructive sleep apnea. Am J Respir Crit Care Med 2003;168(2):238–41.

22. Kushida CA, Morgenthaler TI, Littner MR, et al. Practice parameters for the treatment of snoring and Obstructive Sleep Apnea with oral appliances: an update for 2005. Sleep 2006;29(2):240–3.

23. Practice parameters for the treatment of snoring and obstructive sleep apnea with oral appliances. American Sleep Disorders Association. Sleep 1995;18(6):511–3.

24. Sutherland K, Vanderveken OM, Tsuda H, et al. Oral appliance treatment for obstructive sleep apnea: an update. J Clin Sleep Med 2014;10(2):215–27.

25. Raphaelson MA, Alpher EJ, Bakker KW, et al. Oral appliance therapy for obstructive sleep apnea syndrome: progressive mandibular advancement during polysomnography. Cranio 1998;16(1):44–50.

26. Tsai WH, Vazquez JC, Oshima T, et al. Remotely controlled mandibular positioner predicts efficacy of oral appliances in sleep apnea. Am J Respir Crit Care Med 2004;170(4):366–70.

27. Gindre L, Gagnadoux F, Meslier N, et al. Mandibular advancement for obstructive sleep apnea: dose effect on apnea, long-term use and tolerance. Respiration 2008;76(4):386–92.

28. Almeida FR, Parker JA, Hodges JS, et al. Effect of a titration polysomnogram on treatment success with a mandibular repositioning appliance. J Clin Sleep Med 2009;5(3):198–204.

29. Aarab G, Lobbezoo F, Hamburger HL, et al. Effects of an oral appliance with different mandibular protrusion positions at a constant vertical dimension on obstructive sleep apnea. Clin Oral Investig 2010; 14(3):339–45.

30. Dort L, Remmers J. A combination appliance for obstructive sleep apnea: the effectiveness of mandibular advancement and tongue retention. J Clin Sleep Med 2012;8(3):265–9.

31. Giles TL, Lasserson TJ, Smith BH, et al. Continuous positive airways pressure for obstructive sleep apnoea in adults. Cochrane Database Syst Rev 2006;(3):CD001106.

32. Lim J, Lasserson TJ, Fleetham J, et al. Oral appliances for obstructive sleep apnoea. Cochrane Database Syst Rev 2006;(1):CD004435.

33. Schwartz M, Acosta L, Hung YL, et al. Effects of CPAP and mandibular advancement device treatment in obstructive sleep apnea patients: a systematic review and meta-analysis. Sleep Breath 2018; 22(3):555–68.

34. Zhang M, Liu Y, Liu Y, et al. Effectiveness of oral appliances versus continuous positive airway pressure in treatment of OSA patients: an updated meta-analysis. Cranio 2018;1–18.

35. Dieltjens M, Verbruggen AE, Braem MJ, et al. Determinants of objective compliance during oral appliance therapy in patients with sleep-disordered breathing: a prospective clinical trial. JAMA Otolaryngol Head Neck Surg 2015;141(10):894–900.

36. Vanderveken OM, Dieltjens M, Wouters K, et al. Objective measurement of compliance during oral appliance therapy for sleep-disordered breathing. Thorax 2013;68(1):91–6.

37. Sutherland K, Phillips CL, Cistulli PA. Efficacy versus effectiveness in the treatment of obstructive sleep apnea: CPAP and oral appliances. J Dent Sleep Med 2015;2(4):175–81.

38. Lettieri CJ, Almeida FR, Cistulli PA, et al. Oral appliances for the treatment of obstructive sleep apnea-hypopnea syndrome and for concomitant sleep bruxism. In: MH K, T R, WC D, editors. Principles and practice of sleep medicine. 6th edition. Philadelphia: Elsevier; 2017. p. 1445–57.

39. Ahrens A, McGrath C, Hagg U. Subjective efficacy of oral appliance design features in the management of obstructive sleep apnea: a systematic review. Am J Orthod Dentofacial Orthop 2010;138(5): 559–76.

40. Bratton DJ, Gaisl T, Schlatzer C, et al. Comparison of the effects of continuous positive airway pressure and mandibular advancement devices on sleepiness in patients with obstructive sleep apnoea: a network meta-analysis. Lancet Respir Med 2015; 3(11):869–78.

41. Ng A, Gotsopoulos H, Darendeliler AM, et al. Oral appliance therapy for obstructive sleep apnea. Treat Respir Med 2005;4(6):409–22.

42. Blanco J, Zamarron C, Abeleira Pazos MT, et al. Prospective evaluation of an oral appliance in the treatment of obstructive sleep apnea syndrome. Sleep Breath 2005;9(1):20–5.

43. Gauthier L, Laberge L, Beaudry M, et al. Efficacy of two mandibular advancement appliances in the management of snoring and mild-moderate sleep apnea: a cross-over randomized study. Sleep Med 2009;10(3):329–36.

44. Kuhn E, Schwarz EI, Bratton DJ, et al. Effects of CPAP and mandibular advancement devices on

45. Bratton DJ, Gaisl T, Wons AM, et al. CPAP vs mandibular advancement devices and blood pressure in patients with obstructive sleep apnea: a systematic review and meta-analysis. Jama 2015; 314(21):2280–93.

46. de Vries GE, Wijkstra PJ, Houwerzijl EJ, et al. Cardiovascular effects of oral appliance therapy in obstructive sleep apnea: a systematic review and meta-analysis. Sleep Med Rev 2018;40:55–68.

47. Van Haesendonck G, Dieltjens M, Kastoer C, et al. Cardiovascular benefits of oral appliance therapy in obstructive sleep apnea: a systematic review. J Dent Sleep Med 2015;2(1):9–14.

48. Anandam A, Patil M, Akinnusi M, et al. Cardiovascular mortality in obstructive sleep apnoea treated with continuous positive airway pressure or oral appliance: an observational study. Respirology 2013; 18(8):1184–90.

49. Attali V, Chaumereuil C, Arnulf I, et al. Predictors of long-term effectiveness to mandibular repositioning device treatment in obstructive sleep apnea patients after 1000 days. Sleep Med 2016;27-28:107–14.

50. Marklund M, Stenlund H, Franklin KA. Mandibular advancement devices in 630 men and women with obstructive sleep apnea and snoring: tolerability and predictors of treatment success. Chest 2004; 125(4):1270–8.

51. de Almeida FR, Lowe AA, Tsuiki S, et al. Long-term compliance and side effects of oral appliances used for the treatment of snoring and obstructive sleep apnea syndrome. J Clin Sleep Med 2005; 1(2):143–52.

52. Ferguson KA, Cartwright R, Rogers R, et al. Oral appliances for snoring and obstructive sleep apnea: a review. Sleep 2006;29(2):244–62.

53. Araie T, Okuno K, Ono Minagi H, et al. Dental and skeletal changes associated with long-term oral appliance use for obstructive sleep apnea: a systematic review and meta-analysis. Sleep Med Rev 2018;41:161–72.

54. Pliska BT, Nam H, Chen H, et al. Obstructive sleep apnea and mandibular advancement splints: occlusal effects and progression of changes associated with a decade of treatment. J Clin Sleep Med 2014;10(12):1285–91.

55. Chen H, Lowe AA, de Almeida FR, et al. Three-dimensional computer-assisted study model analysis of long-term oral-appliance wear. Part 2. Side effects of oral appliances in obstructive sleep apnea patients. Am J Orthod Dentofacial Orthop 2008; 134(3):408–17.

56. Otsuka R, Almeida FR, Lowe AA. The effects of oral appliance therapy on occlusal function in patients with obstructive sleep apnea: a short-term

prospective study. Am J Orthod Dentofacial Orthop 2007;131(2):176–83.

57. Martinez-Gomis J, Willaert E, Nogues L, et al. Five years of sleep apnea treatment with a mandibular advancement device. Side effects and technical complications. Angle Orthod 2010;80(1):30–6.

58. Fransson AMC, Kowalczyk A, Isacsson G. A prospective 10-year follow-up dental cast study of patients with obstructive sleep apnoea/snoring who use a mandibular protruding device. Eur J Orthod 2017;39(5):502–8.

59. Alessandri-Bonetti G, D'Anto V, Stipa C, et al. Dentoskeletal effects of oral appliance wear in obstructive sleep apnoea and snoring patients. Eur J Orthod 2017;39(5):482–8.

60. Almeida FR, Lowe AA, Sung JO, et al. Long-term sequellae of oral appliance therapy in obstructive sleep apnea patients: Part 1. Cephalometric analysis. Am J Orthod Dentofacial Orthop 2006;129(2):195–204.

61. Doff MH, Hoekema A, Pruim GJ, et al. Long-term oral-appliance therapy in obstructive sleep apnea: a cephalometric study of craniofacial changes. J Dent 2010;38(12):1010–8.

62. Eckert DJ, White DP, Jordan AS, et al. Defining phenotypic causes of obstructive sleep apnea. Identification of novel therapeutic targets. Am J Respir Crit Care Med 2013;188(8):996–1004.

63. Edwards BA, Eckert DJ, Jordan AS. Obstructive sleep apnoea pathogenesis from mild to severe: is it all the same? Respirology 2017;22(1):33–42.

64. Liu Y, Lowe AA, Fleetham JA, et al. Cephalometric and physiologic predictors of the efficacy of an adjustable oral appliance for treating obstructive sleep apnea. Am J Orthod Dentofacial Orthop 2001;120(6):639–47.

65. Okuno K, Pliska BT, Hamoda M, et al. Prediction of oral appliance treatment outcomes in obstructive sleep apnea: a systematic review. Sleep Med Rev 2016;30:25–33.

66. American Sleep Assocociation | sleep apnea oral appliances - research & treatments | 2018. Available at: https://www.sleepassociation.org/sleep-disorders/sleep-apnea/oral-appliance-for-sleep-apnea/. Accessed July 22, 2018.

67. Dieltjens M, Vanderveken OM, Heyning PH, et al. Current opinions and clinical practice in the titration of oral appliances in the treatment of sleep-disordered breathing. Sleep Med Rev 2012;16(2):177–85.

68. Verbruggen AE, Vroegop AV, Dieltjens M, et al. Predicting Therapeutic Outcome of Mandibular Advancement Device Treatment in Obstructive Sleep Apnoea (PROMAD): study design and baseline characteristics. J Dent Sleep Med 2016;3(4):119–38.

69. National Institutes of Health, United States National Library of Medicine, ClinicalTrials.gov. 2018. Available at: https://clinicaltrials.gov/ct2/show/record/NCT01532050. Accessed 26 July, 2018.

70. Alessandri-Bonetti G, Ippolito DR, Bartolucci ML, et al. Cephalometric predictors of treatment outcome with mandibular advancement devices in adult patients with obstructive sleep apnea: a systematic review. Korean J Orthod 2015;45(6):308–21.

71. Guarda-Nardini L, Manfredini D, Mion M, et al. Anatomically based outcome predictors of treatment for obstructive sleep apnea with intraoral splint devices: a systematic review of cephalometric studies. J Clin Sleep Med 2015;11(11):1327–34.

72. Vanderveken OM, Devolder A, Marklund M, et al. Comparison of a custom-made and a thermoplastic oral appliance for the treatment of mild sleep apnea. Am J Respir Crit Care Med 2008;178(2):197–202.

73. Sasao Y, Nohara K, Okuno K, et al. Videoendoscopic diagnosis for predicting the response to oral appliance therapy in severe obstructive sleep apnea. Sleep Breath 2014;18(4):809–15.

74. Vroegop AV, Vanderveken OM, Dieltjens M, et al. Sleep endoscopy with simulation bite for prediction of oral appliance treatment outcome. J Sleep Res 2013;22(3):348–55.

75. Krishnan V, Collop NA, Scherr SC. An evaluation of a titration strategy for prescription of oral appliances for obstructive sleep apnea. Chest 2008;133(5):1135–41.

76. Kuna ST, Giarraputo PC, Stanton DC, et al. Evaluation of an oral mandibular advancement titration appliance. Oral Surg Oral Med Oral Pathol Oral Radiol Endod 2006;101(5):593–603.

77. Petelle B, Vincent G, Gagnadoux F, et al. One-night mandibular advancement titration for obstructive sleep apnea syndrome: a pilot study. Am J Respir Crit Care Med 2002;165(8):1150–3.

78. Dort LC, Hadjuk E, Remmers JE. Mandibular advancement and obstructive sleep apnoea: a method for determining effective mandibular protrusion. Eur Respir J 2006;27(5):1003–9.

79. Remmers J, Charkhandeh S, Grosse J, et al. Remotely controlled mandibular protrusion during sleep predicts therapeutic success with oral appliances in patients with obstructive sleep apnea. Sleep 2013;36(10):1517–25, 1525A.

80. Sutherland K, Ngiam J, Cistulli PA. Performance of remotely controlled mandibular protrusion sleep studies for prediction of oral appliance treatment response. J Clin Sleep Med 2017;13(3):411–7.

81. Kastoer C, Dieltjens M, Oorts E, et al. The use of remotely controlled mandibular positioner as a predictive screening tool for mandibular advancement device therapy in patients with obstructive sleep apnea through single-night progressive titration of the

mandible: a systematic review. J Clin Sleep Med 2016;12(10):1411–21.

82. Denbar MA. A case study involving the combination treatment of an oral appliance and auto-titrating CPAP unit. Sleep Breath 2002;6(3):125–8.

83. El-Solh AA, Moitheennazima B, Akinnusi ME, et al. Combined oral appliance and positive airway pressure therapy for obstructive sleep apnea: a pilot study. Sleep Breath 2011;15(2):203–8.

84. Liu HW, Chen YJ, Lai YC, et al. Combining MAD and CPAP as an effective strategy for treating patients with severe sleep apnea intolerant to high-pressure PAP and unresponsive to MAD. PLoS One 2017; 12(10):e0187032.

85. de Vries GE, Doff MHJ, Hoekema A, et al. Continuous positive airway pressure and oral appliance hybrid therapy in obstructive sleep apnea: patient comfort, compliance, and preference: a pilot study. J Dent Sleep Med 2016;3(1):5–10.

86. Yow M. An overview of oral appliances and managing the airway in obstructive sleep apnea. Semin Orthod 2009;15(2):88–93.

Avoiding and Managing Oral Appliance Therapy Side Effects

Thomas G. Schell, DMD, DABDSM[a,b,*]

KEYWORDS

- Oral appliance therapy • Side effects of OAT • Obstructive sleep apnea • Dental sleep medicine

KEY POINTS

- There is a serious need to consider all potential side effects thoughtfully before commencing individual treatment.
- Although many of these side effects are self-limiting, easily corrected, or innocuous, others are difficult or impossible to correct and can affect the patient in some serious ways.
- If alternative treatment is not acceptable, the carefully weighed risk of no therapy is what allows practitioners to justify these likely problems to coexist with oral appliance therapy.
- As this field evolves, new information is discovered, and new products are introduced at a rather rapid pace, continuing education and prudent practice are critical to ethical care in the practice of dental sleep medicine.

INTRODUCTION

Oral appliance therapy (OAT) is being used more frequently in the management of obstructive sleep apnea (OSA) as an alternative to continuous positive air pressure. As the frequency of OAT use is increasingly more popular and as more patients are consistently adherent to it over longer periods of time, side effects from this therapy are becoming more clinically evident in both frequency and magnitude.

A *side effect* for the purpose of this article represents any untoward or unexpected outcome; one not intended and quite possibly, but not always having a deleterious effect. Side effects from OAT are common and expectable. The extent to which a side effect is intolerable to a patient is a very individual concern and will vary greatly between patients. One patient's limit for an intolerable bite change may well be within the tolerable range for another. All risks of potential side effects should be weighed against the risks of no therapy, provided no alternative treatment is acceptable.

It is critical for providers to get a broad-reaching and objective range of education in this field before commencing in the practice of dental sleep medicine (DSM). Having an understanding of the number of different side effects that potentially occur from OAT use and their ability to affect the patient in many different ways is critically important. Regular ongoing continuing education in an effort to remain abreast of the constantly evolving changes in this field is essential to be able to predict, prevent, and manage these side effects when they do occur.

There has traditionally been a large gap in knowledge regarding side effects from OAT. Most evidence is anecdotal. What limited research exists on this topic can be difficult to locate, understand, and apply in clinical practice for an average

This article originally appeared in December, 2018 issue of *Sleep Medicine Clinics* (Volume 13, Issue 4).
No conflict of interest or funding sources to disclose.
[a] Dr Thomas G Schell and Dr. Patrick C Noble PLLC, 31 Old Etna Road, N1 Lebanon, NH 03770, USA;
[b] Department of Surgery, Dartmouth Geisel School of Medicine, 1 Rope Ferry Road, Hanover, NH 03755-1404, USA
* PO Box 127, Meriden, NH 03770.
E-mail address: tgschell@gmail.com

Sleep Med Clin 15 (2020) 251–260
https://doi.org/10.1016/j.jsmc.2020.02.011
1556-407X/20/© 2020 Elsevier Inc. All rights reserved.

practitioner. Although many of these side effects are self-limiting, easily corrected, or innocuous, others are difficult or impossible to correct and can affect the patient in some serious ways.

Recently, in an effort to bridge this informational gap, a panel of experts was convened by the American Academy of Dental Sleep Medicine (AADSM) Board of Directors to look at side effects from OAT and their management. Until that time, there had not been an analysis performed with recommendations to detail these issues for clinicians. As a key preliminary part of this process, an exhaustive literature review was performed. In addition, a comprehensive survey of a large number of highly regarded providers in the field was conducted. All of this informational data were carefully analyzed. The panel was able to identify and differentiate these various side effects as well as come to agreement on the most appropriate management of each. The consensus article was published in the October 10, 2017, issue of the *Journal of Dental Sleep Medicine*.[1]

This publication represented the first thorough set of clinical guidelines specifically related to side effects and their management. It was put forth to act as a useful reference tool for practitioners and researchers seeking guidance on the management of these issues in the clinical setting. Until such time as we can turn solely to empirical evidence on side effects, any consideration of these issues should rely on the findings of the experts' conference. This article refers to it as the standard of reference to date.

THE SIDE EFFECTS CONSENSUS CONFERENCE: OVERVIEW

Experts from across the field of DSM were selected to act as voting members on a consensus panel using the UCLA/RAND appropriateness of care method. The selected 13-member panel consisted of dentists chosen with specific intention toward their proper protocol for diagnosis, application of treatment, and follow-up of DSM as well as for their experience in temporomandibular joint (TMJ), occlusion and oral health in general.

As an initial part of the process, an exhaustive literature search and review was performed to seek all published evidence of side effects for consideration. This search resulted in 181 articles published through February 2016. A total of 143 of these were subsequently chosen to be included in the study. In addition, a rather detailed survey of the diplomats of the American Board of Dental Sleep Medicine as well as AADSM committee members was performed to seek out side effects

as they presented in clinical experience for review as well. Fifty-one percent of these surveys were returned and reviewed by the panel in addition to the literature.

With the raw data from the literature and the survey at hand, the panel was then able to consolidate the side effects into 5 categories: (1) TMJ issues, (2) problems with intraoral tissues, (3) changes in occlusion, (4) damage to teeth or restorations, and (5) various other appliance issues.

Voting on the appropriateness of each side-effect treatment within each category was accomplished anonymously via e-mail and then again after the careful review of evidence in 2 additional rounds of voting at the face-to-face conference. The RAND process definitively defines the level of agreement on each item under consideration. Only those treatments clearly deemed appropriate after review of the literature and survey results were retained for additional voting and inclusion in the final recommendations. Any treatments deemed either inappropriate or uncertain were dropped from consideration. The final vote was to qualitatively define whether each treatment represented should be considered primarily, as a second-line option, or whether it was uncommon, but still merited appropriate consideration for use by practitioners.

These methodically established recommendations were then endorsed by the AADSM Board of Directors for publication in the *Journal of Dental Sleep Medicine*. It was noted that this should not be considered an exhaustive list of choices in the management of side effects. While addressing the breadth of common side effects and their management, these recommendations should also be used with clinical expertise and judgment gained through rigorous training in DSM. These can then be adapted in the most appropriate and specific way for any given patient and situation.

CONSENT

As with any medical procedure that carries some risk for unexpected or untoward results, a detailed informed consent process is critical to ensuring both proper education to the patient and protection for the practitioner. Written informed consents should be both easy to read and understand by the average patient population. This also must be detailed enough to not miss the significant risk associated with any unwanted side effects. Most experienced practitioners will inform their patients that they will likely experience some side effects. It is the degree to which they can be tolerated that should be weighed against alternative treatment or the risk of no treatment at all. These written informed consent documents should be explained verbally and signed with a witness before beginning any treatment. One popular site in the marketplace offers 36 specific informed consent, informed-refusal, and release-of-liability documents for practitioners providing OAT; this implies the broad-reaching significance of these concerns.

PRETREATMENT RECORDS

To identify and be able to measure any side effects, it is necessary that each practitioner gather detailed pretreatment records of the patient in both anatomic position and function. This would take the form of (but is not necessarily limited to) cast models, photos of the patient's occlusion in habitual position, and a physical bite record. Additionally, pretreatment measurements of overjet and overbite, interproximal contacts, and interocclusal contacts using thin shim stock would be important to have on record in any ongoing evaluation of potential changes. Finally, pretreatment assessment of the TMJ and muscles of the head and neck as well as the periodontium also should be recorded. These can include records of maximum interincisal opening, both lateral and anterior excursion, as well as qualitative objective evaluation of the joint using visual and bimanual palpation. Audio analysis can be useful as well, using stethoscope and/or Doppler ultrasound. Deviations or shifts in both the path of opening and closing, carefully noting any clicks, pops, and crepitus also can be helpful if evaluating changes in comfort or function during treatment. Preoperative radiographic imaging of the TMJ is also important as a tool to rule out disease and potentially uncover any pathologic change over the course of treatment.

RECALL AND FOLLOW-UP

It is very important to discover progressive side effects early to have the best chance to correct them, or at least to limit their negative effect. This requires early and frequent recall initially and regular follow-up thereafter; on a frequency of at least once per year unless there have been signs of changes that would warrant more frequent evaluation. Any side effect encountered must be detailed in its effect, its management, and throughout its resolution. Here is where baseline records are indispensable. Any side effect must be immediately disclosed to the patient and a detailed discussion of all conceivable consequences of such a change take place. If the decision is made with the patient to discontinue OAT, then alternative treatment options should then be discussed with the patient and documented. In this instance, communication with, and referral back to the managing physician is necessary to be sure that the patient does not go without care. This also needs to be documented in the patient record.

The various different side effects identified by the panelists at the consensus conference are listed in **Box 1**. These side effects were each defined and management protocol was explained for each in the publication.

In addition to the specific management plan recommended by the experts, there were a number of common management considerations that had a

---

Box 1
Side effects

Temporomandibular joint–related side effects
- Transient morning jaw pain
- Persistent temporomandibular joint pain
- Tenderness in muscles of mastication
- Joint sounds

Intraoral tissue–related side effects
- Soft tissue and tongue irritation
- Gingival irritation
- Excessive salivation/drooling
- Dry mouth

Occlusal changes
- Altered occlusal contacts/bite changes
- Incisor changes
- Decreased overjet and overbite
- Alterations in positions of mandibular canines and molars
- Interproximal gaps

Damage to teeth or restorations
- Tooth mobility
- Tooth fractures or damage to dental restorations

Appliance issues
- Appliance breakage
- Allergies to appliance material
- Gagging
- Anxiety

From Sheats RD, Schell TG, Blanton AO, et al. Management of side effects of oral appliance therapy for sleep disordered breathing. J Dent Sleep Med 2017;4(4):113; with permission.

broad-reaching application to many if not all of these side effects. These follow here as choices that should be considered in many common circumstances and will be listed out individually again in each of the specific side-effect recommendations where they apply.

COMMON MANAGEMENT CONSIDERATIONS
Palliative Care

"Palliative care is supportive in nature and intended to manage patient discomfort during the healing phase. It may include any/all of the following options: reassurance, rest, ice, soft diet, topical or systemic pain relief products or anti-inflammatory medications, massage, and physiotherapy."[1]

Watchful Waiting

"Watchful waiting is the ongoing process of careful and diligent observation, with the possibility of additional assessment along the way, in an effort to better understand the side-effect process. Documentation of the process must be included in the patient's record and follow-up of concerns at subsequent visits should occur and be recorded regarding persistence, resolution or management of side effects."[1]

Morning Occlusal Guide

"Morning occlusal guide encompasses many custom-made appliances and prefabricated devices used in the effort to reposition the mandible into its habitual pretreatment position. These devices may function by using biting forces to reseat the condyles to help reestablish/maintain the appropriate occlusal relationship in the morning following each night of OAT. Some of these custom devices may function by reversing changes that may have occurred in tooth position or work to exercise or stretch muscles of mastication as well. They are intended to address the occlusal discrepancy noted after removal of the appliance each morning."[1]

"Before the patient begins using the oral appliance, the morning occlusal guide is fabricated chair-side or by a laboratory, and is often made of hard acrylic, thermoplastic, or compressible materials. The guide must be adapted to the patient's maxillary and mandibular teeth in habitual occlusion or to dental casts in maximum intercuspation."[1]

"Intended to address the occlusal discrepancy noted after the removal of the oral appliance each morning, morning occlusal guides also help patients to monitor their condition by allowing them to ascertain whether their mandible is correctly aligned every morning. Each morning after the sleep appliance is worn, the patient should bite into the guide until the maxillary and mandibular teeth are fully seated for as long as it takes the teeth to reestablish occlusion. In the event that the patient is unable to attain proper habitual occlusion, the patient should contact the oral appliance provider."[1]

It is important to note that despite widespread use of morning repositioners or occlusal guides, there is no clinical evidence that links these with any specific success at either preventing or managing side effects of OAT.

Daytime Intraoral Orthotic

"The daytime intraoral orthotic encompasses many custom appliances and prefabricated devices that are retained by either the maxillary or mandibular dentition/implants. These devices are intended to deprogram masticatory muscles, reseat the mandibular condyles, and/or reduce the magnitude and frequency of bruxism events as well as its consequences. Distinctive from the morning occlusal guide, this device is intended for more active therapy of preexisting or iatrogenically created conditions affecting the TMJ or the masticatory musculature."[1]

Verification and/or Correction of Midline Position

"Verification and/or correction of midline position describes an effort to ascertain and maintain the appropriate lateral position of the mandible in its forward position, often similar in lateral dimensions to the nonprotruded (nontreatment) position."[1]

Verification and/or Correction of Occlusion

"Verification and/or correction of occlusion describes an effort to ascertain balanced occlusal forces on the oral appliance both bilaterally and anteriorly-posteriorly. This balance may be altered as the mandible is advanced or as muscles alternatively relax or contract with use. This may encompass consideration of changes to the vertical dimension of the oral appliance."[1]

Habitual Occlusion

"Habitual occlusion refers to the position of closure between the dental arches in which the patient feels the teeth fit most comfortably with minimal feeling of stress in the muscles and joints."[1]

"Note: the term "habitual occlusion" refers to the patient's most comfortable position of jaw closure at any specific time. Many terms have been used to describe the interarch relationship of the maxilla and mandible, often with the intent of providing a reproducible position for restorative purposes. Terms such as centric relation, centric occlusion, maximum intercuspation, bite of convenience, and intercuspation position have also been used. This article favors the term 'habitual occlusion' because as many as 85% of the patients using OAT for more than 5 years demonstrate altered occlusal relationships from baseline."[1,2]

Isometric and Passive Jaw-Stretching Exercises

"Isometric and passive jaw-stretching exercises include instructing patients to move the mandible against resistance both vertically and laterally and to stretch the mandibular range of motion assisted by the fingers, targeting the masticatory muscles. Examples include instructing a patient to move the mandible against gentle resistance both vertically and laterally within their physiologic range of motion and using finger pressure to stretch the lateral pterygoid, temporalis, and master muscles. These have been shown to decrease the level of discomfort and improve adherence to OAT.[3] Duration and frequency of exercises will be dependent on the ease with which the patient is able to reestablish occlusion."[1]

Conservative Titration

"Conservative titration refers to the minimal amount of advancement of the appliance required to manage sleep disordered breathing. Aarab and colleagues[4] demonstrated that the number of side effects increases as protrusion exceeds 50% from baseline. Moreover, research reveals that 50% and 75% protrusion can be equally effective in groups of patients with mild to moderate OSA."[1,5]

SIDE-EFFECT RECOMMENDATIONS
Here Follows the Specific Recommendations of the Consensus Panel Followed by Some Key Bulleted Points for Each

Section 1: temporomandibular joint–related side effects
Care must be taken to differentiate the various different terms used to describe problems with the TMJ and associated musculature by the various different groups of practitioners involved in this field. It is also important to note here that myofascial pain and TMJ degeneration were not discovered in the research evaluated on this topic and were not included as specific side effects under consideration for this reason.

Transient morning jaw pain "Watchful waiting, palliative care, isometric contraction and passive jaw exercise, and decreasing the titration rate are considered first line of treatment to manage transient jaw pain."[1]

- This discomfort is considered mild and transient during the day following the use of OAT
- Usually originating from the muscles of mastication, this is unlikely to cause OAT abandonment
- Conservative titration should be adhered to
- Active surveillance is indicated to rule out pain originating from the joint(s)
- Reassurance, muscle massage, application of heat, and relaxation techniques are suggested[6,7]
- Isometric contraction and jaw exercises have been shown to be effective in relieving muscle discomfort[7]
- Decreasing titration rate may help alleviate symptoms[4]
- If symptoms continue, worsen during the day, last more than a few weeks, or interfere with normal function they should be considered *persistent* (see the next section)

Persistent temporomandibular joint pain " Palliative care, isometric contraction, and passive jaw-stretching exercises, verifying or correcting midline positions, appliance adjustment, decreasing the titration rate, decreasing advancement, and conducting a temporomandibular disorder (TMD) workup and management are considered first line of treatment to manage persistent TMJ pain. Placing posterior stops or anterior discluding elements, decreasing wearing time, and temporarily discontinuing use of OAT are considered second-line treatment. If these treatment options are insufficient or inappropriate, using a daytime intraoral orthotic, prescribing a steroid dose pack, recommending a different oral appliance (OA) design, referring to a dental specialist or additional health care provider, and permanently discontinuing OAT also may be appropriate."[1]

- Conservative titration should be adhered to (see common management techniques)
- Patients should be reassured that both TMJ baseline discomfort and discomfort associated with OA use is likely to decrease with time and continued use of the oral appliance[7–10]
- Proper documentation throughout resolution is important
- Rest, soft diet, and anti-inflammatory medications should be considered

- Isometric contraction and jaw exercises have been shown to be effective in relieving muscle discomfort[7]
- Decreasing the advancement rate may help speed relief of TMJ symptoms, but should be weighed against the decreasing therapeutic effect of the appliance
- In appliances in which there are both left and right advancement mechanisms, ensure that these advancements have been applied in even value
- As mentioned in the consensus paper, "refractory temporomandibular symptoms related to OAT are uncommon"[1]
- Consider an appliance that allows more jaw movement
- Consider placing posterior or anterior acrylic stops
- Decrease the time of appliance wear
- Limited steroid dose pack prescription where indicated
- If the previous items are ineffective or inapplicable, consider discontinuation of OAT; any decision to abandon OAT needs to be done in conjunction with the patient's physician to be sure that replacement therapy is planned

Tenderness in the muscles of mastication " Palliative care, watchful waiting, verifying or correcting midline positions, use of a morning occlusal guide, and isometric contraction and passive jaw-stretching exercises are considered first line of treatment to manage tenderness in the muscles of mastication. Decreasing OA advancement, vertical dimension, and the rate of forward titration; modifying the acrylic; and temporarily discontinuing use of OAT are considered second-line treatments. If these treatment options are insufficient or inappropriate, recommending a different OA design, referring to a dental specialist or additional health care provider, and permanently discontinuing OAT also may be appropriate. In very rare instances, increasing OA advancement may be indicated."[1]

- Muscle massage, application of heat (or ice if inflammation is present)
- Isometric and/or relaxation techniques[7]
- Balance left and right protrusive forces
- Morning occlusal guide
- Conservative titration should be adhered to
- Decrease the rate of titration or overall advancement position; care to balance against the decreasing therapeutic effect[4,11]
- Decrease vertical dimension of appliance
- Allow for more lateral movement of the mandible

- Temporarily discontinue OAT (then potentially restart in a more retruded position and advancing more slowly)
- Rarely, in some specific cases, advancement might achieve better resolution of OSA and quiet muscular activity
- Selective serotonin reuptake inhibitors also have the ability to affect changes on the tonicity of the muscles of mastication. These should be managed in conjunction with the treating physician if they are interfering with the patient's ability to tolerate treatment
- Consider referral to additional medical specialist, including a physical therapist, or a dentist with advanced training in TMD
- If the previous items are ineffective or inapplicable, consider discontinuation of OAT; any decision to abandon OAT needs to be done in conjunction with the patient's physician to be sure that replacement therapy is planned

Joint sounds "Watchful waiting is considered first line of treatment to manage joint sounds caused as a result of using OAs. If these treatment options are insufficient or inappropriate, temporary or permanent discontinuation of the OAT can also be considered as a treatment option."[1]

- These side effects are usually transient and resolve with time
- If these sounds coincide with persistent pain, it may be necessary to abandon OAT; as usual, the practitioner must be certain alternative therapy is planned
- Conservative titration should be adhered to

Section 2: intraoral tissue–related side effects
Soft tissue and tongue irritation "Palliative care and appliance modification are considered first line of treatment to manage soft tissue and tongue irritation side effects. Temporarily discontinuing use of the OA is considered a second-line treatment. If these treatment options are insufficient or inappropriate, orthodontic wax and switching to a different OA design also may be considered appropriate."[1]

- These are most commonly due to mechanical trauma
- Topical agents and/or appliance modifications are suggested
- Consider a switch to different OA design
- If the preceding items are ineffective or inapplicable, consider discontinuation of OAT; any decision to abandon OAT needs to be done in conjunction with the patient's physician to be sure that replacement therapy is planned

Gingival irritation "Modification of the appliance and palliative care are considered first-line treatment to manage gingival irritation. Discontinuing use of OAT temporarily is considered second-line treatment."[1]

- Appliance modifications
- Commonly due to mechanical trauma
- If the previous items are ineffective or inapplicable, consider discontinuation of OAT; any decision to abandon OAT needs to be done in conjunction with the patient's physician to be sure that replacement therapy is planned.

Excessive salivation "Watchful waiting is considered first line of treatment to manage excessive salivation/drooling. Modification to the appliance is considered second-line treatment. If these treatment options are insufficient or inappropriate, prescribing medications to decrease salivary input also may be appropriate."[1]

- Modification to the appliance should be considered after a period of watchful waiting, as this is normal and expectable for the first few weeks.
- This may include, but is not limited to decreasing vertical dimension to allow for better lip seal with the appliance in place.
- Mouth shields and oral obturators can be added to the appliance to help with the oral seal.

Dry mouth "Palliative care, watchful waiting, and decreasing vertical dimension of the device to encourage lip seal, are considered first line of treatment to manage dry mouth. Modification of the appliance and techniques for discouraging mouth breathing are considered second-line treatment. If these treatment options are insufficient or inappropriate, avoiding commercial mouth rinses with alcohol or peroxide, mouth-taping, and referring to an additional health care provider may also be considered appropriate."[1]

- Decreasing the vertical dimension can improve lip seal and discourage mouth breathing
- Ensure adequate hydration
- Limit over-the-counter substances that contribute to dry mouth
- Check with the physician to evaluate prescriptions that might cause xerostomia
- Consult with the otolaryngologist if nasal patency is problematic

Section 3: occlusal changes
Altered occlusal contacts/bite changes "Watchful waiting, jaw-stretching exercises, and use of a morning occlusal guide are considered first line of treatment to manage altered occlusal contacts or bite changes. Chewing hard gum in the mornings and making modifications to the appliance are considered second-line treatment. If these treatment options are insufficient or inappropriate, discontinuing OAT temporarily or permanently may also be appropriate."[1]

- Adhere to conservative titration: greater titration increases the magnitude of force that in turn increases potential side effects[4,12,13]
- Posterior open bites occur commonly[7,14–19]
- Patients easily tolerate these changes and commonly are unaware of them[4,7,16,20,21]
- Morning occlusal guides are recommended
- Jaw-stretching exercises to help reseat the condyle and relieve muscle stiffness[22]
- Modify ill-fitting appliance
- If the previous items are ineffective or inapplicable, consider discontinuation of OAT; any decision to abandon OAT needs to be done in conjunction with the patient's physician to be sure that replacement therapy is planned
- Inform patient of change, continue with "watchful waiting"

Incisor changes "Watchful waiting, use of a morning occlusal guide. and modification to the appliance are considered first line of treatment to manage incisor angulation and position changes. If these treatment options are insufficient or inappropriate, recommending a different OA design and discontinuing OAT permanently may also be appropriate treatment options."[1]

- Anterior crossbites occur in 62% of all patients after 11 years[23] (at least 1, but commonly 4 teeth)
- Some tooth movements are not detrimental and could be considered beneficial
- Inform patient of change, continue with "watchful waiting"
- Relieve acrylic if necessary
- Proper documentation is important, the use of serial casts and measurements is advised
- Use of a morning occlusal guide is recommended

Decreased overjet and overbite "Watchful waiting, isometric contraction and passive jaw-stretching exercises, and use of a morning occlusal guide are considered first line of treatment to manage decreased overjet and overbite. Chewing hard gum in the morning is considered a second-line treatment."[1]

- More than 85% of all patients will experience some change[2]
- Some bite changes are not considered detrimental and may actually be considered beneficial
- Patients commonly are unaware of these changes
- Inform patient of change, continue with "watchful waiting"
- Morning occlusal guides are recommended
- Isometric passive jaw-stretching exercises to aid in reestablishing normal occlusion[22]

Alterations in positions of the mandibular canines and molars "Watchful waiting and use of a morning occlusal guide are considered first line of treatment to manage altered positions of mandibular canines and molars."[1]

- Mesial shift of mandibular canines and molars have been noted in as many as 27% of patients after just a few years[11,17,24]
- Multiple clinical evaluations during the first year of use
- Regular follow-up at yearly intervals[25]
- Inform patient of change, continue with "watchful waiting"
- Some tooth movements are not detrimental and could be considered beneficial
- Morning occlusal guides may help reestablish pretreatment occlusion

Interproximal gaps "Watchful waiting, use of a morning occlusal guide, adjusting ball clasps, and making modifications to the appliance are considered first line of treatment to manage interproximal gaps. If these treatment options are insufficient or inappropriate, use of a distal wraparound retainer and restoration of contact areas may be appropriate."[1]

- Common occurrence, especially in the mandible of patients with angle class I[2,26]
- Can lead to decay and or periodontal disease if not corrected
- Morning occlusal guide recommended
- Inform patient of change, continue with "watchful waiting"
- Reduction of the interproximal acrylic, removal of ball clasps, and/or addition of material in careful application to specific areas may be considered
- Distal wraparound spring may be considered

Section 4: damage to teeth or restorations
Tooth mobility "Palliative care and modifying the appliance are considered first line of treatment to manage tooth mobility. Decreasing the titration

rate is considered second-line treatment. If these treatment options are insufficient or inappropriate, daytime/fixed splinting of teeth also may be appropriate."[1]

- Palliative care where necessary
- Modification of the appliance if applicable
- Decrease the titration rate
- Daytime or fixed splinting of the teeth
- Consider a switch to different OA design
- If the previous items are ineffective or inapplicable, consider discontinuation of OAT; any decision to abandon OAT needs to be done in conjunction with the patient's physician to be sure that replacement therapy is planned

Tooth fractures or damage to dental restorations "Modifying the appliance and referral to a general/restorative dentist are considered first line of treatment to manage tooth fractures or damage to dental restorations. If these treatment options are insufficient or inappropriate, recommending a different OA design also may be appropriate."[1]

- Modify the appliance where appropriate
- Refer to the primary care dentist where necessary
- Consider a switch to different OA design

Section 5: appliance issues
Appliance breakage "Repairing or replacing the appliance is considered first line of treatment to manage appliance breakage. If these treatment options are insufficient or inappropriate, recommending a different OA design also may be appropriate."[1]

- A 2-year study demonstrated a 60% breakage rate with 40% of patients needing a new appliance[21]
- Frequent fracture of acrylic, particularly in patients with bruxism
- Breakage commonly in the telescoping mechanism of a Herbst appliance[27]

Allergies to appliance materials "Removing the allergenic material and temporary discontinuation of OA use are considered first line of treatment to manage allergies to appliance material. If these treatment options are insufficient or inappropriate, referring to another health care provider also may be considered as a treatment option."[1]

- Under cured methyl methacrylate, acrylic can more likely cause reaction by leaking monomer via porosity of the appliance
- Pressure and heat curing of methyl methacrylate may decrease sensitivity reaction

- Nickel, a common allergen, is a common component of stainless steel hardware

Gagging "Modifications to the appliance are considered first line of treatment to manage gagging. Deprogramming the gag reflex is considered second-line treatment. If these treatment options are insufficient or inappropriate, recommendation of a different OA design also may be appropriate."[1]

- Allow for freedom of movement, especially uninhibited opening and lateral movement
- Consider thinner, less bulky appliances with more tongue space to facilitate swallowing
- Cognitive behavioral therapy/desensitizing techniques may help

Anxiety "Watchful waiting and use of desensitization techniques are considered first line of treatment to manage anxiety. If these treatment options are insufficient or inappropriate, recommending a different OA design and referring to a different health care provider also may be appropriate."[1]

- Wear the appliance for some time before bedtime for desensitization
- Choose appliances that allow for free lateral and vertical movement
- Choose appliances with less bulk

Additional concerns There remains one additional serious negative "effect" of OAT that warrants discussion here. Although not a side effect per se, this negative effect could very well be the most significant unintended consequence of OAT, and the most threatening to our patients' well-being. The sheer bulk of the OA as it is introduced into an already crowded oral environment has the potential to increase the apnea pressure, at least until forward posture through titration can compensate. This does not necessarily need to be accompanied by any worsening overt signs or symptoms. Although likely to help substantially, by no means is OAT a guarantee for improvement of OSA; not all patients in the available research studies demonstrate positive effect. Finding atypical responders is not infrequent and should caution all practitioners' activity. There also exist a certain number of patients who worsen past a certain point of titration, thus missing what is commonly referred to as the "sweet spot" of maximum efficacy. As has been stated many times, adherence to conservative titration is important.

It is critical to make sure that proper follow-up with a physician is encouraged for the objective measure of the presence, absence, and severity of residual apnea. The diagnosis of this disease belongs in the hands of those legally licensed and responsible for it. Without this objective analysis, we may have not only failed to help alleviate disease, but could have actually introduced more harm than had we not intervened. Keep in mind that Home Sleep Apnea Testing is not nearly as predictable as a full polysomnography, especially in mild and moderate OSA. The American Dental Association Principles of Ethics and Code of Professional Conduct insists on 3 important factors: veracity, nonmaleficence, and beneficence. The principle of veracity implies that objective measures of OAT titration success need to be accurate in all the ranges of OSA. The remaining 2 factors insist that in an attempt to help a patient we take care to do no harm.

SUMMARY

As previously mentioned, there is a serious need to consider all potential side effects thoughtfully before commencing individual treatment. Although many of these side effects are self-limiting, easily corrected, or innocuous, others are difficult or impossible to correct and can affect the patient in some serious ways. If alternative treatment is not acceptable, the carefully weighed risk of no therapy is what allows practitioners to justify these likely problems to coexist with OAT. As this field evolves, new information is discovered and new products are introduced at a rather rapid pace, continuing education and prudent practice is critical to ethical care in the practice of DSM.

REFERENCES

1. Sheats RD, Schell TG, Blanton AO, et al. Management of side effects of oral appliance therapy for sleep disordered breathing. J Dent Sleep Med 2017;04(04):111–25.
2. Almeida FR, Lowe AA, Otsuka R, et al. Long-term sequelae of oral appliance therapy in obstructive sleep apnea patients: part 2. Study-model analysis. Am J Orthod Dentofacial Orthop 2006;129(2): 205–13.
3. Cunali PA, Almeida FR, Santos CD, et al. Mandibular exercises improve mandibular advancement device therapy for obstructive sleep apnea. Sleep Breath 2011;15(4):717–27.
4. Aarab G, Lobbezoo F, Hamburger HL, et al. Effects of an oral appliance with different mandibular protrusion positions at a constant vertical dimension on obstructive sleep apnea. Clin Oral Investig 2010; 14(3):339–45.
5. Tegelberg A, Walker-Engstrom ML, Vestling O, et al. Two different degrees of mandibular advancement

with a dental appliance in treatment of patients with mild to moderate obstructive sleep apnea. Acta Odontol Scand 2003;61(6):356–62.

6. Chen H, Lowe AA. Updates in oral appliance therapy for snoring and obstructive sleep apnea. Sleep Breath 2013;17(2):473–86.

7. Perez CV, de Leeuw R, Okeson JP, et al. The incidence and prevalence of temporomandibular disorders and posterior open bite in patients receiving mandibular advancement device therapy for obstructive sleep apnea. Sleep Breath 2013;17(1): 323–32.

8. Cohen-Levy J, Garcia R, Petelle B, et al. Treatment of the obstructive sleep apnea syndrome in adults by mandibular advancement device: the state of the art. Int Orthod 2009;7(3):287–304.

9. Fransson AM, Tegelberg A, Leissner L, et al. Effects of a mandibular protruding device on the sleep of patients with obstructive sleep apnea and snoring problems: a 2-year followup. Sleep Breath 2003; 7(3):131–41.

10. Doff MH, Veldhuis SK, Hoekema A, et al. Long-term oral appliance therapy in obstructive sleep apnea syndrome: a controlled study on temporomandibular side effects. Clin Oral Investig 2012;16(3):689–97.

11. Chen H, Lowe AA, de Almeida FR, et al. Three-dimensional computer-assisted study model analysis of long-term oral-appliance wear. Part 2. Side effects of oral appliances in obstructive sleep apnea patients. Am J Orthod Dentofacial Orthop 2008; 134(3):408–17.

12. Cohen-Levy J, Petelle B, Pinguet J, et al. Forces created by mandibular advancement devices in OSAS patients: a pilot study during sleep. Sleep Breath 2013;17(2):781–9.

13. Tegelberg A, Wilhelmsson B, Walker-Engstrom ML, et al. Effects and adverse events of a dental appliance for treatment of obstructive sleep apnoea. Swed Dent J 1999;23(4):117–26.

14. Vezina JP, Blumen MB, Buchet I, et al. Does propulsion mechanism influence the long-term side effects of oral appliances in the treatment of sleep-disordered breathing? Chest 2011;140(5):1184–91.

15. Rose EC, Schnegelsberg C, Staats R, et al. Occlusal side effects caused by a mandibular advancement appliance in patients with obstructive sleep apnea. Angle Orthod 2001;71(6):452–60.

16. Rose EC, Staats R, Virchow C Jr, et al. Occlusal and skeletal effects of an oral appliance in the treatment

of obstructive sleep apnea. Chest 2002;122(3): 871–7.

17. Ueda H, Almeida FR, Lowe AA, et al. Changes in occlusal contact area during oral appliance therapy assessed on study models. Angle Orthod 2008; 78(5):866–72.

18. Marklund M, Legrell PE. An orthodontic oral appliance. Angle Orthod 2010;80(6):1116–21.

19. Doff MH, Hoekema A, Wijkstra PJ, et al. Oral appliance versus continuous positive airway pressure in obstructive sleep apnea syndrome: a 2-year follow-up. Sleep 2013;36(9):1289–96.

20. Marklund M, Sahlin C, Stenlund H, et al. Mandibular advancement device in patients with obstructive sleep apnea: long-term effects on apnea and sleep. Chest 2001;120(1):162–9.

21. Battagel JM, Kotecha B. Dental side-effects of mandibular advancement splint wear in patients who snore. Clin Otolaryngol 2005;30(2):149–56.

22. Ueda H, Almeida FR, Chen H, et al. Effect of 2 jaw exercises on occlusal function in patients with obstructive sleep apnea during oral appliance therapy: a randomized controlled trial. Am J Orthod Dentofacial Orthop 2009;135(4):430.e1–7 [discussion: 430–31].

23. Pliska BT, Nam H, Chen H, et al. Obstructive sleep apnea and mandibular advancement splints: occlusal effects and progression of changes associated with a decade of treatment. J Clin Sleep Med 2014;10(12):1285–91.

24. Almeida FR, Lowe AA, Sung JO, et al. Long-term sequelae of oral appliance therapy in obstructive sleep apnea patients: part 1. Cephalometric analysis. Am J Orthod Dentofacial Orthop 2006;129(2): 195–204.

25. AADSM treatment protocol: oral appliance therapy for sleep disordered breathing: an update for 2013. American Academy of Dental Sleep Medicine Web site; 2013. Available at: https://aadsm.org/docs/JDSM.04.04.pdf. Accessed August 23, 2017.

26. Doff MH, Finnema KJ, Hoekema A, et al. Long-term oral appliance therapy in obstructive sleep apnea syndrome: a controlled study on dental side effects. Clin Oral Investig 2013;17(2):475–82.

27. Martinez-Gomis J, Willaert E, Nogues L, et al. Five years of sleep apnea treatment with a mandibular advancement device. Side effects and technical complications. Angle Orthod 2010;80(1):30–6.

Positional Therapy for Positional Obstructive Sleep Apnea

Mok Yingjuan, MBBS, MRCP[a],*, Wong Hang Siang, MBBS, MRCP[a],
Tan Kah Leong Alvin, MBChB, MRCS[b], Hsu Pon Poh, MBBS, MD[b]

KEYWORDS

- Positional sleep apnea • Positional therapy • Obstructive sleep apnea • Positional device

KEY POINTS

- A significant proportion of patients with obstructive sleep apnea (OSA) have positional OSA, where breathing abnormalities are reduced in a nonsupine sleeping position.
- Positional therapy is an attractive strategy for such patients, especially given the well-known challenges of standard continuous positive airway pressure (CPAP) treatment.
- The traditional "Tennis Ball Technique," however, failed to achieve widespread adoption due to poor patient tolerance and adherence.
- Recently, more sophisticated vibratory positional therapy devices have been developed with studies demonstrating efficacy and better patient tolerance compared with traditional methods.
- With the goal toward personalized treatment of OSA, positional therapy remains an active area of research. There are currently ongoing well-designed randomized controlled trials comparing the new positional devices with gold standard CPAP or as part of combination therapy.

INTRODUCTION

Positional obstructive sleep apnea (POSA) describes the condition in a group of patients with obstructive apneas and hypopneas that occur more frequently in certain sleep positions, notably in the supine position (Fig. 1). For these patients with POSA, positional therapy (PT) becomes an additional viable option for treatment. One of the earliest definitions of POSA was by Cartwright,[1] who proposed an overall apnea-hypopnea index (AHI) of more than 5 per hour and the supine apnea index to be at least twice that of the nonsupine apnea index. Since then, the criteria to diagnose POSA have been further modified with additional factors but retaining Cartwright's[1] criteria as the basic finding.

Depending on the diagnostic criteria used, patients with POSA make up 53.0% to 77.4% of those diagnosed with obstructive sleep apnea (OSA) following polysomnography (PSG).[2–5] Some Asian studies have demonstrated a higher prevalence of POSA. Teerapraipruk and colleagues[6] found the prevalence of POSA to be 67% in their study from Thailand. Three studies from South Korea showed that their prevalence of POSA was even higher at 74.7%,[7] 75.6%,[4] and 77.4%.[3]

This article originally appeared in March, 2019 issue of *Sleep Medicine Clinics* (Volume 14, Issue 1).
Disclosure Statement: The authors have no conflict of interests to declare.
[a] Department of Respiratory and Critical Care Medicine, Changi General Hospital, 2 Simei Street 3, Singapore 529889; [b] Department of Otorhinolaryngology, Head and Neck Surgery, Changi General Hospital, 2 Simei Street 3, Singapore 529889
* Corresponding author.
E-mail address: ying_juan_mok@cgh.com.sg

sleep.theclinics.com

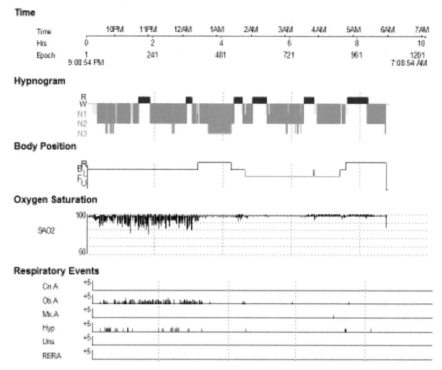

Fig. 1. Sleep study graphical summary of a subject with POSA.

TYPES OF CLASSIFICATION OF POSITIONAL OBSTRUCTIVE SLEEP APNEA

Presently, there are no universally accepted criteria used to diagnose POSA.

The most common criteria used to diagnose POSA are Cartwright's[1] rule of AHI more than 5 per hour and a supine apnea index being at least twice that of nonsupine apnea index, published in 1984.

In 2005, Mador and colleagues[5] modified the definition of POSA. Although he too defined POSA as a total AHI more than 5 per hour with a more than 50% reduction in the nonsupine AHI when compared with the supine AHI, he further classified patients with POSA into 2 groups: supine-predominant OSA (nonsupine AHI equal or more than 5 per hour) and supine-isolated OSA (nonsupine AHI <5 per hour), with at least 15 minutes of sleep in both positions.

More recently, in 2015, Frank and colleagues[8] proposed a new classification system called the Amsterdam Positional OSA Classification (APOC). The aim of this classification is to identify suitable candidates for PT in POSA. According to the APOC criteria, patients need to be diagnosed with OSA and must spend more than 10% of the total sleep time in both the best sleeping position (BSP) and worst sleeping position (WSP). The

patients with POSA are then classified into 3 categories as follows:

1. APOC I: BSP AHI less than 5
2. APOC II: BSP AHI in a lower OSA severity category
3. APOC III: Overall AHI of at least 40 and at least a 25% lower BSP AHI

Using the APOC helps to discriminate between the true patient with POSA who is cured with PT (APOC I), patients who can benefit from PT but are not cured (APOC II or III), and finally patients with nonpositional OSA. Patients in APOC II or III may benefit from combination therapies and may be eligible for lower continuous positive airway pressure (CPAP) requirements and less invasive surgery. This classification system has a better sensitivity, specificity, positive-predictive, and negative predictive value when compared with the classification of Cartwright[1] and Mador and colleagues.[5]

CLINICAL CHARACTERISTICS

Patients with POSA have certain distinctive clinical characteristics that differ from patients with non-positional OSA. Patients with POSA tend to be younger, have a lower body mass index (BMI), a smaller neck and waist circumference, as well as a lower prevalence of hypertension. They also score lower in Mallampati scores, Berlin questionnaires, STOP questionnaires, and Epworth Sleepiness Scale (ESS). When comparing polysomnographic data with patients with nonpositional OSA, patients with POSA sleep more in the nonsupine position, have a longer duration of total sleep time, better sleep efficiency, less wake after sleep onset, lower arousal index, lower AHI, and lower oxygen desaturation index (ODI). Patients with POSA have a higher proportion of stage 3 and rapid eye movement sleep when compared with their nonpositional counterparts.[1]

Mador and colleagues[5] showed that POSA was present in 49.5% of patients with mild OSA, 19.4% of patients with moderate OSA, and 6.5% of those with severe OSA. Mo and colleagues[7] showed in their Asian series that POSA was present in 87% of patients with mild OSA, 84.2% of patients with moderate OSA, and 43.1% of patients with severe OSA.

Studies also have demonstrated that patients with POSA have a lower snoring frequency, higher mean oxygen saturation, and higher nadir oxygen saturation when compared with patients with nonpositional OSA.[6]

PATHOGENESIS

The pharyngeal critical closing pressure (PCrit) measures the pressure at which the upper airway collapses. A higher PCrit indicates that an airway is more collapsible. It has been demonstrated that PCrit is higher in the supine position when compared with the lateral position, indicating a higher collapsibility of the upper airway when supine.[9]

There are several explanations for the improvement in OSA in the nonsupine position when compared with supine.

Studies have shown that in the supine posture, retropalatal anteroposterior diameter and pharyngeal cross-sectional areas are reduced significantly.[10,11] This increases the likelihood of upper airway obstruction. Effects of gravity play a likely role in changing airway dimensions. Nonsupine posture reduces the directional effect of gravity on pharyngeal structures like the soft palate and tongue when compared with the supine posture. This is supported by a study on astronauts in weightlessness, which showed that AHI is lower in the absence of gravity compared with normal gravity.[12]

Lung volume has also been shown to affect the collapsibility of the upper airway, thereby influencing the pathogenesis of OSA. Stanchina and colleagues[13] showed that reducing lung volumes result in increased inspiratory airflow resistance and increased genioglossus muscle activation, causing the pharynx to be more collapsible. The effect of increased lung volume in decreasing upper airway collapsibility has been attributed to the former's effect on caudal trachea.[14] In the clinical setting, increasing BMI has an effect on reducing lung volume. Studies have shown that when patients change position to the supine posture, there is a reduction in total lung capacity, functional residual capacity, and vital capacity with a resultant increase in pulmonary flow-resistance and reduction in lung compliance.[15]

WHAT IS POSITIONAL THERAPY?

PT is defined as any technique used to avoid the worst sleeping position causing POSA. The worst sleeping position usually refers to the supine position.

The tennis ball technique (TBT) is the classic traditional PT in which a tennis ball–sized material is placed in a pocket stitched into the back of a patient's nightwear. TBT works by causing discomfort when sleeping on the back, forcing the patient to roll into a nonsupine position.

In 1984, a letter written by a patient's wife describing how she cured his snoring was first published in the journal *CHEST*. She sewed a pocket into the back of his T-shirt and inserted a hollow, lightweight plastic ball. By wearing this modified T-shirt during sleep, the patient stopped snoring and his daytime sleepiness resolved. Since then, various modifications of the TBT technique have been described over the years.

EFFICACY OF "TENNIS BALL TECHNIQUE" POSITIONAL THERAPY

De Vries and colleagues[16] evaluated the efficacy of TBT in a single-arm study of 53 patients, in whom 40 patients had a follow-up polysomnogram (PSG) (**Table 1**). The TBT mimickers included a commercial fabricated waistband as well as self-made constructions in the treatment of POSA. Overall AHI was found to decrease significantly after a median treatment time interval of 12 weeks (median AHI: 14.5–5.9/h, *P*<.001).

Jackson and colleagues[17] compared the use of a sleep position modification device (active group) to sleep hygiene advice (control group) in the treatment of POSA in a 4-week randomized controlled trial. Eighty-six subjects completed the trial, of which 47 were in the active group and 39 were in the control group. Both the supine sleep time and AHI were reduced significantly from baseline in the active group as compared with the control

Table 1
Trials using traditional positional therapy strategies

Author, Year	Design	Subjects and Sample Size, n	Intervention	Control	Follow-up Duration	Outcomes
de Vries et al,[16] 2015	Retrospective observational	Supine AHI 2x ≥ nonsupine AHI n = 40	TBT	NA	Median interval of 12 wk	AHI, compliance
Jackson et al,[17] 2015	Randomized controlled trial	Total AHI ≥10 supine AHI 2x ≥ nonsupine AHI n = 86	Sleep position modification device	Sleep hygiene	4 wk	Supine sleep time, AHI, quality of life, daytime sleepiness, mood, symptoms, neuropsychological measures, blood pressure
Zuberi et al,[18] 2004	Single arm	RDI >5/h n = 22	SONA pillow	NA	1 night without and 1 night with SONA pillow	RDI, SaO₂, snoring
Bidarian-Moniri et al,[19] 2015	Single arm	Mild to severe OSA n = 14	Pillow for prone positioning	NA	4 wk	AHI, ODI, supine sleep time, compliance
Loord et al,[20] 2007	Single arm	Supine AHI >15, lateral AHI <5 n = 23	"Positioner"	NA	3 mo	AHI, ESS, snoring
Berger et al,[21] 1997	Single arm	Total RDI ≥10; supine RDI 2x ≥ nonsupine RDI n = 13	TBT	NA	1 mo	Blood pressure

TBT vs CPAP

Jokic et al,[22] 1999	Randomized crossover	Lateral AHI <15/h; supine AHI ≥ 2x lateral AHI n = 13	Tennis ball in a backpack	CPAP	2 wk per arm	ESS, AHI, minimum SaO_2, sleep quality, MWT, psychometric test battery, mood scales, QOL, treatment preference
Skinner et al,[23] 2008	Randomized crossover trial	AHI >5/h; supine AHI 2x ≥AHI in other positions n = 20	Thoracic antisupine band	Nasal CPAP	1 mo per arm, with 1 wk washout	AHI, ESS, adherence, sleep quality and QOL, adverse effects
Permut et al,[24] 2010	Randomized crossover trial	Nonsupine AHI <5/h; supine AHI 2x ≥ nonsupine AHI n = 38	Zzoma Positional sleeper	CPAP	1 night per arm	AHI, total sleep time, supine sleep time, minimum SaO_2, treatment preference

Abbreviations: AHI, apnea-hypopnea index; CPAP, continuous positive airway pressure; ESS, Epworth sleepiness scale; MWT, maintenance of wakefulness; NA, not applicable; PT, positional therapy; QOL, quality of life; RDI, respiratory disturbance index; SaO_2, oxygen saturation; TBT, tennis ball technique.

group. However, no significant differences were seen in quality of life, daytime sleepiness, mood, neuropsychological measures, or blood pressure between both groups.

POSITIONAL THERAPY VERSUS CONTINUOUS POSITIVE AIRWAY PRESSURE

Jokic and colleagues[22] compared CPAP and PT in 13 patients with POSA in a randomized crossover trial. PT took the form of a soft ball placed in a backpack, a variation of the classic "TBT." Patients were randomized to either the PT or the CPAP intervention arm for 2 weeks before crossing over to the other arm for another 2 weeks. PT was shown to be effective in reducing sleep time in the supine position. PT was also able to decrease AHI, although a lower AHI was achieved with CPAP. In addition, minimum oxygen saturation was higher in the CPAP arm. Interestingly, no significant difference was found in terms of sleep architecture, daytime sleepiness, mood, or quality of life assessments. Of note, more patients preferred CPAP to PT (7 vs 4 respectively), with 2 having no preference.

Skinner and colleagues[23] conducted a similar study that compared 20 subjects with mild to moderate POSA in a randomized crossover trial. Subjects were randomized to a thoracic antisupine band as PT or nasal CPAP (nCPAP) for 1 month before crossing over to the opposite arm after a 1-week washout period. PT reduced mean AHI from 22.7 to 12.0 events per hour; however, more patients using nCPAP achieved treatment success compared with PT (16/18 vs 13/18, $P<.004$), defined as an AHI ≤ 10 events per hour. Mean AHI was also significantly lower in nCPAP compared with PT (4.9 vs 12.0, $P = .02$). Again, there was no significant difference in daytime sleepiness or quality of life indices between the 2 arms. However, as the primary outcome was AHI, the study may not be powered to detect differences in measures of symptoms and quality of life. It is noteworthy that subjective adherence was higher in PT and fewer side events were reported compared with nCPAP.

In another crossover trial, by Permut and colleagues,[24] 38 patients with POSA were randomized to 1 night of sleep study with CPAP therapy followed by another night of sleep study with the Zzoma Positional Sleeper or vice versa. The Zzoma Positional Sleeper (**Fig. 2**) was made up of semi-rigid foam worn on the back like a backpack attached with a Velcro belt. PT using the Zzoma Positional Sleeper was shown to be as efficacious as CPAP at normalizing AHI to less than 5

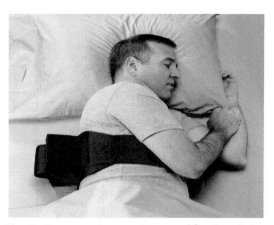

Fig. 2. Zzoma, a sleep position modification device that prevents a user from sleeping in the supine position. (*Courtesy of* ZzOMA, Bala Cynwyd, PA; with permission.)

events per hour (92% vs 97% of study subjects in the groups respectively, $P = .16$).

OTHER POSITIONAL THERAPY TECHNIQUES

Techniques other than TBT have been studied over the years. Zuberi and colleagues[18] evaluated the efficacy of the SONA pillow in the treatment of 22 subjects with OSA. The SONA pillow was a specially designed inclined pillow that allowed one to place one's arm under the head while sleeping in a lateral recumbent position. In subjects with mild to moderate OSA, mean Respiratory Disturbance Index (RDI) was shown to decrease significantly from 17 events per hour to less than 5 events per hour while using the SONA Pillow ($P<.0001$). Bidarian-Moniri and colleagues[19] assessed the effectiveness of prone positioning through the combination of a mattress and pillow and again demonstrated a reduction in overall AHI in patients with OSA. Of note, however, both studies included all patients with OSA and no analysis was performed on treatment efficacy for patients with positional versus nonpositional OSA.

Loord and colleagues[20] conducted a trial in 2006 on 23 patients with POSA using a device called a "Positioner." It was a soft vest attached to a board placed under the pillow that prevents the patient from sleeping on the back; 18 patients completed the study. After 3 months of treatment, 61% of patients had a reduction in AHI to less than 10 per hour. Mean ESS however, decreased only from 12.3 to 10.2.

COMPLIANCE TO TRADITIONAL POSITIONAL THERAPY

Despite its apparent efficacy, PT has not been widely adopted in part due to the poor treatment adherence observed.

In a study by Oksenberg and colleagues,[25] TBT compliance was recorded at only 38% (19/50) at 6-month follow-up. In a longer term study by Bignold and colleagues,[26] fewer than 10% of patients were using their PT device after 30 months. In a more recent study in 2015 by de Vries and colleagues[16] on TBT, although short-term compliance appeared to be good (mean PT usage 7.2 hours per night), long-term compliance was again poor, with 65% of patients having stopped their PT usage after a mean of 13 months. Of note, PT compliance was measured with self-reported questionnaires in the studies.

In 2012, Heinzer and colleagues[27] objectively measured treatment compliance in 16 subjects at 3 months with a built-in actigraphy within a TBT device. Actigraphy recordings demonstrated that the patients used the device 73.7% $\pm$ 29.3% of the nights (range 9%–100%) for an average of 8.0 $\pm$ 2.0 hours per night (range 3.8–10.6 hours). Ten patients used PT for more than 80% of the nights with 13 using more than 60% of the nights.

LIMITATIONS OF POSITIONAL THERAPY TRIALS

Most studies performed with the traditional PT have significant limitations. Many are underpowered, have different definitions of POSA, and different outcome measures. Treatment adherence was mostly measured through subjective reporting by patients, potentially leading to reporting bias. There is also a lack of trials evaluating clinical outcomes with PT therapy in the treatment of POSA. A study by Berger and colleagues[21] in 1997 had been the only trial assessing the effect of TBT on blood pressure as the primary outcome.

NEW POSITIONAL THERAPY DEVICES

Recent technological advances have renewed interest in PT for the treatment of POSA. In the past few years, more sophisticated PT devices have been developed and they appeared to be better than the traditional PT strategies. The new devices are the Night Shift,[28] Sleep Position Trainer (SPT),[29] and BuzzPOD.[30] The small Night Shift device (**Fig. 3**) is worn at the back of the neck with a latex-free silicone rubber strap that is secured using a magnetic clasp. The SPT (**Fig. 4**) and BuzzPOD (**Fig. 5**) are small devices placed on the sternum or chest and secured in place with a chest strap. An in-built accelerometer in these devices ascertains the neck position (Night Shift) or body position (SPT and BuzzPOD) of the user during sleep. When a supine position is

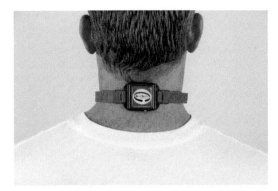

Fig. 3. Night Shift, a neck-worn vibrating PT device. (*Courtesy of* Night Shift, Carlsbad, CA; with permission.)

detected, the devices vibrate with increasing intensity until the patient changes to a nonsupine position. Of the 3 devices, the Night Shift is currently the only one approved by the US Food and Drug Administration for the treatment POSA.

EFFICACY OF THE NEW POSITIONAL THERAPY DEVICES

In 2011, Bignold and colleagues[30] first evaluated a novel position monitoring device with an in-built supine avoidance vibratory alarm in a randomized controlled crossover trial of 15 patients with POSA (**Table 2**). Subjects were randomized to the vibratory positional therapy device or no treatment for 1 week before crossing over to opposite arm after a 1-week washout period. This device significantly reduced mean percentage of supine sleep time and mean AHI (25–13.7 events per hour, $P = .03$).

In 2013, van Maanen and colleagues[29] demonstrated the ability of the SPT device to significantly reduce median percentage of supine sleeping time and median AHI in 31 subjects with POSA after 4 weeks of treatment in a single-arm study. ESS was found to be significantly decreased and the Functional Outcomes of Sleep Questionnaire (FOSQ) scores improved significantly.

In a more recent randomized controlled trial in 2017, Laub and colleagues[31] compared the use of the SPT device (52 subjects) versus no treatment (49 subjects) in patients with POSA. The reduction in mean total AHI with SPT was shown to remain significant after 6 months. Daytime sleepiness also improved after 6 months of SPT treatment.

The evaluation of a small vibrating neck-worn apparatus was first performed by van Maanen and colleagues[32] in 2012 on 30 patients with POSA. Mean AHI was decreased from 27.7 $\pm$ 2.4 per hour to 12.8 $\pm$ 2.2 per hour ($P<.05$).

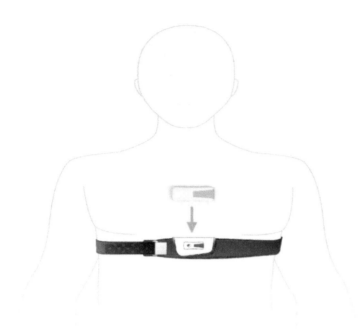

Fig. 4. NightBalance Sleep Position Trainer, a chest-worn vibratory PT device. (*Courtesy of* Night Balance BV, Delft, Netherlands; with permission.)

Subsequently in 2014, Levendowski at al[28] demonstrated that after a 4-week use of the neck-worn Night Shift PT device, the overall AHI of 30 patients with POSA decreased from 24.7 ± 14.7 per hour to 7.5 ± 7.7 per hour (P<.00001). This study also showed a significant improvement in sleep architecture and Patient Health Questionnaire-9 depression score (P = .027).

NEW POSITIONAL THERAPIES VERSUS TENNIS BALL TECHNIQUE

In 2015, Eijsvogel and colleagues[33] compared the efficacy of the SPT device with that of the

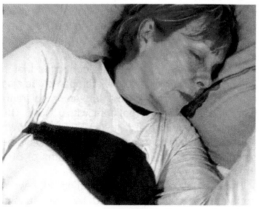

Fig. 5. BuzzPod, a chest-worn vibratory PT device. (*Courtesy of* BuzzPod, Victoria, Australia; with permission.)

traditional TBT in patients with POSA. Both therapies (29 patients in SPT arm and 26 patients in TBT arm) reduced supine sleep position to a median of 0% (minimum-maximum: SPT 0.0% to 67%, TBT 0.0% to 38.9%). Treatment success was defined as AHI less than 5 per hour and appeared to be higher in the SPT group (68.0%) compared with the TBT group (42.9%) although this was not statistically significant. Greater improvements were seen in the SPT arm compared with the TBT arm with regard to sleep quality, total QSQ (Quebec Sleep Questionnaire) scores, the QSQ domains of nocturnal symptoms, and social interactions.

NEW POSITIONAL THERAPY DEVICES VERSUS CONTINUOUS POSITIVE AIRWAY PRESSURE

To date, there are no published data from a randomized controlled trial comparing the new vibratory PT devices with the gold standard CPAP in the treatment of POSA. Three crossover randomized controlled trials are currently ongoing to compare the efficacy of these new vibratory PT devices to CPAP in POSA patients (**Table 3**).

The POSAtive study (ClinicalTrials.gov: NCT03061071)[34] is a multicenter trial in Europe that compares the Nightbalance SPT with autoCPAP. A total of 120 subjects with POSA will be randomized to either treatment for 6 weeks, before crossing over to the alternative treatment arm. The primary outcomes to be studied are treatment adherence and AHI.

Table 2
Trials using new vibratory positional therapy devices

Author, Year	Design	Subjects and Sample Size, n	Intervention	Control	Follow-up Duration	Outcomes
Levendowski et al,[28] 2014	Single arm	Overall AHI ≥5; overall AHI 1.5x ≥ nonsupine AHI n = 30	Neck-worn vibrating device (Night Shift)	NA	4 wk	AHI, % time SaO₂<90%, depression score, sleep architecture
van Maanen et al,[29] 2013	Single arm	supine AHI 2x ≥ nonsupine AHI n = 36	SPT	NA	1 mo	AHI, sleep efficiency, ESS, functional outcomes of sleep questionnaire, compliance
Bignold et al,[30] 2011	Randomized controlled crossover trial	Total AHI >5/h; nonsupine AHI <15/h; supine AHI 2x ≥ nonsupine AHI n = 15	A position monitoring and supine alarm device	No treatment	1 wk per arm with 1 wk washout	AHI, snoring frequency, supine sleep time
Laub et al,[31] 2017	Randomized controlled trial	Supine AHI 2x ≥ nonsupine AHI; supine AHI ≥10 per h; nonsupine AHI <10 per h n = 101	SPT	No treatment	2 mo and 6 mo	Supine sleep time, AHI, ESS, compliance
van Maanen et al,[32] 2012	Single arm	AHI >5; supine AHI 2x ≥ nonsupine AHI n = 30	Neck-worn vibrating device	NA	1 night with no device, 1 night with device on, 1 night with device off	AHI, supine sleep time
Eijsvogel et al,[33] 2015	Prospective randomized trial	Nonsupine AHI <10/ h; supine AHI 2x ≥ nonsupine AHI n = 55	SPT	TBT	1 mo	Supine sleep time, AHI, ESS, sleep quality, QSQ, compliance

Abbreviations: AHI, apnea-hypopnea index; ESS, Epworth sleepiness scale; NA, not applicable; PT, positional therapy; QSQ, Quebec sleep questionnaire; SaO₂, oxygen saturation; SPT, sleep position trainer; TBT, tennis ball technique.

Table 3
Comparing the new positional therapy devices and other obstructive sleep apnea treatment modalities

Author, Year	Design	Subjects and Sample Size, n	Intervention A	Intervention B	Follow-up Duration	Outcomes
ClinicalTrials.gov Identifier: NCT03061071,[34] Ongoing	Multicenter randomized crossover trial	Total AHI >15, or 10< AHI <15 with ESS >10; supine AHI 2x ≥ nonsupine AHI, nonsupine AHI <10 (<5 in mild patients) n = 200	Sleep Position Trainer	Automated CPAP	6 wk	Primary outcomes: adherence, AHI Secondary outcomes: ESS, FOSQ, SF36, patient satisfaction, sleep parameters, mean disease alleviation
ACTRN12613001242718,[35] Ongoing	Randomized crossover trial	ESS: ≥8; AHI >10, nonsupine AHI <10; Supine AHI 2x ≥ nonsupine AHI n = 140	BuzzPOD supine avoidance device	CPAP	8 wk	Primary outcomes: Change in ESS Secondary outcomes: AHI, snoring, sleep quality, QOL, adherence, patient and partner satisfaction
ClinicalTrials.gov Identifier: NCT03125512,[40] Ongoing	Randomized crossover trial	ESS: ≥10; AHI >10, nonsupine AHI <10; Supine AHI 2x ≥nonsupine AHI n = 40	Night Shift Positional Device	Automated CPAP	8 wk	Primary outcomes: Difference in ESS Secondary outcomes: Treatment preference, AHI, FOSQ, SF36, sleep quality, mood and QOL questionnaires
Comparing the new PT devices and Oral Appliance						
Benoist et al,[36] 2017	Prospective multicenter randomized controlled trial	AHI ≥ 5 ≤ 30; Supine AHI 2x ≥ nonsupine AHI n = 99	SPT	Oral appliance therapy	3 mo	Primary outcome: AHI Secondary outcomes: ODI, sleepiness, sleep quality, adherence, mean disease alleviation, QOL, side effects

Study	Study design	Population	Intervention	Comparator	Follow-up	Outcomes
Maurits et al,[41] 2018	(12-mo follow-up of the above trial)	n = 99	SPT	Oral appliance therapy	12 mo	
The new PT devices as part of combination therapy						
Dieltjens et al,[37] 2015	Randomized crossover trial	n = 20	SPT	Oral mandibular device + SPT	1 night per arm	Primary outcome: AHI Secondary outcomes: supine sleeping time, patient preference, sleep study parameters
Benoist et al,[38] 2017	Prospective single-arm study	Subjects with residual positional OSA after surgery n = 33	Sleep Position Trainer	NA	3 mo	AHI, sleep position parameters, daytime sleepiness, compliance, mean disease alleviation, QOL
ClinicalTrials.gov NCT02553902,[39] Ongoing	Multicenter randomized clinical trial	Moderate positional OSA (15< AHI <30); supine AHI 2x ≥ nonsupine AHI n = 200	Sleep Position Trainer + MAD	CPAP	3, 6, and 12 mo	AHI, compliance, QOL, economic evaluation, cardiovascular parameters

Abbreviations: AHI, apnea-hypopnea index; CPAP, continuous positive airway pressure; ESS, Epworth sleepiness scale; FOSQ, functional outcomes of sleep questionnaire; NA, not applicable; ODI, oxygen desaturation index; PT, positional therapy; QOL, quality of life; SF36, 36-item short form health survey; SPT, sleep position trainer.

The second study (ClinicalTrials.gov: NCT03125512) is a crossover randomized controlled trial currently being conducted in Singapore, a multiethnic Asian country. This study compares the Night Shift PT device with autoC-PAP. A total of 40 subjects with POSA and significant daytime sleepiness (defined as an ESS ≥10) will be randomized to either treatment for 8 weeks before crossing over to the alternative arm with a 1-week washout period in-between. The primary outcome is the difference in daytime sleepiness between the 2 arms after 8 weeks of device use. We look forward to its results, as studies on the new PT devices have mostly been conducted in the white population.

The SUPA OSA Trial[35] is a multicenter randomized controlled trial being conducted in South Australia that compares the BuzzPOD device with CPAP in the treatment of POSA. Due to recruitment challenges in meeting the original target sample size of 280 patients, the study was redesigned to become a crossover trial with a revised target sample size of 140. Subjects with POSA and ESS score ≥8 will be randomized to either treatment for 8 weeks, before crossing over to the opposite treatment arm after a 1 week washout interval. The primary outcome is the change in daytime sleepiness.

NEW POSITIONAL THERAPY DEVICES VERSUS ORAL APPLIANCE THERAPY

Benoist and colleagues[36] recently published their results from a multicenter, prospective randomized controlled trial that compared the SPT with oral appliance therapy (OAT) for the treatment of POSA. In this study, 99 subjects with mild to moderate POSA were randomized to either SPT or OAT for 3 months and 81 subjects completed the study. In the intention-to-treat (ITT) analysis, both SPT and OAT decreased the median AHI (SPT: 13.0–7.0/h, OAT: 11.7–9.1/h) and there were no significant differences between the 2 groups at 3 months ($P = .535$). Similarly, no between-group difference in AHI reduction at 3 months was observed in the per-protocol analysis. Mean adherence on per-protocol analysis was comparable between both interventions (SPT: 89.3% vs OAT: 81.3%) although adjusted adherence on ITT analysis was higher in SPT compared with OAT (SPT: 88.4%, OAT: 60.5%). There was no significant difference in mean disease alleviation. The investigators concluded that SPT and OAT were equivalent in the treatment of mild to moderate POSA with regard to AHI reduction. Of note, the OAT group reported a higher frequency of adverse events (n = 26, 26.8%) compared with the SPT group

(n = 13, 13.4%). In addition, 15 of the 18 subjects who dropped out of the study came from the OAT intervention arm.

NEW POSITIONAL THERAPY DEVICES AS PART OF COMBINATION THERAPY

Dieltjens and colleagues[37] conducted a crossover randomized controlled trial to evaluate the efficacy of the SPT device in combination with mandibular advancement device (MAD) for the treatment of residual POSA. This study included patients with OSA who had undergone treatment with mandibular advancement device, but demonstrated residual POSA on PSG. The inclusion criteria were a residual AHI between 5 and 50 per hour and a supine AHI ≥2x nonsupine AHI. Of note, another inclusion criterion was the amount of supine sleeping time must be at least 20% of total sleep time during the PSG while wearing the MAD. Twenty patients with residual OSA on MAD were randomized to either SPT only or combination therapy with both MAD and SPT for a single-night PSG. They subsequently cross over to the opposite arm for a second PSG. The results demonstrated that the combination of MAD and SPT was most effective in reducing median overall AHI (from 20.9/h to 5.5/h) although individually, MAD and SPT were also able to significantly reduce AHI from baseline (to 11.6/h and 12.8/h, respectively). With combination therapy, 95% of subjects achieved treatment success, defined as a minimum of 50% or more reduction in overall AHI. Seven of 15 subjects indicated preference for combination therapy. Further studies would be required to evaluate longer term efficacy and treatment adherence.

Benoist and colleagues[38] evaluated the role of positional therapy in subjects with residual POSA despite surgery. In a prospective single-arm study, 33 subjects with residual POSA after upper airway surgery were treated with the SPT for 3 months. Of note, 76% of the subjects had failed CPAP treatment and 48.5% had failed oral appliance therapy before study participation. A decrease in overall AHI of at least 50% was deemed to be a positive treatment response, and treatment success was achieved if overall AHI was reduced to less than 5 per hour. The results revealed that PT was able to further decrease the median postoperative AHI from 18.3 per hour to 12.5 per hour and the ESS from 10 to 7 after 3 months; 37.5% (n = 12) and 31.3% (n = 10) of the subjects had treatment response and treatment success, respectively. Mean disease alleviation (MDA) with PT was shown to be 41.3%, thereby increasing the overall MDA to 65.6% when combined with surgery.

Nevertheless, 20 subjects remained as nonresponders and further research is warranted to identify predictors of treatment response to PT. When compared with responders, nonresponders were found to have a higher AHI, supine AHI, nonsupine AHI, and ODI. The investigators hypothesized that one of the reasons for nonresponse to PT treatment could be the disparity in head position when the trunk is lateral, given that the positional device is worn on the chest.

There is currently an ongoing multicenter randomized controlled trial in Europe (ClinicalTrials.gov NCT02553902)[39] that aims to compare combination therapy with the gold standard CPAP for the treatment of POSA. A total of 200 patients with moderate POSA will be randomized to either the gold standard CPAP or combination therapy comprising both the SPT and mandibular advancement device. The study will evaluate treatment efficacy, adherence, quality of life indices, cardiovascular parameters, and cost-effectiveness.

COMPLIANCE WITH THE NEW POSITIONAL THERAPY DEVICES

Treatment adherence with the new vibratory positional devices has generally appeared to be high, possibly due to enhanced patient comfort with their petite design. In a study by Van Maanen and colleagues[29] using the Sleep Position Trainer, a treatment adherence rate of as high as 92.7% was reported at 1 month. Treatment adherence was defined as more than 4 hours of device use per day during 7 days a week. In the 2 studies by Benoist and colleagues[36,38] mentioned previously, treatment adherence was 89.3%[36] and 89.0%,[38] respectively, at 3 months, when defined as mean daily device use of at least 4 hours per night for a minimum of 5 days a week.

Van Maanen and colleagues[42] were the first to report the long-term compliance rate of the SPT device in a multicenter prospective cohort study of 145 subjects. At 6 months, 106 subjects had available device data and 71.2% achieved regular use of their device, defined as more than 4 hours. Over 5 days per week, 64.4% of subjects used more than 4 hours of their device/night across all nights. Subsequently, in an even longer follow-up study of 12 months by de Ruiter and colleagues,[41] 29 patients assigned SPT who completed follow-up were found to have an average device use per night of 5.2 hours; 82% used their PT device for more than 4 hours over 7 days per week.

Overall, the results of these studies are promising, although they were mainly performed with the SPT device. It remains to be seen if comparable results can be achieved with other new vibratory PT devices.

SUMMARY AND FUTURE DIRECTIONS

Significant progress in positional therapy has been made with the recent advent of new vibratory PT devices. Studies have demonstrated that these new PT devices are efficacious in reducing overall AHI and better tolerated by patients. Short-term and long-term treatment adherence also appears to be markedly higher compared with traditional positional therapy methods.

Nevertheless, more research is required to determine if the new PT devices can be offered as first-line treatment to patients with positional OSA. Most of the latest evidence has been limited to a single PT device and further studies would be necessary to evaluate if the results are generalizable to all devices. Most studies have also been conducted in the Caucasian population, and these positive results would need to be replicated in other ethnic groups in which genetic, anatomic, and societal traits are likely to differ.

In addition, there is currently a lack of high-quality evidence comparing these new devices with the gold standard CPAP in the treatment of positional OSA. Three randomized controlled trials are under way to address this important clinical question and we look forward to their results. PT as part of combination therapy in the personalized treatment of OSA is also another active area of research. It is hoped that these latest advances in positional therapy may offer an equivalent treatment alternative to many patients with positional OSA who are struggling with CPAP.

REFERENCES

1. Cartwright RD. Effect of sleep position on sleep apnea severity. Sleep 1984;7(2):110–4.
2. Oulhaj A, Al Dhaheri S, Su BB, et al. Discriminating between positional and non-positional obstructive sleep apnea using some clinical characteristics. Sleep Breath 2017;21(4):877–84.
3. Kim KT, Cho YW, Kim DE, et al. Two subtypes of positional obstructive sleep apnea: supine-predominant and supine-isolated. Clin Neurophysiol 2016;127(1):565–70.
4. Lee SA, Paek JH, Chung YS, et al. Clinical features in patients with positional obstructive sleep apnea according to its subtypes. Sleep Breath 2017; 21(1):109–17.
5. Mador MJ, Kufel TJ, Magalang UJ, et al. Prevalence of positional sleep apnea in patients undergoing polysomnography. Chest 2005;128(4):2130–7.

6. Teerapraipruk B, Chirakalwasan N, Simon R, et al. Clinical and polysomnographic data of positional sleep apnea and its predictors. Sleep Breath 2012; 16(4):1167–72.

7. Mo JH, Lee CH, Rhee CS, et al. Positional dependency in Asian patients with obstructive sleep apnea and its implication for hypertension. Arch Otolaryngol Head Neck Surg 2011;137(8):786–90.

8. Frank MH, Ravesloot MJ, van Maanen JP, et al. Positional OSA part 1: towards a clinical classification system for position-dependent obstructive sleep apnoea. Sleep Breath 2015;19(2):473–80.

9. Penzel T, Moller M, Becker HF, et al. Effect of sleep position and sleep stage on the collapsibility of the upper airways in patients with sleep apnea. Sleep 2001;24(1):90–5.

10. Yildirim N, Fitzpatrick MF, Whyte KF, et al. The effect of posture on upper airway dimensions in normal subjects and in patients with the sleep apnea/hypopnea syndrome. Am Rev Respir Dis 1991;144(4): 845–7.

11. Jan MA, Marshall I, Douglas NJ. Effect of posture on upper airway dimensions in normal human. Am J Respir Crit Care Med 1994;149(1):145–8.

12. Elliott AR, Shea SA, Dijk DJ, et al. Microgravity reduces sleep-disordered breathing in humans. Am J Respir Crit Care Med 2001;164(3):478–85.

13. Stanchina ML, Malhotra A, Fogel RB, et al. The influence of lung volume on pharyngeal mechanics, collapsibility, and genioglossus muscle activation during sleep. Sleep 2003;26(7):851–6.

14. Kairaitis K, Byth K, Parikh R, et al. Tracheal traction effects on upper airway patency in rabbits: the role of tissue pressure. Sleep 2007;30(2):179–86.

15. Behrakis PK, Baydur A, Jaeger MJ, et al. Lung mechanics in sitting and horizontal body positions. Chest 1983;83(4):643–6.

16. de Vries GE, Hoekema A, Doff MH, et al. Usage of positional therapy in adults with obstructive sleep apnea. J Clin Sleep Med 2015;11(2):131–7.

17. Jackson M, Collins A, Berlowitz D, et al. Efficacy of sleep position modification to treat positional obstructive sleep apnea. Sleep Med 2015;16(4): 545–52.

18. Zuberi NA, Rekab K, Nguyen HV. Sleep apnea avoidance pillow effects on obstructive sleep apnea syndrome and snoring. Sleep Breath 2004;8(4): 201–7.

19. Bidarian-Moniri A, Nilsson M, Attia J, et al. Mattress and pillow for prone positioning for treatment of obstructive sleep apnoea. Acta Otolaryngol 2015; 135(3):271–6.

20. Loord H, Hultcrantz E. Positioner–a method for preventing sleep apnea. Acta Otolaryngol 2007; 127(8):861–8.

21. Berger M, Oksenberg A, Silverberg DS, et al. Avoiding the supine position during sleep lowers 24 h blood pressure in obstructive sleep apnea (OSA) patients. J Hum Hypertens 1997;11(10):657–64.

22. Jokic R, Klimaszewski A, Crossley M, et al. Positional treatment vs continuous positive airway pressure in patients with positional obstructive sleep apnea syndrome. Chest 1999;115(3):771–81.

23. Skinner MA, Kingshott RN, Filsell S, et al. Efficacy of the 'tennis ball technique' versus nCPAP in the management of position-dependent obstructive sleep apnoea syndrome. Respirology 2008;13(5):708–15.

24. Permut I, Diaz-Abad M, Chatila W, et al. Comparison of positional therapy to CPAP in patients with positional obstructive sleep apnea. J Clin Sleep Med 2010;6(3):238–43.

25. Oksenberg A, Silverberg D, Offenbach D, et al. Positional therapy for obstructive sleep apnea patients: a 6-month follow-up study. Laryngoscope 2006; 116(11):1995–2000.

26. Bignold JJ, Deans-Costi G, Goldsworthy MR, et al. Poor long-term patient compliance with the tennis ball technique for treating positional obstructive sleep apnea. J Clin Sleep Med 2009;5(5):428–30.

27. Heinzer RC, Pellaton C, Rey V, et al. Positional therapy for obstructive sleep apnea: an objective measurement of patients' usage and efficacy at home. Sleep Med 2012;13(4):425–8.

28. Levendowski DJ, Seagraves S, Popovic D, et al. Assessment of a neck-based treatment and monitoring device for positional obstructive sleep apnea. J Clin Sleep Med 2014;10(8):863–71.

29. van Maanen JP, Meester KA, Dun LN, et al. The sleep position trainer: a new treatment for positional obstructive sleep apnoea. Sleep Breath 2013;17(2): 771–9.

30. Bignold JJ, Mercer JD, Antic NA, et al. Accurate position monitoring and improved supine-dependent obstructive sleep apnea with a new position recording and supine avoidance device. J Clin Sleep Med 2011;7(4):376–83.

31. Laub RR, Tonnesen P, Jennum PJ. A Sleep Position Trainer for positional sleep apnea: a randomized, controlled trial. J Sleep Res 2017;26(5):641–50.

32. van Maanen JP, Richard W, Van Kesteren ER, et al. Evaluation of a new simple treatment for positional sleep apnoea patients. J Sleep Res 2012;21(3): 322–9.

33. Eijsvogel MM, Ubbink R, Dekker J, et al. Sleep position trainer versus tennis ball technique in positional obstructive sleep apnea syndrome. J Clin Sleep Med 2015;11(2):139–47.

34. ClinicalTrials.gov. Bethesda (MD): National Library of Medicine (US). 2000 Feb 29-. Identifier NCT03061071, The POSAtive Study: Study for the Treatment of Positional Obstructive Sleep Apnea. 2017. Available at: https://www.clinicaltrials.gov/ct2/show/NCT03061071?cond=positional+obstructive+sleep+apnea&rank=4. Accessed July 1, 2018.

35. Australian New Zealand Clinical Trials Registry: Sydney (NSW): NHMRC Clinical Trials Centre, University of Sydney (Australia); 2005-. Identifier. ACTRN1 2613001242718. Does a supine-avoidance device achieve a similar reduction in sleepiness as usual CPAP treatment in patients with supine-predominant obstructive sleep apnoea? 2013. Available at: http://www.anzctr.org.au/TrialSearch.aspx?searchTxt=SUPA+OSA&isBasic=True. Accessed July 1, 2018.

36. Benoist L, de Ruiter M, de Lange J, et al. A randomized, controlled trial of positional therapy versus oral appliance therapy for position-dependent sleep apnea. Sleep Med 2017;34: 109–17.

37. Dieltjens M, Vroegop AV, Verbruggen AE, et al. A promising concept of combination therapy for positional obstructive sleep apnea. Sleep Breath 2015; 19(2):637–44.

38. Benoist LBL, Verhagen M, Torensma B, et al. Positional therapy in patients with residual positional obstructive sleep apnea after upper airway surgery. Sleep Breath 2017;21(2):279–88.

39. ClinicalTrials.gov. Bethesda (MD):National Library of Medicine (US). 2000 Feb 29-. Identifier NCT02553902, Economic evaluation of treatment modalities for position dependent obstructive sleep apnea; 2015. Available at: https://www.clinicaltrials.gov/ct2/show/NCT02553902?term=NCT02553902&rank=1. Accessed July 1, 2018.

40. ClinicalTrials.gov. Bethesda (MD): National Library of Medicine (US). 2000 Feb 29-. Identifier NCT03125512, Positional Therapy Versus CPAP for Positional OSA; 2017. Available at: https://www.clinicaltrials.gov/ct2/show/NCT03125512?cond=positional+obstructive+sleep+apnea&rank=5. Accessed July 1, 2018.

41. de Ruiter MHT, Benoist LBL, de Vries N, et al. Durability of treatment effects of the Sleep Position Trainer versus oral appliance therapy in positional OSA: 12-month follow-up of a randomized controlled trial. Sleep Breath 2018;22(2):441–50.

42. van Maanen JP, de Vries N. Long-term effectiveness and compliance of positional therapy with the sleep position trainer in the treatment of positional obstructive sleep apnea syndrome. Sleep 2014;37(7): 1209–15.

Pharmacologic and Nonpharmacologic Treatment of Restless Legs Syndrome

Galia V. Anguelova, MD, MSc, Monique H.M. Vlak, MD, PhD, Arthur G.Y. Kurvers, MD, Roselyne M. Rijsman, MD, PhD*

KEYWORDS

- Restless legs syndrome • Therapy • Treatment • Pharmacologic • Nonpharmacologic
- Augmentation

KEY POINTS

- There is limited evidence for nonpharmacologic treatment in primary restless legs syndrome (RLS): pneumatic compression, near-infrared light spectroscopy, and transcranial magnetic stimulation.
- In moderate to severe RLS, pharmacologic treatment may be considered, starting with iron supplemention if applicable.
- There is strong evidence for both α2δ ligands and dopamine agonists in the therapy for RLS.
- When single-drug therapy with an α2δ ligand or dopamine agonist is insufficient, a combination of both may be considered or oxycodone/naloxone.
- To treat augmentation, a low dose or longer-acting dopaminergic drug may be chosen, or a switch to an α2δ ligand or oxycodone/naloxone may be considered.

INTRODUCTION

Restless legs syndrome (RLS) is a sleep-related disorder defined by an urgency to move the legs, usually combined with uncomfortable or unpleasant sensations, which occurs or worsens during rest, usually in the evening or at night, and disappears with movement of the legs.[1] It occurs in 5% to 15% of European and North American adults, 2% to 3% with moderate to severe symptoms, twice as often in women as in men, and has a mean onset age between 30 and 40 years.[1] RLS can be classified as idiopathic or primary, and secondary to comorbid conditions (eg, renal disease, polyneuropathy).[1] The pathophysiology of RLS is still unclear. However, dopaminergic dysfunction and iron deficiency have been suggested to play an essential role, possibly interacting with each other as well.[1] Glutamate, adenosine, and opiate systems are also considered to play a role in the pathophysiology.[1] This article provides an updated practical guide for the treatment of primary RLS in adults. Iron deficiency is included in our definition of primary RLS because of its essential role in the pathophysiology. Treatment of periodic limb movements was beyond the focus of this article. The available evidence is reviewed for pharmacologic as well as nonpharmacologic treatment options.

Disclosure: The authors declare that they have no conflict of interest. This research received no specific grant from any funding agency in the public, commercial, or not-for-profit sectors.
This article originally appeared in June, 2018 issue of *Sleep Medicine Clinics* (Volume 13, Issue 2).
Center for Sleep and Wake Disorders, Haaglanden Medical Center, The Hague, The Netherlands
* Corresponding author. Center for Sleep and Wake disorders, Haaglanden Medical Center, PO 432, The Hague 2501 CK, The Netherlands.
E-mail address: r.rijsman@haaglandenmc.nl

Sleep Med Clin 15 (2020) 277–288
https://doi.org/10.1016/j.jsmc.2020.02.013
1556-407X/20/© 2020 Elsevier Inc. All rights reserved.

METHODS

This article was written in continuation of the 2016 RLS guidelines by the American Academy of Neurology (AAN).[2] The authors performed a PubMed search for articles on treatment of primary RLS using MeSH (Medical Subject Headings) terms and keywords with a start date of 1 January 2015, because the AAN guideline included articles published until the 15 July 2015.[2] Our search was last performed on 15 October 2017. Details on the search strategy are given in **Box 1**.

The titles and abstracts of the eligible articles were screened. The authors only included studies that met the following criteria: (1) original article; (2) on treatment of primary RLS (including iron deficiency–related RLS); (3) in humans; (4) published in English. Case reports were excluded. We focused primarily on the effect on RLS symptoms and periodic limb movements. A standardized tool to report RLS symptom severity is the International Restless Legs Syndrome Study Group rating scale (IRLS), which measures symptoms in the past week with 10 items each graded from 0 to 4 with increasing severity (with a maximum score of 40).[2] Because international guidelines no longer recommend the use of pergolide for RLS, we did not include new studies on pergolide alone. Acupuncture, Chinese herbs, meditation, music, and prayer were considered outside the scope of our review.

Additional articles found in the references of articles identified through our database search were also reviewed if considered relevant according to the criteria mentioned earlier. Relevant articles were classified according to their risk of bias (increasing from I to IV) and subsequent recommendations were made according to the criteria described by the AAN guideline (level A, B, C, and U in decreasing order of evidence level).[2] Studies published after the 2016 AAN guideline are discussed in detail. For studies already described in the 2016 AAN guideline, we refer to the AAN guideline.

RESULTS
Pharmacologic Treatment Options

Table 1 shows the pharmacologic agents effective in RLS treatment with at least evidence level C with their initial and usual daily dose, pharmacokinetics, specific considerations, and side effects.

Dopamine precursors
Levodopa Levodopa was one of the first drugs studied for treating RLS. There are 4 class III studies showing a benefit of levodopa (100–200 mg) on RLS severity (level C).[2] Also a possible effect on the periodic limb movement index (PLMI) was found based on 3 class III studies (level C).[2] Augmentation (discussed later) is a major problem with long-term daily use of levodopa in RLS. It occurs in 40% to 60% of patients after 6 months of follow-up, but augmentation rates as high as 71% have been reported.[3]

Non–ergot-derived dopamine agonists
Pramipexole Pramipexole is a dopamine agonist which is excreted by the kidney. There is level A evidence that pramipexole improves RLS symptoms based on 3 class I studies and 6 class II studies.[2] Improvement of PLMI was seen in 3 class II studies giving level B evidence.[2] Two open-label studies reported that efficacy on RLS symptoms continues up to 1 year.[4,5] A study comparing pramipexole with dual-release levodopa/benserazide found that both drugs are effective in reducing RLS symptoms and PLMI, but levodopa had a higher rate of augmentation (21%) compared with pramipexole (6%).[6]

Ropinirole Ropinirole was effective in improving RLS symptoms up to 6 months according to 2 class I studies and up to 1 year according to 2 class I studies (level B).[2] Ropinirole also improves PLMI according to 2 class I studies (level A).[2] Ropinirole is a dopamine agonist primarily metabolized by the liver, mainly via the cytochrome P (CYP) 1A2 enzyme but also via CYP3A. Substances that inhibit and promote those enzymes can interact with ropinirole.[7]

Rotigotine Rotigotine is a dopaminergic agonist delivered through a transdermal patch allowing a continuous release and thus maintaining stable concentrations that mimic physiologic striatal dopamine receptor function.[8–10] Because of the transdermal delivery, rotigotine is especially useful in patients with daytime symptoms, patients with swallowing difficulties, and patients undergoing surgery.[11] Rotigotine has been shown to reduce RLS symptoms up to 6 months in 2 class I and 3 class II studies (level A) and reduce PLMI in 1 class I study (level B).[2] Our search strategy identified 1 new class I study that has been published since the AAN guideline in 2016.[12] This study randomized 150 patients to receive an optimal dose of rotigotine (1–3 mg) or placebo (randomization 2:1). Although rotigotine was effective in improving IRLS scores at 4 weeks of treatment, there was no superiority compared with placebo (least square mean with 95% confidence intervals [CIs] from an ANCOVA [Analysis of Covariance] model −0.27, 95% CI, −3.0–2.4; $P = .8451$). Long-term efficacy was studied in 3 noncomparative

Box 1
PubMed search strategy

- Dopamine agonists ("Dopamine Agonists"[Mesh] OR "Dopamine Agonists" [Pharmacological Action] OR (dopamin* AND agonist*) OR "Levodopa"[Mesh] OR levodopa*[tiab] OR "pramipexole" [Supplementary Concept] OR pramipexol*[tiab] OR "ropinirole" [Supplementary Concept] OR ropinirol* [tiab] OR "rotigotine" [Supplementary Concept] OR Rotigotin*[tiab] OR "Pergolide"[Mesh] OR Pergolid*[tiab] OR "cabergoline" [Supplementary Concept] OR Cabergolin*[tiab]) AND ("Restless Legs Syndrome"[Mesh] OR "rls"[ti] OR rls'*[ti] OR (restles*[ti] AND leg*[ti]) OR restless leg*[tiab] OR ekbom*[tiab]) NOT ("Animals"[Mesh] NOT "Humans"[Mesh]) AND 2015/01:3000/01 [dp]

- α2δ ligands (alpha-2-delta[tiab] OR alpha2delta[tiab] OR α2δ[tiab] OR α-2-δ[tiab] OR "gabapentin" [Supplementary Concept] OR gabapentin*[tiab] OR "Pregabalin"[Mesh] OR pregabalin*[tiab] OR "1-(((alpha-isobutanoyloxyethoxy)carbonyl)aminomethyl)-1-cyclohexaneacetic acid" [Supplementary Concept] OR "Cyclohexanecarboxylic Acids"[Mesh] OR "gamma-Aminobutyric Acid"[Mesh]) AND ("Restless Legs Syndrome"[Mesh] OR "rls"[ti] OR rls'*[ti] OR (restles*[ti] AND leg*[ti]) OR restless leg*[tiab] OR ekbom*[tiab]) NOT ("Animals"[Mesh] NOT "Humans"[Mesh]) AND 2015/01:3000/01 [dp]

- Specific N-methyl-ᴅ-aspartate receptor agonists and drugs acting on AMPA-receptors ("traxoprodil mesylate" [Supplementary Concept] OR Traxoprodil*[tiab] OR "ifenprodil" [Supplementary Concept] OR Ifenprodil*[tiab] OR "aniracetam" [Supplementary Concept] OR Aniracetam*[tiab] OR "Kynurenic Acid"[Mesh] OR Kynurenic acid*[tiab] OR Kynurenate[tiab] OR "perampanel" [Supplementary Concept] OR Perampanel*[tiab] OR "tezampanel" [Supplementary Concept] OR Tezampanel*[tiab]) AND ("Restless Legs Syndrome"[Mesh] OR "rls"[ti] OR rls'*[ti] OR (restles*[ti] AND leg*[ti]) OR restless leg*[tiab] OR ekbom*[tiab]) NOT ("Animals"[Mesh] NOT "Humans"[Mesh]) AND 2015/01:3000/01 [dp]

- Opioids ("Analgesics, Opioid"[Mesh] OR "Analgesics, Opioid" [Pharmacological Action] OR "Narcotics" [Pharmacological Action] OR Opiate[tiab] OR opioid*[tiab] OR "Tramadol"[Mesh] OR tramadol[tiab] OR tramdol[tiab] OR "Morphine"[Mesh] OR morphin*[tiab] OR "Oxycodone"[Mesh] OR Oxycodon*[tiab] OR "Fentanyl"[Mesh] OR Fentanyl[tiab] OR "Naloxone"[Mesh] OR Naloxon*[tiab] OR "Methadone"[Mesh] OR Methadon*[tiab] OR "Ketamine"[Mesh] OR Ketamin*[tiab] OR "Tilidine"[Mesh] OR Tilidine[tiab]) AND ("Restless Legs Syndrome"[Mesh] OR "rls"[ti] OR rls'*[ti] OR (restles*[ti] AND leg*[ti]) OR restless leg*[tiab] OR ekbom*[tiab]) NOT ("Animals"[Mesh] NOT "Humans"[Mesh]) AND 2015/01:3000/01 [dp]

- Iron ("Iron"[Mesh] OR "ferric carboxymaltose" [Supplementary Concept] AND ferric carboxymaltose [tiab] OR iron carboxymaltose[tiab] OR "ferrous sulfate" [Supplementary Concept] OR ferrous sulfate [tiab] OR iron sulfate[tiab] OR ferric sulfate[tiab] OR ferrous sulphate[tiab] OR iron sulphate[tiab] OR ferric sulphate[tiab] OR "ferric oxide, saccharated" [Supplementary Concept] OR iron-saccharate[tiab] OR iron sucrose[tiab] OR "saccharated iron oxide"[tiab] OR ferric saccharate[tiab] OR ferri saccharate [tiab] OR "ferric gluconate" [Supplementary Concept] AND "Bioferrico" [Supplementary Concept] OR ferric gluconate[tiab] OR iron gluconate[tiab] OR ferrous gluconate[tiab] OR ferrigluconate[tiab] OR "Iron-Dextran Complex"[Mesh] OR Iron Dextran[tiab] OR ferridextran[tiab] OR "Ferrosoferric Oxide"[Mesh] OR Ferrosoferric Oxide[tiab] OR ferumoxytol[tiab] OR ferriferrous oxide[tiab] OR "iron isomaltoside 1000" [Supplementary Concept] OR iron isomaltoside[tiab]) AND ("Restless Legs Syndrome"[Mesh] OR "rls"[ti] OR rls'*[ti] OR (restles*[ti] AND leg*[ti]) OR restless leg*[tiab] OR ekbom*[tiab]) NOT ("Animals"[Mesh] NOT "Humans"[Mesh]) AND 2015/01:3000/01 [dp]

- Other medication ("Melatonin"[Mesh] OR melatonin*[tiab] OR "Glucosamine"[Mesh] OR Glucosamine[tiab] OR 2-Amino-2-Deoxyglucose[tiab] OR Hespercorbin[tiab] OR dona[tiab] OR xicil[tiab] OR "Magnesium"[Mesh] OR magnesium*[tiab] OR "Creatine"[Mesh] OR creatin*[tiab] OR "coenzyme Q10" [Supplementary Concept] OR coenzyme Q10[tiab] OR co-enzyme Q10[tiab] OR "CoQ 10"[tiab] OR "CoQ10"[tiab] OR ubidecarenone[tiab] OR ubiquinone[tiab] OR Bio-Quinone Q10 [tiab] OR ubisemiquinone radical[tiab] OR Q-ter[tiab] OR ubisemiquinone[tiab]) AND ("Restless Legs Syndrome"[Mesh] OR "rls"[ti] OR rls'*[ti] OR (restles*[ti] AND leg*[ti]) OR restless leg*[tiab] OR ekbom*[tiab]) NOT ("Animals"[Mesh] NOT "Humans"[Mesh]) AND 2015/01:3000/01 [dp]

  ○ Benzodiazepines ("Benzodiazepines"[Mesh] OR Benzodiazepin*[tiab] OR "Clonazepam"[Mesh] OR clonazepam*[tiab] OR "zolpidem" [Supplementary Concept] OR zolpidem*[tiab]) AND ("Restless Legs Syndrome"[Mesh] OR "rls"[ti] OR rls'*[ti] OR (restles*[ti] AND leg*[ti]) OR restless leg* [tiab] OR ekbom*[tiab]) NOT ("Animals"[Mesh] NOT "Humans"[Mesh]) AND 2015/01:3000/01 [dp]

  ○ Antiepileptics ("Anticonvulsants" [Pharmacological Action] OR "Anticonvulsants"[Mesh] OR anticonvuls*[tiab] OR anti-convuls*[tiab] OR antiepileptic*[tiab] OR anti-epileptic*[tiab] OR "Carbamazepine"[Mesh] OR Carbamazepin*[tiab] OR "etiracetam" [Supplementary Concept] OR etiracetam [tiab] OR Levetiracetam[tiab] OR "Valproic Acid"[Mesh] OR Valproic acid*[tiab] OR Tegretol[tiab]

OR Carbazepin[tiab] OR Epitol[tiab] OR Finlepsin[tiab] OR Neurotol[tiab] OR Amizepine[tiab] OR keppla[tiab] OR Propylisopropylacetic Acid[tiab] OR 2 Propylpentanoic Acid[tiab] OR Divalproex [tiab] OR Depakene[tiab] OR Depakine[tiab] OR Convulsofin[tiab] OR Depakote[tiab] OR Vupral [tiab] OR Divalproex Sodium[tiab] OR Valproate[tiab] OR Ergenyl[tiab] OR Dipropyl Acetate[tiab]) AND ("Restless Legs Syndrome"[Mesh] OR "rls"[ti] OR rls'*[ti] OR (restles*[ti] AND leg*[ti]) OR restless leg*[tiab] OR ekbom*[tiab]) NOT ("Animals"[Mesh] NOT "Humans"[Mesh]) AND 2015/01:3000/01 [dp]

Nonpharmacologic treatment options

- Sleep hygiene ("Sleep Hygiene"[Mesh] OR sleep hygiene[tiab] OR sleep habit*[tiab]) AND ("Restless Legs Syndrome"[Mesh] OR "rls"[ti] OR rls'*[ti] OR (restles*[ti] AND leg*[ti]) OR restless leg*[tiab] OR ekbom*[tiab]) NOT ("Animals"[Mesh] NOT "Humans"[Mesh]) AND 2015/01:3000/01 [dp]

- Caffeine and alcohol intake and smoking ("coffee"[MeSH Terms] OR "Caffeine"[Mesh] OR coffee [tiab] OR Caffeine[tiab] OR "Alcohol Drinking"[Mesh] OR "alcoholic beverages"[MeSH Terms] OR alcohol*[tiab]) AND ("Restless Legs Syndrome"[Mesh] OR "rls"[ti] OR rls'*[ti] OR (restles*[ti] AND leg*[ti]) OR restless leg*[tiab] OR ekbom*[tiab]) NOT ("Animals"[Mesh] NOT "Humans"[Mesh]) AND 2015/01:3000/01 [dp]

- Mental activity ("Mental Processes"[Mesh] OR "mental activity"[tiab] OR "Reading"[Mesh] OR reading[tiab] OR read[tiab] OR card game*[tiab] OR brain teaser*[tiab] OR chess[tiab] OR computer work[tiab]) AND ("Restless Legs Syndrome"[Mesh] OR "rls"[ti] OR rls'*[ti] OR (restles*[ti] AND leg*[ti]) OR restless leg*[tiab] OR ekbom*[tiab]) NOT ("Animals"[Mesh] NOT "Humans"[Mesh]) AND 2015/ 01:3000/01 [dp]

- Physical activity (including yoga) (Aerobic*[tiab] OR "Exercise Therapy"[MeSH] OR "Exercise"[MeSH] OR exercise[tiab] OR "Yoga"[Mesh] OR yoga[tiab] OR "Resistance Training"[Mesh] OR resistance training[tiab] OR "Weight Lifting"[Mesh] OR Weight lifting[tiab] OR weight bearing[tiab] OR "Bicycling"[Mesh] OR bicycl*[tiab] OR cycling[tiab] OR cycle[tiab]) AND ("Restless Legs Syndrome"[Mesh] OR "rls"[ti] OR rls'*[ti] OR (restles*[ti] AND leg*[ti]) OR restless leg*[tiab] OR ekbom*[tiab]) NOT ("Animals"[Mesh] NOT "Humans"[Mesh]) AND 2015/01:3000/01 [dp]

- Pneumatic compression ("Intermittent Pneumatic Compression Devices"[Mesh] OR ((Pneumatic[tiab] OR mechanical[tiab]) AND compression[tiab]) OR IPC[tiab]) AND ("Restless Legs Syndrome"[Mesh] OR "rls"[ti] OR rls'*[ti] OR (restles*[ti] AND leg*[ti]) OR restless leg*[tiab] OR ekbom*[tiab]) NOT ("Animals"[Mesh] NOT "Humans"[Mesh]) AND 2015/01:3000/01 [dp]

- Tactile stimulus (including hot baths, massage and vibratory pads) ("Vibration"[Mesh] OR vibrat* [tiab] OR pad[tiab] OR pads[tiab] OR "Balneology"[Mesh] OR "Hydrotherapy"[Mesh] OR "Hot Temperature"[Mesh] OR "Hot Springs"[Mesh] OR bath*[tiab] OR "Massage"[Mesh] OR massage*[tiab] OR bodywork*[tiab]) AND ("Restless Legs Syndrome"[Mesh] OR "rls"[ti] OR rls'*[ti] OR (restles*[ti] AND leg*[ti]) OR restless leg*[tiab] OR ekbom*[tiab]) NOT ("Animals"[Mesh] NOT "Humans"[Mesh]) AND 2015/01:3000/01 [dp]

- Current or magnetic stimulus ((("Transcranial Direct Current Stimulation"[Mesh] OR tsDCS*[tiab] OR tDCS*[tiab] OR ((transcranial[tiab] OR cathodal[tiab] OR anodal[tiab] OR electric*[tiab]) AND stimul*[tiab]) OR "Transcutaneous Electric Nerve Stimulation"[Mesh] OR TENS[tiab] OR tsDCS[tiab] OR ((Percutaneous[tiab] OR Transcutaneous[tiab] OR transdermal[tiab] OR cutaneous[tiab]) AND (Electric[tiab] OR electrical[tiab] OR electrostimulation[tiab] OR stimul*[tiab])) OR ("Transcranial Magnetic Stimulation"[Mesh] OR Transcranial Magnetic Stimulation*[tiab] OR rTMS[tiab] OR TMS [tiab] OR "Cortical Excitability"[Mesh] OR Cortical Excitability[tiab])) AND ("Restless Legs Syndrome"[Mesh] OR "rls"[ti] OR rls'*[ti] OR (restles*[ti] AND leg*[ti]) OR restless leg*[tiab] OR ekbom*[tiab]) NOT ("Animals"[Mesh] NOT "Humans"[Mesh]) AND ("2015/01/01"[PDAT]: "3000/12/31"[PDAT])

- Light stimulus ("Infrared Rays"[Mesh] OR near-infrared light[tiab] OR NIR[tiab] OR near-infrared ray* [tiab] OR "Phototherapy"[Mesh] OR phototherap*[tiab] OR light therap*[tiab] OR phototherap* [tiab] OR photoradiation therap*[tiab] OR heliotherap*[tiab] OR) AND ("Restless Legs Syndrome"[Mesh] OR "rls"[ti] OR rls'*[ti] OR (restles*[ti] AND leg*[ti]) OR restless leg*[tiab] OR ekbom*[tiab]) NOT ("Animals"[Mesh] NOT "Humans"[Mesh]) AND 2015/01:3000/01 [dp]

- Cognitive therapy ("Adaptation, Psychological"[Mesh] OR "Cognitive Therapy"[Mesh] OR (cogniti* [ti] AND therap*[ti]) OR psychotherap*[tiab] OR "Mindfulness"[Mesh] OR mindful*[tiab]) AND ("Restless Legs Syndrome"[Mesh] OR "rls"[ti] OR rls'*[ti] OR (restles*[ti] AND leg*[ti]) OR restless leg*[tiab] OR ekbom*[tiab]) NOT ("Animals"[Mesh] NOT "Humans"[Mesh]) AND 2015/01:3000/01 [dp]

- Vitamins ("Vitamins"[Pharmacological Action] OR vitamin*[tiab] OR ascorbic acid[tiab] OR cholecalciferol[tiab] OR calcitriol[tiab] OR calciol[tiab] OR "Calcium"[Mesh] OR "Calcium Carbonate"[Mesh] OR calcium[tiab] OR tocopherol[tiab] OR alpha-tocopherol[tiab] OR beta-tocopherol[tiab] OR gamma-tocopherol[tiab] OR "Vitamin B 6"[Mesh] OR "Vitamin B 12"[Mesh] OR "Vitamin B Complex"[Mesh] OR "Vitamin B Complex" [Pharmacological Action] OR "Folic Acid"[Mesh] OR folic acid[tiab] OR folvite[tiab] OR folacin[tiab] OR folate[tiab]) AND ("Restless Legs Syndrome"[Mesh] OR "rls"[ti] OR rls'*[ti] OR (restles*[ti] AND leg*[ti]) OR restless leg*[tiab] OR ekbom*[tiab]) NOT ("Animals"[Mesh] NOT "Humans"[Mesh]) AND 2015/01:3000/01 [dp]

extension studies that found continued efficacy up to 5 years.[13-15]

Piribedil There is insufficient evidence (level U) for the effectiveness of piribedil on RLS symptoms based on 1 open-label class IV study in which RLS symptoms improved in a group of 13 patients with a median dose of 50 mg of piribedil daily.[16]

Ergot-derived dopamine agonists
Both pergolide (1 class I study and 2 class II studies) and cabergoline (2 class I studies) have been shown to be effective in treating RLS (level A).[2] However, all ergot-derived dopamine agonists have been associated with severe life-threatening side effects, including fibrosis and valvulopathy. International guidelines do not recommend the use of pergolide, which is no longer available in the United States for RLS.[2,17,18] European RLS guidelines also no longer recommend cabergoline for treating patients with RLS.[18] In the United States, cabergoline is only suggested as an option when other recommended agents have been tried first and failed, and on the condition that close clinical follow-up is provided.[17]

α2δ Ligands
Gabapentin enacarbil Gabapentin enacarbil is a slow-release prodrug of gabapentin. It is absorbed by active transport in the gut and then converted to gabapentin. Four class I studies show that gabapentin enacarbil is effective in moderate to severe RLS in treating daytime symptoms (level A).[2] It is likely to be effective for at least 6 months (1 class II study).[2] The IRLS score had improved by 15.5 points at 24 weeks. Relapses were less common in the active treatment arm compared with the placebo arm (9% vs 23%; P = .02). There is insufficient evidence based on 1 class III study (level U) for gabapentin enacarbil to have any significant effect on PLMI, although it is likely to improve other sleep measures based on 1 class I and 1 class III study.[2]

Pregabalin Pregabalin is effective in the treatment of moderate to severe primary RLS up to 1 year when dosed 150 to 450 mg/d (level B). This advice is based on 1 class I study: at 52 weeks pregabalin

significantly reduced IRLS scores compared with pramipexole.[2] Pregabalin is likely to improve PLMI (2 class II studies), also likely to improve some other sleep measures (1 class I study, 2 class II studies), and likely to improve subjective sleep (1 class I study, 3 class II studies).[1,2] Compared with pramipexole, pregabalin is more likely to improve subjective sleep outcomes (based on 2 class II studies).[2]

Gabapentin There is 1 class III study showing an effect of gabapentin at 6 weeks.[2] However, no long-term studies were performed (level U).[19] Unlike gabapentin enacarbil, the absorption of gabapentin is variable, which makes it more difficult to select the optimal dose.

Specific N-methyl-ᴅ-aspartate (NMDA) receptor agonists and drugs acting on α-amino-3-hydroxy-5-methyl-4-isoxazolepropionic acid (AMPA) receptors α2δ Ligands reduce glutamatergic transmission. Therefore, other drugs with a similar effect are being studied, such as AMPA-type glutamate receptor antagonists. One class IV study showed that perampanel (a selective noncompetitive AMPA-type glutamate receptor antagonist) administered 2 to 4 mg orally daily significantly improves IRLS scores after 2 months (longer follow-up is currently investigated by the same study group) and decreases PLMI and the periodic limb movement arousal index.[20]

Opioids
In 1 class II study, prolonged-release oxycodone/naloxone improved, for example, IRLS scores compared with placebo after 12 weeks (level C).[2] One class III crossover study showed that oxycodone improved RLS symptoms and PLMI compared with placebo (level C).[2] There is insufficient evidence (level U) for both methadone (1 class III and 1 class IV study), tramadol (1 class IV study), and intrathecal morphine (1 class IV study).[2] There was also insufficient evidence (level U) for dihydrocodeine, propoxyphene, and tilidine (2 class IV studies).[2] Two studies have reported augmentation after RLS treatment with tramadol, whereas it has not been reported with other opioids.[21,22]

Table 1
Pharmacologic treatment options for primary restless legs syndrome with a focus on restless legs syndrome symptoms

Medication	Level of Evidence	Initial Daily Dose (mg)	Usual Dose Range	$T_{1/2}$ (h)	T_{max}	Specific Considerations	Side Effects
Carbidopa/levodopa	C	125	25/100 mg PO	1.5	10–30 min	Occasional use	Headache, muscle cramps, confusion, somnolence, dizziness, depression, palpitations, orthostatic hypotension, gastrointestinal symptoms
Pramipexole	B	0.125	0.125 mg PO up to 0.5–0.75 mg 2–3 h before bedtime Dose increasing every 4–7 d	8–12, regular; 24, extended release	1–3 h, regular; 6 h, extended release	Chronic therapy; can be used for patients with medications that affect hepatic enzymes	Nausea, sleepiness and insomnia, fatigue, vivid dreams, confusion, visual hallucinations, headache, postural hypotension, impulse control disorder
Ropinirole	B	0.25(−0.5)	0.25–0.5 mg PO in the evening during the first week up to 4 mg PO	1.5–2.5, regular; 6–10, extended release	1.5 h	Chronic therapy; can be used for patients with decreased renal function	Nausea, somnolence, fatigue, depression, impulse control disorder

Drug							Adverse effects
Rotigotine	A	1	1–3 mg/24 h transdermal Dose increasing every 7 d	5–7		1–3 h	Chronic therapy; round-the-clock symptoms or swallowing difficulties — Allergic reactions at the application site, nausea, headache, fatigue, orthostatic hypotension, sleepiness, impulse control disorders
Gabapentin enacarbil	A	600	600–1200 mg PO	5.1–6	5–7.3 h	—	Somnolence, dizziness
Pregabalin	B	75	150–450 mg PO	6	1 h	—	Unsteadiness, daytime sleepiness
Oxycodone/ naloxone prolonged release	C	5/2.5	5/2.5–40/20 mg PO	4.1–17.2	1.3–5.3 h	To consider in refractory RLS	Fatigue, constipation, nausea, headache, hyperhidrosis, somnolence, dry mouth, pruritus, OSAS
Ferrous sulfate	C	325	325 mg PO twice daily with 100 mg vitamin C	6	4 h	—	Nausea, sickness, and constipation
Ferric carboxymaltose	A	—	1000 mg IV	7–12	15 min–1.2 h	—	Nausea, headache

Abbreviations: IV, intravenous; OSAS, obstructive sleep apnea syndrome; PO, medication administered orally; T_{max}, time to maximum plasma concentration; $T_{1/2}$, elimination half-life.

Iron

One class II study found that oral iron as ferrous sulfate 325 mg combined with vitamin C 100 mg twice a day was effective for treating RLS in patients with a serum ferritin level of less than or equal to 75 μg/L (level C).[23] Two class I studies found that ferric carboxymaltose 1000 mg is effective for the treatment of moderate to severe RLS in patients with a serum ferritin level less than 300 μg/L and a transferrin saturation of less than 45% (level A).[23] One class I study using iron sucrose 200 mg and 1 class II study using iron sucrose 500 mg found no effect on RLS symptoms or PLMI (level B).[23] Expert consensus considered iron sucrose to be effective for treatment of RLS but less so than ferric carboxymaltose or low-molecular-weight iron dextran.[23] There is insufficient evidence for the efficacy of low-molecular-weight iron dextran for the treatment of RLS (2 class IV studies, level U).[23] Expert consensus, however, points at substantial clinical experience that shows it to be effective. There is insufficient evidence for the efficacy of iron gluconate (1 class IV study, level U).[23] No studies were available to evaluate the efficacy of ferumoxytol or isomaltoside for the treatment of RLS. Expert consensus was that 1000 mg of these formulations given intravenously as a single dose or as 2 divided doses is possibly effective for RLS.[23] In a class III study, oral iron 150 mg was compared with bupropion 300 mg and ropinirole 0.25 to 0.5 mg. IRLS score reduction was seen in all groups, but most in the ropinirole group.[24]

Other medications

There is insufficient evidence (level U) for the use of clonidine (1 class III study),[2] selenium (1 class III study and 1 class IV study),[2,25] botulinum toxin A (1 class III study),[2] oxcarbazepine (1 class IV study),[26] carbamazepine (1 class III study),[2] valproic acid (1 class III study),[2] levetiracetam (1 class IV study),[27] and clonazepam (2 contradictory class III studies).[2]

Valerian (1 class II study) is possibly ineffective (level C).[2] Since the 2016 AAN guideline, a new class III study has supported bupropion efficacy, because it improved RLS symptoms significantly at 6 weeks compared with baseline. A group of 30 patients treated with 300 mg of bupropion (initial 5 days with a 150 mg dose) was also compared with 30 patients treated with ropinirole (0.25–0.5 mg), but there was no placebo group.[24] A lower than recommended ropinirole dose was used in this study and it is unclear how randomization, blinding, and allocation concealment were performed. Therefore, this class III study should be viewed as a noninferiority study assuming ropinirole as the standard treatment, and bupropion was inferior to ropinirole. Based on this class III study and a class II study included in the AAN guideline, bupropion is possibly ineffective (level C).[2,24]

Augmentation

A well-known side effect of levodopa and dopamine agonist is augmentation. Augmentation is characterized by an advance of the RLS symptoms compared with the onset time before starting the medication, a shorter latency of symptoms at rest, a spread of symptoms to other parts of the body, or a greater intensity of the symptoms. Another key symptom of augmentation is the paradoxic effect on RLS symptoms after changing the dose: dose increase causes symptom worsening, and dose reduction improvement. The time of onset of the paradoxic effect after dose change is considered, by expert opinion, drug dependent: several days after change of levodopa and weeks to months after change of the longer-acting dopamine agonists. These characteristics were outlined by the Max Planck Institute (MPI) diagnostic criteria in 2007.[28] Because the MPI definition criteria have shown some shortcomings in the everyday clinical setting, the International RLS Task Force (IRLSTF) has established consensus-based recommendation for screening for augmentation in the clinical setting to facilitate the identification of augmentation (**Box 2**).[29]

Box 2
International Restless Legs Syndrome Study Group Task Force screening questions for augmentations in the clinical setting

1. Do RLS symptoms appear earlier than when the drug was first started?

2. Are higher doses of the drug now needed, or do you need to take the medicine earlier, to control the RLS symptoms, compared to the original effective dose?

3. Has the intensity of symptoms worsened since starting the medication?

4. Have symptoms spread to other parts of the body (eg, arms) since starting the medication?

From Garcia-Borreguero D, Silber MH, Winkelman JW, et al. Guidelines for the first-line treatment of restless legs syndrome/Willis-Ekbom disease, prevention and treatment of dopaminergic augmentation: a combined task force of the IRLSSG, EURLSSG, and the RLS-foundation. Sleep Med 2016;21:4; with permission.

Augmentation is seen in all dopaminergic drugs but is most prevalent in levodopa (up to 73%) and less in dopamine agonists. Prevalence rates for dopamine agonist–related augmentation vary from less than 10% in the short term to 42% to 68% after approximately 10 years of treatment.[29] Seventy-six percent of all patients treated with dopaminergic agents showed indications for partial or full augmentation, with a yearly incidence rate of approximately 8%.[30] The prevalence of augmentation seems to be lower in the longer-acting dopamine agonists (rotigotine and cabergoline) compared with the short-acting dopamine agonists (ropinirole and pramipexole). Other possible risk factors for the development of augmentation are low ferritin levels, having more frequent and more severe RLS symptoms pretreatment, greater discomfort with RLS symptoms before treatment, comorbid asthma, older age, longer treatment duration, development of tolerance on dopaminergic medication, positive family history of RLS, fewer out-patient clinic visits, and lack of any neuropathy. Polysomnographic analysis does not seem useful to identify augmentation and immobilization tests might be promising.[29]

It is important to rule out augmentation mimics before diagnosing augmentation, such as the natural waxing and waning course of RLS. Other causes of RLS progression to distinguish from augmentation are iron deficiency, poor RLS medication adherence, lifestyle changes (eg, more immobile), use of RLS exacerbating medications (eg, antihistamines, selective serotonin reuptake inhibitors), and other physiologic or comorbid conditions (eg, pregnancy and renal failure). In addition, tolerance and end-of-dose exacerbation must be distinguished from augmentation, although tolerance is likely to precede augmentation and could therefore be recognized as a possible indicator to develop augmentation in the further course of the treatment. Several consensus-based measures are suggested to prevent and treat augmentation (**Fig. 1**).[29]

Nonpharmacologic Treatment Options

Evidence level B was found for the effectiveness of pneumatic compression (1 class I and 1 class IV study)[2,31] and near-infrared light spectroscopy (NIRS) (2 class II studies and 1 new class IV

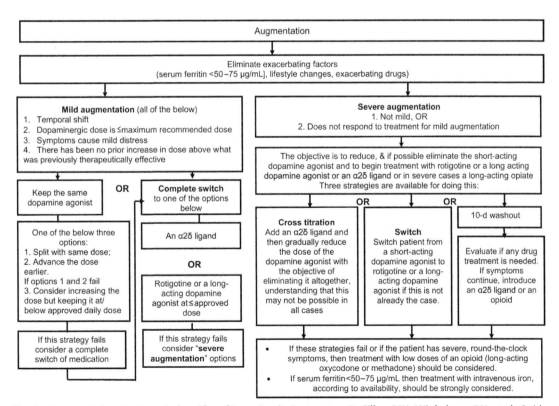

Fig. 1. Augmentation treatment algorithm. (*From* Garcia-Borreguero D, Silber MH, Winkelman JW, et al. Guidelines for the first-line treatment of restless legs syndrome/Willis-Ekbom disease, prevention and treatment of dopaminergic augmentation: a combined task force of the IRLSSG, EURLSSG, and the RLS-foundation. Sleep Med 2016;21:7; with permission.)

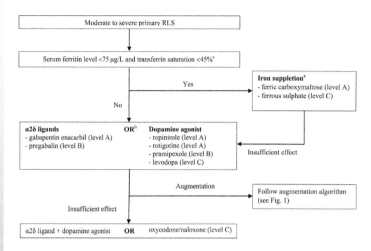

Fig. 2. Pharmacologic treatment algorithm in primary RLS. [a] Consider intravenous iron when serum ferritin level is less than 100 µg/L and transferrin saturation less than 45%. [b] The choice for an α2δ ligand or dopamine agonist may be based on considerations regarding patient characteristics (see **Table 1**), comorbidities, and the risk of augmentation with dopaminergic treatment.

study).[2,32] Transcranial direct current stimulation (1 class I study)[2] is probably ineffective (level B). Repetitive transcranial magnetic stimulation is possibly effective based on 1 class II study and 2 new class IV studies[2,33,34] and vibratory treatment (2 class II studies and 1 class IV study)[2,35] possibly ineffective (level C). There is insufficient evidence (level U) for an effect on RLS symptoms of sleep hygiene improvement, change in caffeine or alcohol intake or smoking, mental activity, massage, hot baths, vitamins, aerobics/lower body training (1 class III study),[36] straight leg traction (1 class IV study),[37] yoga (1 class III study),[38] whole-body vibration (1 class III study),[39] transcutaneous spinal direct current stimulation (1 class III study),[40] posterior tibial nerve stimulation (1 class IV study),[41] enhanced external counterpulsation (1 class IV study),[42] and cognitive behavior therapy (1 class IV study).[43]

SUMMARY

For nonpharmacologic treatment options, there is some evidence for the effectiveness of pneumatic compression, NIRS, and possibly transcranial magnetic stimulation. For all other nonpharmacologic treatment options, including lifestyle changes, there is insufficient evidence.

In moderate to severe primary RLS, pharmacologic treatment can be considered (**Fig. 2**).[2] The first step of pharmacologic treatment is iron suppletion if applicable. Dopamine agonists and α2δ ligands are both effective for the treatment of RLS.[2] Considering the risk of augmentation with dopaminergic treatment and clinical consensus,[2,19] an α2δ ligand may be preferred to a dopamine agonist as first-line treatment.[2] The choice of treatment may also depend on comorbidity, although recommendations are mainly based on clinical consensus.[19] In patients with comorbid insomnia, painful RLS, comorbid pain syndrome, history of impulse control disorder, and comorbid anxiety, an α2δ ligand can be preferred, whereas, in patients with excessive weight or comorbid depression, a dopamine agonist can be the preferred drug.[19] When prescribing dopaminergic drugs, a low dose or longer-acting version may reduce the risk of augmentation. Rotigotine could also be preferred for patients with round-the-clock symptoms or in case of swallowing difficulties. Levodopa can be considered only in patients who need occasional treatment during periods of prolonged forced immobilization or with intermittent or sporadic RLS. When single-drug therapy is insufficient, a combination of an α2δ ligand and a dopamine agonist may be considered, based on clinical consensus. In otherwise refractory primary RLS, oxycodone/naloxone may be considered.[2] If augmentation has already occurred, there are several consensus-based strategies to address, including reducing the dopamine agonist dose or switching to a longer-lasting version or an α2δ ligand.

Most new trials are now focusing on nondopaminergic treatment options, and future studies will include intravenous iron treatments and substances that act on adenosine and glutamate.[1]

ACKNOWLEDGMENTS

The authors thank T. Visser and A. van der Velden for their support with the PubMed search strategy.

REFERENCES

1. Garcia-Borreguero D, Cano-Pumarega I. New concepts in the management of restless legs syndrome. BMJ 2017;356:j104.

2. Winkelman JW, Armstrong MJ, Allen RP, et al. Practice guideline summary: treatment of restless legs syndrome in adults: report of the Guideline Development, Dissemination, and Implementation Subcommittee of the American Academy of Neurology. Neurology 2016;87(24):2585–93.

3. Garcia-Borreguero D, Benitez A, Kohnen R, et al. Augmentation of restless leg syndrome (Willis-Ekbom disease) during long-term dopaminergic treatment. Postgrad Med 2015;127(7):716–25.

4. Inoue Y, Kuroda K, Hirata K, et al. Long-term open-label study of pramipexole in patients with primary restless legs syndrome. J Neurol Sci 2010;294(1–2):62–6.

5. Partinen M, Hirvonen K, Jama L, et al. Open-label study of the long-term efficacy and safety of pramipexole in patients with restless legs syndrome (extension of the PRELUDE study). Sleep Med 2008;9(5):537–41.

6. Bassetti CL, Bornatico F, Fuhr P, et al. Pramipexole versus dual release levodopa in restless legs syndrome: a double blind, randomised, cross-over trial. Swiss Med Wkly 2011;141:w13274.

7. Kvernmo T, Hartter S, Burger E. A review of the receptor-binding and pharmacokinetic properties of dopamine agonists. Clin Ther 2006;28(8):1065–78.

8. Boroojerdi B, Wolff HM, Braun M, et al. Rotigotine transdermal patch for the treatment of Parkinson's disease and restless legs syndrome. Drugs Today (Barc) 2010;46(7):483–505.

9. Elshoff JP, Braun M, Andreas JO, et al. Steady-state plasma concentration profile of transdermal rotigotine: an integrated analysis of three, open-label, randomized, phase I multiple dose studies. Clin Ther 2012;34(4):966–78.

10. Benitez A, Edens H, Fishman J, et al. Rotigotine transdermal system: developing continuous dopaminergic delivery to treat Parkinson's disease and restless legs syndrome. Ann N Y Acad Sci 2014;1329:45–66.

11. Hogl B, Oertel WH, Schollmayer E, et al. Transdermal rotigotine for the perioperative management of restless legs syndrome. BMC Neurol 2012;12:106.

12. Garcia-Borreguero D, Allen R, Hudson J, et al. Effects of rotigotine on daytime symptoms in patients with primary restless legs syndrome: a randomized, placebo-controlled study. Curr Med Res Opin 2016;32(1):77–85.

13. Oertel W, Trenkwalder C, Benes H, et al. Long-term safety and efficacy of rotigotine transdermal patch for moderate-to-severe idiopathic restless legs syndrome: a 5-year open-label extension study. Lancet Neurol 2011;10(8):710–20.

14. Oertel WH, Benes H, Garcia-Borreguero D, et al. One year open-label safety and efficacy trial with rotigotine transdermal patch in moderate to severe idiopathic restless legs syndrome. Sleep Med 2008;9(8):865–73.

15. Hogl B, Oertel WH, Stiasny-Kolster K, et al. Treatment of moderate to severe restless legs syndrome: 2-year safety and efficacy of rotigotine transdermal patch. BMC Neurol 2010;10:86.

16. Evidente VG. Piribedil for restless legs syndrome: a pilot study. Mov Disord 2001;16(3):579–81.

17. Aurora RN, Kristo DA, Bista SR, et al. The treatment of restless legs syndrome and periodic limb movement disorder in adults–an update for 2012: practice parameters with an evidence-based systematic review and meta-analyses: an American Academy of Sleep Medicine Clinical Practice Guideline. Sleep 2012;35(8):1039–62.

18. Garcia-Borreguero D, Ferini-Strambi L, Kohnen R, et al. European guidelines on management of restless legs syndrome: report of a joint task force by the European Federation of Neurological Societies, the European Neurological Society and the European Sleep Research Society. Eur J Neurol 2012;19(11):1385–96.

19. Garcia-Borreguero D, Kohnen R, Silber MH, et al. The long-term treatment of restless legs syndrome/Willis-Ekbom disease: evidence-based guidelines and clinical consensus best practice guidance: a report from the International Restless Legs Syndrome Study Group. Sleep Med 2013;14(7):675–84.

20. Garcia-Borreguero D, Cano I, Granizo JJ. Treatment of restless legs syndrome with the selective AMPA receptor antagonist perampanel. Sleep Med 2017;34:105–8.

21. Vetrugno R, La Morgia C, D'Angelo R, et al. Augmentation of restless legs syndrome with long-term tramadol treatment. Mov Disord 2007;22(3):424–7.

22. Earley CJ, Allen RP. Restless legs syndrome augmentation associated with tramadol. Sleep Med 2006;7(7):592–3.

23. Allen RP, Picchietti DL, Auerbach M, et al. Evidence-based and consensus clinical practice guidelines for the iron treatment of restless legs syndrome/Willis-Ekbom disease in adults and children: an IRLSSG task force report. Sleep Med 2018;41:27–44.

24. Vishwakarma K, Kalra J, Gupta R, et al. A double-blind, randomized, controlled trial to compare the efficacy and tolerability of fixed doses of ropinirole, bupropion, and iron in treatment of restless legs syndrome (Willis-Ekbom disease). Ann Indian Acad Neurol 2016;19(4):472–7.

25. Ulfberg J, Stehlik R, Mitchell U. Treatment of restless legs syndrome/Willis-Ekbom disease with selenium. Iran J Neurol 2016;15(4):235–6.

26. Jimenez-Trevino L. Oxcarbazepine treatment of restless legs syndrome: three case reports. Clin Neuropharmacol 2009;32(3):169–70.

27. Della Marca G, Vollono C, Mariotti P, et al. Levetiracetam can be effective in the treatment of restless legs syndrome with periodic limb movements in sleep: report of two cases. J Neurol Neurosurg Psychiatry 2006;77(4):566–7.

28. Garcia-Borreguero D, Allen RP, Kohnen R, et al. Diagnostic standards for dopaminergic augmentation of restless legs syndrome: report from a World Association of Sleep Medicine-International Restless Legs Syndrome Study Group consensus conference at the Max Planck Institute. Sleep Med 2007;8(5):520–30.

29. Garcia-Borreguero D, Silber MH, Winkelman JW, et al. Guidelines for the first-line treatment of restless legs syndrome/Willis-Ekbom disease, prevention and treatment of dopaminergic augmentation: a combined task force of the IRLSSG, EURLSSG, and the RLS-foundation. Sleep Med 2016;21:1–11.

30. Allen RP, Ondo WG, Ball E, et al. Restless legs syndrome (RLS) augmentation associated with dopamine agonist and levodopa usage in a community sample. Sleep Med 2011;12(5):431–9.

31. Eliasson AH, Lettieri CJ. Sequential compression devices for treatment of restless legs syndrome. Medicine (Baltimore) 2007;86(6):317–23.

32. Guffey JS, Motts S, Barymon D, et al. Using near infrared light to manage symptoms associated with restless legs syndrome. Physiother Theory Pract 2016;32(1):34–44.

33. Liu C, Dai Z, Zhang R, et al. Mapping intrinsic functional brain changes and repetitive transcranial magnetic stimulation neuromodulation in idiopathic restless legs syndrome: a resting-state functional magnetic resonance imaging study. Sleep Med 2015;16(6):785–91.

34. Lin YC, Feng Y, Zhan SQ, et al. Repetitive transcranial magnetic stimulation for the treatment of restless legs syndrome. Chin Med J (Engl) 2015;128(13):1728–31.

35. Montagna P, Sassoli de Bianchi L, Zucconi M, et al. Clonazepam and vibration in restless legs syndrome. Acta Neurol Scand 1984;69(6):428–30.

36. Aukerman MM, Aukerman D, Bayard M, et al. Exercise and restless legs syndrome: a randomized controlled trial. J Am Board Fam Med 2006;19(5):487–93.

37. Dinkins EM, Stevens-Lapsley J. Management of symptoms of restless legs syndrome with use of a traction straight leg raise: a preliminary case series. Man Ther 2013;18(4):299–302.

38. Innes KE, Selfe TK, Agarwal P, et al. Efficacy of an eight-week yoga intervention on symptoms of restless legs syndrome (RLS): a pilot study. J Altern Complement Med 2013;19(6):527–35.

39. Mitchell UH, Hilton SC, Hunsaker E, et al. Decreased symptoms without augmented skin blood flow in subjects with RLS/WED after vibration treatment. J Clin Sleep Med 2016;12(7):947–52.

40. Heide AC, Winkler T, Helms HJ, et al. Effects of transcutaneous spinal direct current stimulation in idiopathic restless legs patients. Brain Stimul 2014;7(5):636–42.

41. Rozeman AD, Ottolini T, Grootendorst DC, et al. Effect of sensory stimuli on restless legs syndrome: a randomized crossover study. J Clin Sleep Med 2014;10(8):893–6.

42. Rajaram SS, Rudzinskiy P, Walters AS. Enhanced external counter pulsation (EECP) for restless legs syndrome (RLS): preliminary negative results in a parallel double-blind study. Sleep Med 2006;7(4):390–1.

43. Hornyak M, Grossmann C, Kohnen R, et al. Cognitive behavioural group therapy to improve patients' strategies for coping with restless legs syndrome: a proof-of-concept trial. J Neurol Neurosurg Psychiatry 2008;79(7):823–5.

Drugs Used in Parasomnia

Paola Proserpio, MD[a], Michele Terzaghi, MD[b], Raffaele Manni, MD[b],
Lino Nobili, MD, PhD[a,c],*

KEYWORDS

- Disorders of arousal • REM behavior disorder • Sleep-related eating disorder • Sleep enuresis
- Benzodiazepines • Clonazepam • Melatonin • Antidepressant drugs

KEY POINTS

- Nonrapid eye movement (NREM) parasomnias, especially during childhood, are often benign conditions, and pharmacologic therapy is usually unnecessary.
- There are no properly powered randomized controlled studies evaluating the efficacy of pharmacologic therapy for NREM parasomnias.
- The most commonly used drugs for NREM parasomnias are intermediate- and long-acting benzodiazepines and antidepressants. Anecdotal cases reported the efficacy of melatonergic agents and hydroxytryptophan.
- The pharmacologic treatment of rapid eye movement sleep behavior disorder is symptomatic, and the most commonly used drugs are clonazepam and melatonin.

INTRODUCTION

Parasomnias are defined as "undesirable physical events or experiences that occur during entry into sleep, within sleep, or during arousal from sleep."[1] Depending on the sleep stage of occurrence, they are classified as nonrapid eye movement (NREM)-related parasomnias (confusional arousals, sleepwalking, sleep terrors, and sleep-related eating disorder), rapid eye movement (REM)-related parasomnias (REM sleep behavior disorder [RBD], recurrent isolated sleep paralysis, and nightmare disorder), and other parasomnias (exploding head syndrome [EHS], sleep-related hallucinations, and sleep enuresis [SE]).[1]

Parasomnias are not generally associated with a primary complaint of insomnia or excessive sleepiness, although this last one may be present in some of them. On the other hand, parasomnias can be associated with possible resulting injuries, adverse health, and negative psychosocial effects. Moreover, the clinical consequences of parasomnias can affect the patient, parents, or both.

Parasomnias, especially disorders of arousal (DOA) during childhood, are often relatively benign and transitory and do not usually require a pharmacologic therapy. A relevant aspect in both NREM and REM parasomnia treatment is to prevent sleep-related injuries by maintaining a safe environment. Physicians should always evaluate the possible presence of favoring and precipitating factors (sleep disorders and drugs). A pharmacologic treatment may be indicated in case of frequent, troublesome, or particularly dangerous events. The aim of this article is to review current available evidence on pharmacologic treatment of different forms of parasomnia.

NON RAPID EYE MOVEMENT PARASOMNIAS
Disorder of Arousal from Non Rapid Eye Movement Sleep

DOA are the subgroup of parasomnias arising from NREM sleep, encompassing confusional arousals, sleep terrors, and sleep walking.[1] They are most prevalent during childhood and normally cease

This article originally appeared in June, 2018 issue of *Sleep Medicine Clinics* (Volume 13, Issue 2).
[a] Department of Neuroscience, Centre of Sleep Medicine, Centre for Epilepsy Surgery, Niguarda Hospital, Piazza Ospedale Maggiore, Milan 3-20162, Italy; [b] Sleep Medicine and Epilepsy, IRCCS Mondino Foundation, Via Mondino, Pavia 2-27100, Italy; [c] Department of Neuroscience (DINOGMI), University of Genoa, Child neuropsychiatry, Gaslini Institute, Via Gerolamo Gaslini, Genoa 5-16147, Italy
* Corresponding author. Department of Neuroscience, Centre of Sleep Medicine, Niguarda Hospital, Piazza Ospedale Maggiore, Milan 3-20162, Italy
E-mail address: lino.nobili@unige.it

by adolescence, but onset or persistence during adulthood is well recognized.[2] More than one type may coexist within the same patient.[3] Many clinical features are common to these manifestations.[4,5] First, they generally occur during deep NREM sleep (N3) and, thus, most often take place in the first third of the night. During the episode, patients are usually unresponsive to the environment and completely or partially amnestic after the event. A positive family history is frequently found in DOA. Finally, any factor that deepens (sleep deprivation, stress, febrile illness, medications, alcohol) or fragments sleep (external or internal stimuli, sleep disorders, mental activity) may increase the occurrence of DOA.

DOA are generally considered benign phenomena. However, especially in adults, they can be characterized by complex behavior with potentially violent or injurious features[6] or be associated with significant functional impairment, such as daytime sleepiness, fatigue, and distress.[7] Therefore, evaluation and treatment are recommended in these cases, especially when violent manifestations are frequent or very disturbing for the patient or other family members.

The management of DOA is not well codified. No drug has yet been approved, and there are no properly powered randomized controlled studies evaluating the efficacy of behavioral or pharmacologic interventions for DOA.[8] Current treatment recommendations are based on scarce evidence derived from expert opinions, case reports, and only few case series. To date, the largest retrospective case series, analyzing treatment options and efficacy in DOA, refers to a population of 103 adults.[9]

Only recently, a self-administered scale has been developed with the aim of providing a valid and reliable tool able to assess the diagnosis and severity of NREM parasomnia as well as to monitor the efficacy of treatment.[10] Considering that evidence is lacking for off-label use of pharmacologic agents, clinicians may wish to ensure that patients are fully informed about all therapeutic options.[8]

Nonpharmacologic treatment

As previously discussed, if the episodes are rare, or not associated with harm potential, treatment is often unnecessary. Management includes reassuring patients about the usual benign nature of the episodes. Parents or bed partners should be instructed to keep calm and not to insist in trying to awaken the patient because this may aggravate or lengthen the episodes.[11] Precautions should be taken to ensure a safe sleep environment. Simple safety measures can include the removal of obstructions in the bedroom, securing windows,

sleeping on the ground floor, and installing locks or alarms on windows, doors, and stairways.[4,11]

Every priming or triggering factor should be investigated and avoided. For instance, every effort should be made to ensure regular and adequate sleep routines, to prevent sleep loss or disruption of the sleep-wake cycle. Sleep disorders (sleep apnea or periodic leg movements) must be recognized and treated.[12] Moreover, patients should avoid the intake of drugs or substances that could favor the occurrence of episodes (alcohol, hypnotics, antipsychotics, antidepressants, antihistamines).

Some investigators proposed "scheduled awakenings" in the case of DOA occurring nightly and consistently at or around the same time each night.[13] In adults, a psychological approach may be considered (hypnosis, relaxation therapy, or cognitive behavioral therapy), although studies evaluating its efficacy have provided contrasting results.[14,15]

Pharmacologic treatment

The main indications for a pharmacologic treatment in patients with DOA encompass the following: (1) persistence of frequent episodes despite resolution and removal of all potential predisposing and precipitating factors; (2) high risk of injury for the patient or the family; (3) significant functional impairment (such as insomnia, daytime sleepiness, weight gain from nocturnal eating); (4) potential legal consequences related to sexual or violent behavior.

As illustrated above, if drug therapy is planned, patients or their parents should be advised that drugs for DOA are considered "off label" and, if the decision is to prescribe, a patient's written consent is recommended.

Benzodiazepines Intermediate and long-acting agents in the benzodiazepine class of sedative hypnotics (BZD) are the most frequently used treatment of DOA,[4,11,16] although they have never been approved for this indication. They act by increasing the chloride conductance through GABA A receptors,[17] thus inducing a hypnotic-sedative effect. It is worth reminding that BDZ may have muscle-relaxing properties and should be used with caution if comorbid sleep-disordered breathing is suspected. The use of BZD in the treatment of DOA is apparently paradoxic, considering that other sedative-hypnotics such as non-BZD receptor agonists can induce amnestic nocturnal behavior.[18] The exact mechanism by which BZD suppress DOA is unknown. Probably, their effectiveness may be related to sedative effects or to decreases in slow-wave sleep.[19] Alternatively, they may work through the suppression of cortical arousals.[16]

Among the BZD class, clonazepam at 0.5 to 2 mg is the most common medication used in the treatment of DOA. However, studies (mainly conducted in adults) in the last 2 decades showed conflicting results. To date, only small case series, analyzing the efficacy of BDZ in children,[20] have been published. In 1989, Schenck and colleagues[21] studied 100 consecutive adults referred to their sleep disorders center for repeated nocturnal injury. All patients underwent full polysomnographic recordings. Fifty-four of these patients were diagnosed with either sleep terrors or sleepwalking. Clonazepam was prescribed for 28 of these patients and a rapid and sustained response was observed in 83.6% of them. A few years later, the same group published the results of a study designed to look for safety and abuse of BZDs taken for sleep disorders.[22] They analyzed 170 adults with sleep-related injuries of whom 69 had either sleepwalking or sleep terrors and were treated with BDZ, essentially clonazepam (n = 58) but also alprazolam. Most patients (86%) reported good control after an average follow-up of 3.5 years. The mean dose for clonazepam at the end of the study was 1.10 ± 0.96 mg. Interestingly, the risk of dosage escalation was low. In a more recent case series, Attarian and Zhu[9] analyzed the response to various therapeutic modalities in 103 adults with DOA. They found that clonazepam (0.5–2 mg) was used in 55% of the patients with a high response to treatment (73.7%).

Conversely, in another report, 5 patients with sleepwalking treated with clonazepam reported persistence of nocturnal episodes after 1 year of follow-up.[15]

Clonazepam has also been used successfully in somnambulism induced by neuroleptics,[23] and in DOA with behaviors such as driving and sleep violence.[22,24]

Anecdotal data have shown that patients with DOA respond to diazepam (2 to 5 mg).[25] However, in a small double-blind placebo-controlled crossover study of diazepam in sleepwalking, results failed to show significant difference between placebo and diazepam,[26] although investigators stated that in some participants, there was an alleviation of self-reported symptoms. Other BZDs that have been shown to be effective include triazolam (0.25 mg) at bedtime[27] and flurazepam.[28]

Antidepressant drugs Antidepressant drugs are occasionally effective in the treatment of DOA.[4,29] In the already mentioned recent largest case series study,[9] 4 patients responded to sertraline and 2 responded to clomipramine.

Anecdotal data reported efficacy of tricyclic antidepressant (imipramine or clomipramine) and trazodone. For instance, 2 patients with a history of sleep terrors and sleepwalking, in both of whom diazepam therapy failed, responded well to imipramine.[30] Conversely, trazodone provided a remarkable relief of symptoms in a 7-year-old girl who suffered from a severe sleep terror disorder, previously treated unsuccessfully with imipramine.[31]

Serotoninergic antidepressants, especially paroxetine, have been reported to be particularly effective in the treatment of sleep terrors. Indeed, a small case series showed a significant reduction of sleep terror events in 6 patients.[32] The investigators suggested that selective serotonin reuptake inhibitors (SSRI) may improve sleep terrors by virtue of serotonergic effects on the mesencephalic periaqueductal gray matter. Considering sleepwalking, a single case report showed the efficacy of paroxetine,[33,34] whereas other evidence reported a paroxetine inducing somnambulism.[35]

The mechanism by which antidepressant medications would influence DOA remains unclear, especially in light of these contradictory results. Indeed, the different efficacy of serotonin in sleepwalking and sleep terrors could suggest possible distinct pathophysiologic mechanisms at the basis of these manifestations.[4]

Other drugs Single case reports have shown the efficacy of other pharmacologic treatments, such as melatonin, hydroxytryptophan, and ramelteon.

Melatonin (N-acetyl-5-methoxytryptamine) is an endogenous hormone produced by the pineal gland and released exclusively at night. Exogenous melatonin supplementation is well tolerated and has no significant adverse effects and a low potential for dependence. Melatonin has been shown to synchronize the circadian rhythms and improve the onset, duration, and quality of sleep. Thus, melatonin seems to represent an alternative treatment of sleep disorders with significantly less side effects.[36] Moreover, melatonin has been shown to be particularly useful for treatment of sleep disorders in children with neurodevelopmental disabilities.[37] To date, only 2 case reports showed its efficacy in the treatment of DOA. In particular, Jan and colleagues[38] described a 12-year-old patient affected by Asperger syndrome and a chronic sleep-phase onset delay in whom melatonin was effective in the treatment of sleepwalking and sleep terror episodes. However, its efficacy could be related mainly to the correction of the circadian disorder and the consequent improvement of the underlying sleep deprivation. More recently, Özcan and Dönmez[39] reported the efficacy of treatment with melatonin for 2 weeks in a 36-month-old patient with sleep terror.

An open pharmacologic trial conducted in 45 children with sleep terror demonstrated the efficacy of L-5-hydroxytryptophan, a precursor of serotonin, in 83.9% of patients after 6 months of therapy.[40] The investigators hypothesized that this drug could induce a long-term improvement of sleep terrors through a stabilization of the sleep microstructure and a modulation of the arousal level in children.

Finally, Sasayama and colleagues[41] recently reported a boy with attention-deficit/hyperactivity disorder whose night terrors and sleepwalking were effectively treated with ramelteon, a melatonin receptor agonist, probably improving sleep deprivation.

SLEEP-RELATED EATING DISORDER

Sleep-related eating disorder (SRED) is an NREM sleep parasomnia characterized by frequent episodes of dysfunctional and involuntary eating and drinking that occur after an arousal during NREM sleep associated with diminished levels of consciousness and subsequent recall, with problematic health consequences.[1] This sleep disorder generally starts in young adults, with a female predominance.[42] SRED is sometimes associated with the use of psychotropic drugs (triazolam, zolpidem, amitriptyline, olanzapine, and risperidone) and other sleep disorders, including parasomnias, narcolepsy, restless legs syndrome, and periodic leg movements.[43] Thus, the first goal of treatment is to eliminate any precipitating factors and to recognize and treat any comorbid sleep disorders. Indeed, removal of any offending drug together with treatment of sleep disturbances has been shown to resolve many cases of SRED.[43,44] Moreover, the nonpharmacologic treatment plan should also include education regarding proper sleep hygiene, the maintenance of a safe sleep environment, and the limitation of other precipitating factors, such as cigarette smoking or alcohol intake.[45–47]

The preferred drugs used for treatment of SRED are represented by dopamine agonists, BZDs, topiramate, and SSRI.[47,48(p2)]

A randomized, double-blind, placebo-controlled crossover study of pramipexole (0.18–0.36 mg/d) on 11 SRED subjects demonstrated improvement in sleep quality and actigraphic measures.[49] Nevertheless, number and duration of waking episodes related to eating behaviors were unchanged, and no weight loss was observed. A more recent work confirmed the efficacy of dopamine agonist in 3 patients with SRED.[50] Interestingly, other dopaminergic agents, such as carbidopa/L-dopa and bromocriptine as monotherapy, were effective in 25% of the patients with SRED associated with sleepwalking, and in combination with BZDs (mainly clonazepam), opiates, or both in approximately 87% of subjects.[51]

SSRI (fluoxetine, paroxetine, and fluvoxamine) were reportedly effective in 2 different studies.[51,52]

Substantial reduction of sleep-related eating episodes and significant weight loss have been achieved in subjects treated with topiramate, an antiepileptic drug that induces weight loss.[50,53–55] In particular, Winkelman[55] reported that 68% of patients responded to topiramate, with a mean dose of 135 mg/d, but the discontinuation rate was high, because of side effects, including dullness, paresthesia, and daytime sleepiness. In a more recent study, 20 patients with SRED were treated with topiramate, 17 of whom showed cessation or a clear reduction in night eating episodes, whereas 6 (30%) had to discontinue medication because of adverse effects (eg, dizziness, visual problems, and worsening of preexisting depressive symptoms).[50] Physicians should follow up patients regularly with SRED treated with topiramate in order to promptly recognize and treat side effects.[47] It is unclear how topiramate works to decrease SRED manifestations. It was hypothesized that the drug may work by suppressing arousals produced by underlying sleep disorders or by acting as an anorexigenic agent, either through glutamatergic antagonism or serotonergic agonism.[54] Moreover, topiramate has been reported to stimulate insulin release and increase insulin sensitivity, both of which may contribute to appetite regulation and weight loss.[56]

Zapp and colleagues[57] recently described a case of a patient with SRED associated with the use of various antidepressants and sleep apnea that completely vanished after treatment with agomelatine or melatonin extended release.

RAPID EYE MOVEMENT PARASOMNIAS
Rapid Eye Movement Sleep Behavior Disorder

RBD treatment is currently based on a symptomatic approach, because interventions to prevent or slow the conversion toward neurodegenerative diseases in susceptible subjects are not available at the moment.

Sleep-related injuries are frequent and reported in up to 65% of RBD cases,[58–60] so that RBD subjects should be offered a treatment immediately following the diagnosis. Symptomatic treatment is aimed at preventing injuries to the patient and/or to the bed partner by reducing the frequency and severity of dream-enacted behaviors. Effects on dream content and sleep quality should also be considered when optimizing RBD pharmacologic interventions.

In the management of RBD subjects, clinicians should also be aware of the possibility that ongoing pharmacologic treatment with antidepressants, particularly SSRIs, can have an impact on RBD, worsening its manifestations.[61]

Despite the importance of establishing treatment, research found a limited number of drugs effective in RBD, and current knowledge about efficacy and tolerability profile of drugs used in RBD subjects is still based on low-level evidence data based on case reports and case series.[62] Thus, adequately powered controlled trials addressing drug effects in this category are needed.

Clonazepam

The effectiveness of clonazepam on RBD was reported in the seminal paper from Schenck and colleagues,[63] and since then, it has been widely used for RBD treatment as first-choice therapy. Its efficacy is reflected in a complete remission of symptoms in 55% to 90% of RBD subjects.[60] In a recent open-label study of the effect of clonazepam up to 3 mg, the figure of RBD subjects defined as responders (ie, absence of injuries and potential injurious behaviors to self and/or to bed partner) was reported to be 66.7%.[64] Clonazepam doses are between 0.25 and 4.0 mg at bedtime, with 0.5 mg appearing to be a suitable dosage for most of the subjects.[65]

Although RBD symptoms occur after discontinuation of clonazepam,[62] they usually are easily controlled by the resumption of therapy. Tolerance and withdrawal symptoms only rarely occur, even if complaints of insomnia and unsatisfactory sleep quality can be reported.[62] Main side effects, such as early morning sedation, incoordination, falls, confusion, memory impairment, sexual dysfunctions, and worsening of sleep-disordered breathing, can occur.[62] Clonazepam does not influence the occurrence of dreams with emotional or sorrowful content, but results in a reduction of the frequency of nightmares and dreams with violent and frightening content, paralleled by the reduction in potential injurious behaviors.[64] In consideration of the side-effect profile of the drug, caution is needed in elderly subjects for the possibility to impair both postural instability and cognitive performances, up to the occurrence of confusional states in subjects with cognitive decline.[66] Furthermore, clonazepam should be prescribed at the lowest effective dose in patients with sleep apnea, and respiratory pattern should be assessed during treatment.

Melatonin

Exogenous melatonin has been shown as being approximately equally effective at reducing RBD severity in respect to clonazepam.[62,65,67] In a comparative study to clonazepam, melatonin resulted in better tolerability, with subjects taking clonazepam reporting more frequently drowsiness, instability, and neuropsychological impairment.[65] Differently from clonazepam, melatonin has univocal evidence of restoring REM sleep muscle atonia.[68] Melatonin dosages are 2 mg to 12 mg at bedtime. Melatonin at a median dosage of 6 mg proved to be as effective in reducing RBD behavior as clonazepam (0.5 mg).[65] These doses are usually well tolerated, despite dose-dependent side effects, such as morning headache, sleepiness, delusions, and hallucinations.[69]

Because of its profile of effectiveness and tolerability, melatonin is a valid option in RBD subjects and can be preferred to clonazepam in the case of background disease features, consisting of sleep-disordered breathing, disorders of gait and unsteadiness, or cognitive impairment.

Melatonergic agents

On the basis of the effectiveness and tolerability profile of exogenous melatonin, melatoninergic agents are expected to benefit RBD subjects. Effects of ramelteon at doses of 8 mg/d (in improving RBD control in subjects affected by extrapyramidal disorders[70]) were not confirmed on objective polysomnographic assessment of RBD behavior and REM sleep without atonia (RSWA), despite a subjective reduction in dream enactment frequency and severity.[71,72] In the same way, agomelatine (25 mg) proved to improve RBD symptoms in idiopathic RBD, but did not change RBD motor events frequency and RSWA on polysomnographic assessment.[73]

Dopamine agonists

Controversial results were carried out by efforts in treating RBD with pramipexole. Pramipexole was reported to reduce RBD symptoms[74–76] and seems to be effective mainly in the form of RBD with limited loss of atonia.[75] However, no changes were found in RBD subjects with extrapyramidal disorders on clinical or polysomnographic grounds.[77] All in all, pramipexole should be considered when other treatments have failed to control RBD. Since its efficacy in restless legs syndrome, pramipexole can be considered initial treatment of subjects with comorbid restless legs syndrome, but deserves a short-interval follow-up visit to assess RBD evolution.

Acetylcholinesterase inhibitors

Use of acetylcholinesterase inhibitors for RBD treatment is based on the notion that cholinergic mechanisms are central for the initiation and coordination of REM sleep.[78] Furthermore, in dementia with Lewy bodies, in which cholinergic transmission is impaired, administration of acetylcholinesterase inhibitor was reported to potentially restore correct sleep patterns and resolve nocturnal confusional events.[79,80]

However, conflicting data are reported in the literature about acetylcholinesterase inhibitor's efficacy in RBD.

Acetylcholinesterase inhibitors donepezil and rivastigmine were reported to reduce RBD behavior.[62,81–84] On the other hand, no changes in RBD in subjects with comorbid neurodegenerative diseases could be found,[69] and even the occurrence of de novo RBD was reported in a patient with Alzheimer disease.[85] Altogether, considering the limited and conflicting data about the efficacy of acetylcholinesterase inhibitors in RBD, these drugs should be used as a third-line treatment analogously to pramipexole, in cases of clonazepam or melatonin failure. Because the possibility that RBD occurs in the context of cognitive impairment, acetylcholinesterase inhibitors can be used in symptomatic RBD patients requiring concurrent treatment of cognitive impairment or hallucinations (ie, dementia with Lewy bodies and Parkinson disease dementia).

Cannabidiol

There has been evidence that suggests that cannabis may have therapeutic potential in several neurologic disorders, and sleep in particular.[86] Data on the effect of cannabinoids on RBD are limited, but the efficacy of cannabidiol, the nonintoxicating constituent of cannabis, in ameliorating RBD in subjects with Parkinson disease was reported, together with a good tolerability profile.[87]

Miscellaneous

For BZDs other than clonazepam, temazepam as monotherapy or in association to zopiclone,[88,89] triazolam,[60] and alprazolam[22] were used in RBD, suggesting that they may have a class-specific effect. Zopiclone appears to be effective and well tolerated in reducing RBD symptoms.[88] Herbal derivates, as Yi-Gan San[90] or Yokukansan, which contain exactly measured mixtures of dried herbs, can be effective in improving RBD symptoms. Sodium oxybate can be an effective add-on option for the treatment of idiopathic RBD, refractory to conventional therapies, despite a lack of improvement in polysomnographic parameters.[91,92]

Nightmare Disorder

The therapeutic approach to nightmares encompasses nonpharmacologic as well as pharmacologic options. Although psychotherapy and cognitive behavior interventions have traditionally been the treatment of choice, drugs alone or in combination therapy can be used as an alternative to psychological interventions.

In the evaluation of nightmares, it should be kept in mind that numerous drugs can trigger nightmares and vivid dreams, among which are catecholaminergic agents, β-blockers, barbiturates, dopaminergic agents, and alcohol and even some antidepressants. Several drugs classes, including SSRIs, tricyclic antidepressants, antipsychotics, and adrenergic agonists, were studied in nightmare disorder.[93–95] Some lines of evidence show that risperidone, trazodone, clonidine, quetiapine, fluvoxamine, mirtazapine, and terazosin can be helpful.[95] However, data are limited, and the quality of evidence is poor.[62]

Prazosin

Prazosin is a centrally acting selective α1-adrenergic antagonist and has been considered efficacious as pharmacologic treatment of nightmares, especially in cases of posttraumatic nightmares, with a good profile of tolerability.[96–98] The relapse of nightmares following discontinuation of prazosin was reported, showing the need for long-term use.[99] However, recent data put into discussion the results from previous studies,[100] and data showing no effect of prazosin on nightmare frequency were reported.[95]

Cannabinoids

The use of tetrahydrocannabinol in the treatment of nightmares associated with posttraumatic stress disorder was reported to result in the reduction of nightmare recurrence and intensity.[101–104] A good profile of tolerability accompanied the drug,[104] with dry mouth, headache, and dizziness being the more frequently reported symptoms.

RECURRENT ISOLATED SLEEP PARALYSIS

It should be carefully considered whether to pharmacologically treat sleep paralysis episodes or not. Most of the patients with sleep paralysis do not experience clinically significant distress, and basic treatment is avoidance of sleep deprivation and other precipitants. In the case of recurrent sleep paralysis and significant clinical distress, the cost/benefit balance of drug therapy should be considered. A substantial lack of systematic data in this field leads personal experience to have a central role in the choice of the drug.

Pharmacologic intervention is based on the possibility of suppressing REM sleep, and tricyclic antidepressants (clomipramine, imipramine, desmethylimipramine)[105–107] and SSRIs (fluoxetine, femoxetine, and viloxazine)[107–109] can be considered. Sodium oxybate is a possible therapy for sleep paralysis in narcolepsy.[110]

OTHER PARASOMNIAS
Exploding Head Syndrome

EHS is characterized by a "sudden, loud imagined noise or sense of a violent explosion in the head occurring as the patient is falling asleep or waking during the night."[1]

To date, no open or controlled clinical trials for EHS treatment are available, but several case studies of effective treatment have been conducted.[111,112] In many cases, reassurance about the benign nature of EHS could lead to a remission of EHS episodes. Tricyclic antidepressants (clomipramine, amitriptyline) are reported to decrease the frequency and intensity of attacks in some patients.[111,113] Moreover, calcium channel blockers (flunarizine and slow-release nifedipine) may also be useful.[114,115] Finally, anticonvulsants have been prescribed in some cases. Topiramate reduced the intensity of auditory sounds from loud bangs to much softer buzzing sounds, but without a complete remission.[116] Carbamazepine was described to be effective in 3 cases.[112]

Sleep-Related Hallucinations

Sleep-related hallucinations are "hallucinatory experiences that occur at sleep onset (hypnagogic) or on awakening from sleep (hypnopompic)."[1] They can be associated with narcolepsy, but a high prevalence in the normal population is also described. Complex nocturnal visual hallucinations are often associated with different disorders, especially in elderly, such as visual loss (Charles Bonnet syndrome), Lewy body disorders, and pathologic abnormality of the mesencephalon and diencephalon (peduncular hallucinosis).

Little objective information is available regarding the management of sleep-related hallucinations. Reassurance is frequently sufficient. Tricyclic antidepressants have been suggested for hypnagogic and hypnopompic hallucinations.

Sleep Enuresis

SE is characterized by "recurrent involuntary voiding that occurs during sleep. In primary SE, recurrent involuntary voiding occurs at least twice a week during sleep after 5 years of age in a subject who has never been consistently dry during sleep for 6 consecutive months. SE is considered secondary in a child or adult who had previously been dry for 6 consecutive months and then began wetting at least twice a week. Both primary and secondary enuresis must be present for a period of at least 3 months."[1] Moreover, SE is defined as *monosymptomatic* when the subject has no associated daytime symptoms of bladder dysfunction (such as wetting, increased voiding frequency, urgency, jiggling, squatting, and holding maneuvers). However, usually, when a meticulous history is obtained, most children have at least some mild daytime void symptoms, and their SE is classifiable as *non-monosymptomatic*.[117]

The management of SE starts from some simple strategies, such as lifting or wakening, rewarding dry nights, bladder training (including retention control training), and fluid restriction.[117–119] On the other hand, it has been suggested that children should be encouraged to maintain an adequate fluid intake, because fluid restriction can worsen bladder function.[120] Alarm systems that alert and awaken the child if any moisture is detected are considered a first-line treatment, and its effect seems to be more gradual but sustained with respect to drugs.[121]

The established drug treatment for polyuric bedwetting is desmopressin, a synthetic analogue of the pituitary hormone arginine vasopressin, which reduces urine production by increasing water absorption.[119,120] It is available in tablet or fast-melting oral lyophilisate form. Desmopressin should be taken 1 hour before going to sleep. Treatment begins with a 0.2-mg desmopressin tablet or 120 µg of the melt tablet. If the starting dose does not lead to a clinical response, after 14 days the dose can be increased up to 0.4 mg or 240 µg. If treatment is successful, it can continue to be prescribed in 3-month blocks.[119] The sudden discontinuation of desmopressin results in a high recurrence of enuresis.[122] Desmopressin is considered a safe drug. The rare and most severe side effect of oral desmopressin therapy is the risk of "water intoxication" (if medication intake coincides with drinking large volumes) with symptoms of vomiting, headache, decreased consciousness, possible seizures, and hyponatremia. Therefore, fluid intake in the evening should be restricted to 250 mL, and night-time drinking is not recommended. This complication seems to be more frequent during therapy with intranasal formulation of desmopressin.[123] Desmopressin is mostly indicated in children with nocturnal polyuria and normal bladder reservoir function and in those in whom alarm therapy has failed or who are thought to be unlikely to comply with alarm therapy.[124] It is frequently used as a stopgap (sleepovers and school camps) rather than cure for long term. About 30% of children with enuresis are full responders, and 40% have a partial response to desmopressin.[124] However, the long-lasting curative effect is low.[125]

The tricyclic antidepressant imipramine has anticholinergic, antispasmodic, and local anesthetic effects, and possibly a central nervous system effect on voiding, and has been approved for use in treating nocturnal enuresis in children aged 6 years and older.[126] It is effective in about 40% of patients with enuresis, but only 25% of them experience complete dryness once the medication is withdrawn.[127] Side effects encompass cardiac arrhythmias, hypotension, hepatotoxicity, central nervous system depression, interaction with other drugs, and the danger of intoxication by accidental overdose. Therefore, screening for a long QT syndrome with electrocardiogram before starting treatment is recommended.

Anticholinergic drugs are used for SE, mainly for non-monosymptomatic cases.[117–120] They are thought to act by increasing the functional bladder capacity and enabling patients affected to achieve better control over micturition. The anticholinergic drug most frequently used is represented by oxybutynin (0.1–0.3 mg/kg/d), although it has considerable risk of side effects (flushing, blurred vision, constipation, tremor, decreased salivation, and decreased ability to sweat) because of its relatively nonspecific affinity for several cholinergic receptor isoforms. The fourth International Consultation on Incontinence[128] recommended the use of propiverine (0.8–1 mg/kg/d) as first-line medication for non-monosymptomatic SE (level of evidence 1, grade of recommendation B/C). Recent studies have shown the efficacy and safety of other anticholinergic drugs, such as trospium chloride, solifenacin,[129] and tolterodine[130] in children.

Although anticholinergic monotherapy could be ineffective, it can improve treatment response when combined with other established treatments, such as imipramine, desmopressin, or enuresis alarms, particularly in treatment-resistant cases.[131] Indeed, a recent meta-analysis demonstrated that the combination therapy, comprising desmopressin plus an anticholinergic agent, was more effective compared with desmopressin monotherapy for the treatment of SE in children.[132]

REFERENCES

1. American Academy of Sleep Medicine. International classification of sleep disorders-third edition (ICSD-3). Darien (Illinois); 2014.
2. Stallman HM, Kohler M. Prevalence of sleepwalking: a systematic review and meta-analysis. PLoS One 2016;11(11):e0164769.
3. Derry CP, Harvey AS, Walker MC, et al. NREM arousal parasomnias and their distinction from nocturnal frontal lobe epilepsy: a video EEG analysis. Sleep 2009;32(12):1637–44.
4. Howell MJ. Parasomnias: an updated review. Neurotherapeutics 2012;9(4):753–75.
5. Zadra A, Desautels A, Petit D, et al. Somnambulism: clinical aspects and pathophysiological hypotheses. Lancet Neurol 2013;12(3):285–94.
6. Siclari F, Khatami R, Urbaniok F, et al. Violence in sleep. Brain 2010;133(12):3494–509.
7. Lopez R, Jaussent I, Scholz S, et al. Functional impairment in adult sleepwalkers: a case-control study. Sleep 2013;36(3):345–51.
8. Harris M, Grunstein RR. Treatments for somnambulism in adults: assessing the evidence. Sleep Med Rev 2009;13(4):295–7.
9. Attarian H, Zhu L. Treatment options for disorders of arousal: a case series. Int J Neurosci 2013;123(9):623–5.
10. Arnulf I, Zhang B, Uguccioni G, et al. A scale for assessing the severity of arousal disorders. Sleep 2014;37(1):127–36.
11. Attarian H. Treatment options for parasomnias. Neurol Clin 2010;28(4):1089–106.
12. Tinuper P, Bisulli F, Provini F. The parasomnias: mechanisms and treatment: the parasomnias: mechanisms and treatment. Epilepsia 2012;53:12–9.
13. Kotagal S. Treatment of dyssomnias and parasomnias in childhood. Curr Treat Options Neurol 2012;14(6):630–49.
14. Galbiati A, Rinaldi F, Giora E, et al. Behavioural and cognitive-behavioural treatments of parasomnias. Behav Neurol 2015;2015:786928.
15. Guilleminault C, Kirisoglu C, Bao G, et al. Adult chronic sleepwalking and its treatment based on polysomnography. Brain 2005;128(Pt 5):1062–9.
16. Cochen De Cock V. Sleepwalking. Curr Treat Options Neurol 2016;18(2):6.
17. Rudolph U, Möhler H. GABA-based therapeutic approaches: GABAA receptor subtype functions. Curr Opin Pharmacol 2006;6(1):18–23.
18. Dolder CR, Nelson MH. Hypnosedative-induced complex behaviours: incidence, mechanisms and management. CNS Drugs 2008;22(12):1021–36.
19. Mason TBA, Pack AI. Sleep terrors in childhood. J Pediatr 2005;147(3):388–92.
20. Allen RM. Attenuation of drug-induced anxiety dreams and pavor nocturnus by benzodiazepines. J Clin Psychiatry 1983;44(3):106–8.
21. Schenck CH, Milner DM, Hurwitz TD, et al. A polysomnographic and clinical report on sleep-related injury in 100 adult patients. Am J Psychiatry 1989;146(9):1166–73.

22. Schenck CH, Mahowald MW. Long-term, nightly benzodiazepine treatment of injurious parasomnias and other disorders of disrupted nocturnal sleep in 170 adults. Am J Med 1996;100(3):333–7.

23. Goldbloom D, Chouinard G. Clonazepam in the treatment of neuroleptic-induced somnambulism. Am J Psychiatry 1984;141(11):1486.

24. Schenck CH, Mahowald MW. A polysomnographically documented case of adult somnambulism with long-distance automobile driving and frequent nocturnal violence: parasomnia with continuing danger as a noninsane automatism? Sleep 1995;18(9):765–72.

25. Remulla A, Guilleminault C. Somnambulism (sleepwalking). Expert Opin Pharmacother 2004;5(10): 2069–74.

26. Reid WH, Haffke EA, Chu CC. Diazepam in intractable sleepwalking: a pilot study. Hillside J Clin Psychiatry 1984;6(1):49–55.

27. Berlin RM, Qayyum U. Sleepwalking: diagnosis and treatment through the life cycle. Psychosomatics 1986;27(11):755–60.

28. Kavey NB, Whyte J, Resor SR, et al. Somnambulism in adults. Neurology 1990;40(5):749–52.

29. Kierlin L, Littner MR. Parasomnias and antidepressant therapy: a review of the literature. Front Psychiatry 2011;2:71.

30. Cooper AJ. Treatment of coexistent night-terrors and somnambulism in adults with imipramine and diazepam. J Clin Psychiatry 1987;48(5):209–10.

31. Balon R. Sleep terror disorder and insomnia treated with trazodone: a case report. Ann Clin Psychiatry 1994;6(3):161–3.

32. Wilson SJ, Lillywhite AR, Potokar JP, et al. Adult night terrors and paroxetine. Lancet 1997; 350(9072):185.

33. Frölich Alfred Wiater Gerd Lehmkuhl J. Successful treatment of severe parasomnias with paroxetine in a 12-year-old boy. Int J Psychiatry Clin Pract 2001; 5(3):215–8.

34. Lillywhite AR, Wilson SJ, Nutt DJ. Successful treatment of night terrors and somnambulism with paroxetine. Br J Psychiatry 1994;164(4):551–4.

35. Kawashima T, Yamada S. Paroxetine-induced somnambulism. J Clin Psychiatry 2003;64(4):483.

36. Xie Z, Chen F, Li WA, et al. A review of sleep disorders and melatonin. Neurol Res 2017;39(6): 559–65.

37. Jan JE, Freeman RD. Melatonin therapy for circadian rhythm sleep disorders in children with multiple disabilities: what have we learned in the last decade? Dev Med Child Neurol 2004;46(11): 776–82.

38. Jan JE, Freeman RD, Wasdell MB, et al. A child with severe night terrors and sleep-walking responds to melatonin therapy. Dev Med Child Neurol 2004;46(11):789.

39. Özcan Ö, Dönmez YE. Melatonin treatment for childhood sleep terror. J Child Adolesc Psychopharmacol 2014;24(9):528–9.

40. Bruni O, Ferri R, Miano S, et al. l-5-Hydroxytryptophan treatment of sleep terrors in children. Eur J Pediatr 2004;163(7):402–7.

41. Sasayama D, Washizuka S, Honda H. Effective treatment of night terrors and sleepwalking with ramelteon. J Child Adolesc Psychopharmacol 2016; 26(10):948.

42. Winkelman JW, Johnson EA, Richards LM. Sleep-related eating disorder. Handb Clin Neurol 2011; 98:577–85.

43. Inoue Y. Sleep-related eating disorder and its associated conditions: clinical implication of SRED. Psychiatry Clin Neurosci 2015;69(6):309–20.

44. Howell MJ, Schenck CH. Restless nocturnal eating: a common feature of Willis-Ekbom Syndrome (RLS). J Clin Sleep Med 2012;8(4):413–9.

45. Auger RR. Sleep-related eating disorders. Psychiatry (Edgmont) 2006;3(11):64.

46. Brion A, Flamand M, Oudiette D, et al. Sleep-related eating disorder versus sleepwalking: a controlled study. Sleep Med 2012;13(8):1094–101.

47. Chiaro G, Caletti MT, Provini F. Treatment of sleep-related eating disorder. Curr Treat Options Neurol 2015;17(8):361.

48. Howell MJ, Schenck CH. Treatment of nocturnal eating disorders. Curr Treat Options Neurol 2009; 11(5):333–9.

49. Provini F, Albani F, Vetrugno R, et al. A pilot double-blind placebo-controlled trial of low-dose pramipexole in sleep-related eating disorder. Eur J Neurol 2005;12(6):432–6.

50. Santin J, Mery V, Elso MJ, et al. Sleep-related eating disorder: a descriptive study in Chilean patients. Sleep Med 2014;15(2):163–7.

51. Schenck CH, Hurwitz TD, O'Connor KA, et al. Additional categories of sleep-related eating disorders and the current status of treatment. Sleep 1993; 16(5):457–66.

52. Miyaoka T, Yasukawa R, Tsubouchi K, et al. Successful treatment of nocturnal eating/drinking syndrome with selective serotonin reuptake inhibitors. Int Clin Psychopharmacol 2003;18(3):175–7.

53. Martinez-Salio A, Soler-Algarra S, Calvo-Garcia I, et al. Nocturnal sleep-related eating disorder that responds to topiramate. Rev Neurol 2007;45(5): 276–9 [in Spanish].

54. Winkelman JW. Treatment of nocturnal eating syndrome and sleep-related eating disorder with topiramate. Sleep Med 2003;4(3):243–6.

55. Winkelman JW. Efficacy and tolerability of open-label topiramate in the treatment of sleep-related eating disorder: a retrospective case series. J Clin Psychiatry 2006;67(11):1729–34.

56. Wilkes JJ, Nelson E, Osborne M, et al. Topiramate is an insulin-sensitizing compound in vivo with direct effects on adipocytes in female ZDF rats. Am J Physiol Endocrinol Metab 2005;288(3): E617–24.

57. Zapp AA, Fischer EC, Deuschle M. The effect of agomelatine and melatonin on sleep-related eating: a case report. J Med Case Rep 2017; 11(1):275.

58. Comella CL, Nardine TM, Diederich NJ, et al. Sleep-related violence, injury, and REM sleep behavior disorder in Parkinson's disease. Neurology 1998;51(2):526–9.

59. McCarter SJ, St Louis EK, Boswell CL, et al. Factors associated with injury in REM sleep behavior disorder. Sleep Med 2014;15(11):1332–8.

60. Olson EJ, Boeve BF, Silber MH. Rapid eye movement sleep behaviour disorder: demographic, clinical and laboratory findings in 93 cases. Brain J Neurol 2000;123(Pt 2):331–9.

61. Postuma RB, Gagnon J-F, Tuineaig M, et al. Antidepressants and REM sleep behavior disorder: isolated side effect or neurodegenerative signal? Sleep 2013;36(11):1579–85.

62. Aurora RN, Zak RS, Maganti RK, et al. Best practice guide for the treatment of REM sleep behavior disorder (RBD). J Clin Sleep Med 2010;6(1):85–95.

63. Schenck CH, Bundlie SR, Ettinger MG, et al. Chronic behavioral disorders of human REM sleep: a new category of parasomnia. Sleep 1986;9(2): 293–308.

64. Li SX, Lam SP, Zhang J, et al. A prospective, naturalistic follow-up study of treatment outcomes with clonazepam in rapid eye movement sleep behavior disorder. Sleep Med 2016;21:114–20.

65. McCarter SJ, Boswell CL, St Louis EK, et al. Treatment outcomes in REM sleep behavior disorder. Sleep Med 2013;14(3):237–42.

66. Terzaghi M, Sartori I, Rustioni V, et al. Sleep disorders and acute nocturnal delirium in the elderly: a comorbidity not to be overlooked. Eur J Intern Med 2014;25(4):350–5.

67. Kunz D, Mahlberg R. A two-part, double-blind, placebo-controlled trial of exogenous melatonin in REM sleep behaviour disorder. J Sleep Res 2010; 19(4):591–6.

68. Kunz D, Bes F. Melatonin as a therapy in REM sleep behavior disorder patients: an open-labeled pilot study on the possible influence of melatonin on REM-sleep regulation. Mov Disord 1999;14(3): 507–11.

69. Boeve BF, Silber MH, Ferman TJ. Melatonin for treatment of REM sleep behavior disorder in neurologic disorders: results in 14 patients. Sleep Med 2003;4(4):281–4.

70. Nomura T, Kawase S, Watanabe Y, et al. Use of ramelteon for the treatment of secondary REM sleep behavior disorder. Intern Med 2013;52(18):2123–6.

71. Esaki Y, Kitajima T, Koike S, et al. An open-labeled trial of ramelteon in idiopathic rapid eye movement sleep behavior disorder. J Clin Sleep Med 2016; 12(5):689–93.

72. St. Louis EK, McCarter SJ, Boeve BF. Ramelteon for idiopathic REM sleep behavior disorder: implications for pathophysiology and future treatment trials. J Clin Sleep Med 2016;12(05):643–5.

73. Bonakis A, Economou N-T, Papageorgiou SG, et al. Agomelatine may improve REM sleep behavior disorder symptoms. J Clin Psychopharmacol 2012; 32(5):732–4.

74. Fantini ML, Gagnon J-F, Filipini D, et al. The effects of pramipexole in REM sleep behavior disorder. Neurology 2003;61(10):1418–20.

75. Sasai T, Matsuura M, Inoue Y. Factors associated with the effect of pramipexole on symptoms of idiopathic REM sleep behavior disorder. Parkinsonism Relat Disord 2013;19(2):153–7.

76. Schmidt MH, Koshal VB, Schmidt HS. Use of pramipexole in REM sleep behavior disorder: results from a case series. Sleep Med 2006;7(5):418–23.

77. Kumru H, Iranzo A, Carrasco E, et al. Lack of effects of pramipexole on REM sleep behavior disorder in Parkinson disease. Sleep 2008;31(10): 1418–21.

78. McCarley RW. Neurobiology of REM and NREM sleep. Sleep Med 2007;8(4):302–30.

79. Fernandez HH, Wu C-K, Ott BR. Pharmacotherapy of dementia with Lewy bodies. Expert Opin Pharmacother 2003;4(11):2027–37.

80. Terzaghi M, Rustioni V, Manni R, et al. Agrypnia with nocturnal confusional behaviors in dementia with Lewy bodies: immediate efficacy of rivastigmine. Mov Disord 2010;25(5):647–9.

81. Brunetti V, Losurdo A, Testani E, et al. Rivastigmine for refractory REM behavior disorder in mild cognitive impairment. Curr Alzheimer Res 2014;11(3): 267–73.

82. Di Giacopo R, Fasano A, Quaranta D, et al. Rivastigmine as alternative treatment for refractory REM behavior disorder in Parkinson's disease. Mov Disord 2012;27(4):559–61.

83. Massironi G, Galluzzi S, Frisoni GB. Drug treatment of REM sleep behavior disorders in dementia with Lewy bodies. Int Psychogeriatr 2003;15(4):377–83.

84. Ringman JM, Simmons JH. Treatment of REM sleep behavior disorder with donepezil: a report of three cases. Neurology 2000;55(6):870–1.

85. Yeh S-B, Yeh P-Y, Schenck CH. Rivastigmine-induced REM sleep behavior disorder (RBD) in an 88-year-old man with Alzheimer's disease. J Clin Sleep Med 2010;6(2):192–5.

86. Babson KA, Sottile J, Morabito D. Cannabis, cannabinoids, and sleep: a review of the literature. Curr Psychiatry Rep 2017;19(4):23.

87. Chagas MHN, Eckeli AL, Zuardi AW, et al. Cannabidiol can improve complex sleep-related behaviours associated with rapid eye movement sleep behaviour disorder in Parkinson's disease patients: a case series. J Clin Pharm Ther 2014;39(5):564–6.

88. Anderson KN, Shneerson JM. Drug treatment of REM sleep behavior disorder: the use of drug therapies other than clonazepam. J Clin Sleep Med 2009;5(3):235–9.

89. Bonakis A, Howard RS, Ebrahim IO, et al. REM sleep behaviour disorder (RBD) and its associations in young patients. Sleep Med 2009;10(6): 641–5.

90. Jung Y, St Louis EK. Treatment of REM sleep behavior disorder. Curr Treat Options Neurol 2016;18(11):50.

91. Moghadam KK, Pizza F, Primavera A, et al. Sodium oxybate for idiopathic REM sleep behavior disorder: a report on two patients. Sleep Med 2017;32: 16–21.

92. Shneerson JM. Successful treatment of REM sleep behavior disorder with sodium oxybate. Clin Neuropharmacol 2009;32(3):158–9.

93. Detweiler MB, Pagadala B, Candelario J, et al. Treatment of post-traumatic stress disorder nightmares at a Veterans Affairs medical center. J Clin Med 2016;5(12) [pii: E117].

94. Jeffreys M, Capehart B, Friedman MJ. Pharmacotherapy for posttraumatic stress disorder: review with clinical applications. J Rehabil Res Dev 2012;49(5):703–15.

95. Miller KE, Brownlow JA, Woodward S, et al. Sleep and dreaming in posttraumatic stress disorder. Curr Psychiatry Rep 2017;19(10):71.

96. George KC, Kebejian L, Ruth LJ, et al. Meta-analysis of the efficacy and safety of prazosin versus placebo for the treatment of nightmares and sleep disturbances in adults with posttraumatic stress disorder. J Trauma Dissociation 2016;17(4): 494–510.

97. Kung S, Espinel Z, Lapid MI. Treatment of nightmares with prazosin: a systematic review. Mayo Clin Proc 2012;87(9):890–900.

98. Raskind MA, Peterson K, Williams T, et al. A trial of prazosin for combat trauma PTSD with nightmares in active-duty soldiers returned from Iraq and Afghanistan. Am J Psychiatry 2013;170(9): 1003–10.

99. Hudson SM, Whiteside TE, Lorenz RA, et al. Prazosin for the treatment of nightmares related to posttraumatic stress disorder: a review of the literature. Prim Care Companion CNS Disord 2012;14(2) [pii: PCC.11r01222].

100. Khachatryan D, Groll D, Booij L, et al. Prazosin for treating sleep disturbances in adults with posttraumatic stress disorder: a systematic review and meta-analysis of randomized controlled trials. Gen Hosp Psychiatry 2016;39:46–52.

101. Cameron C, Watson D, Robinson J. Use of a synthetic cannabinoid in a correctional population for posttraumatic stress disorder-related insomnia and nightmares, chronic pain, harm reduction, and other indications: a retrospective evaluation. J Clin Psychopharmacol 2014;34(5):559–64.

102. Fraser GA. The use of a synthetic cannabinoid in the management of treatment-resistant nightmares in posttraumatic stress disorder (PTSD). CNS Neurosci Ther 2009;15(1):84–8.

103. Jetly R, Heber A, Fraser G, et al. The efficacy of nabilone, a synthetic cannabinoid, in the treatment of PTSD-associated nightmares: a preliminary randomized, double-blind, placebo-controlled crossover design study. Psychoneuroendocrinology 2015;51:585–8.

104. Roitman P, Mechoulam R, Cooper-Kazaz R, et al. Preliminary, open-label, pilot study of add-on oral Δ9-tetrahydrocannabinol in chronic post-traumatic stress disorder. Clin Drug Investig 2014;34(8): 587–91.

105. Guilleminault C, Raynal D, Takahashi S, et al. Evaluation of short-term and long-term treatment of the narcolepsy syndrome with clomipramine hydrochloride. Acta Neurol Scand 1976;54(1):71–87.

106. Hishikawa Y, Ida H, Nakai K, et al. Treatment of narcolepsy with imipramine (tofranil) and desmethylimipramine (pertofran). J Neurol Sci 1966;3(5): 453–61.

107. Mitler MM, Hajdukovic R, Erman M, et al. Narcolepsy. J Clin Neurophysiol 1990;7(1):93–118.

108. Koran LM, Raghavan S. Fluoxetine for isolated sleep paralysis. Psychosomatics 1993;34(2): 184–7.

109. Schrader H, Kayed K, Bendixen Markset AC, et al. The treatment of accessory symptoms in narcolepsy: a double-blind cross-over study of a selective serotonin re-uptake inhibitor (femoxetine) versus placebo. Acta Neurol Scand 1986;74(4): 297–303.

110. Abad VC, Guilleminault C. New developments in the management of narcolepsy. Nat Sci Sleep 2017;9:39–57.

111. Frese A, Summ O, Evers S. Exploding head syndrome: six new cases and review of the literature. Cephalalgia 2014;34(10):823–7.

112. Sharpless BA. Exploding head syndrome. Sleep Med Rev 2014;18(6):489–93.

113. Sachs C, Svanborg E. The exploding head syndrome: polysomnographic recordings and therapeutic suggestions. Sleep 1991;14(3):263–6.

114. Chakravarty A. Exploding head syndrome: report of two new cases. Cephalalgia 2008;28(4): 399–400.

115. Jacome DE. Exploding head syndrome and idiopathic stabbing headache relieved by nifedipine. Cephalalgia Int J Headache 2001;21(5):617–8.

116. Palikh GM, Vaughn BV. Topiramate responsive exploding head syndrome. J Clin Sleep Med 2010; 6(4):382–3.

117. Harari MD. Nocturnal enuresis: nocturnal enuresis. J Paediatr Child Health 2013;49(4):264–71.

118. Jain S, Bhatt GC. Advances in the management of primary monosymptomatic nocturnal enuresis in children. Paediatr Int Child Health 2016;36(1):7–14.

119. Kuwertz-Bröking E, von Gontard A. Clinical management of nocturnal enuresis. Pediatr Nephrol 2017. [Epub ahead of print].

120. Caldwell PHY, Deshpande AV, Gontard AV. Management of nocturnal enuresis. BMJ 2013; 347(oct29 11):f6259.

121. Glazener CMA, Evans JHC, Peto RE. Alarm interventions for nocturnal enuresis in children. Cochrane Database Syst Rev 2005;(2):CD002911.

122. Hjalmas K, Arnold T, Bower W, et al. Nocturnal enuresis: an international evidence based management strategy. J Urol 2004;171(6 Pt 2): 2545–61.

123. Robson WLM, Leung AKC, Norgaard JP. The comparative safety of oral versus intranasal desmopressin for the treatment of children with nocturnal enuresis. J Urol 2007;178(1):24–30.

124. Neveus T, Eggert P, Evans J, et al. Evaluation of and treatment for monosymptomatic enuresis: a standardization document from the International Children's Continence Society. J Urol 2010;183(2): 441–7.

125. Glazener CM, Evans JH. Desmopressin for nocturnal enuresis in children. Cochrane Database Syst Rev 2002;(3):CD002112.

126. Nevéus T. Nocturnal enuresis-theoretic background and practical guidelines. Pediatr Nephrol 2011;26(8):1207–14.

127. Caldwell PHY, Sureshkumar P, Wong WCF. Tricyclic and related drugs for nocturnal enuresis in children. Cochrane Database Syst Rev 2016;(1): CD002117.

128. International Consultation on Incontinence, Abrams P, Cardozo L, et al, editors. Incontinence. 4th edition. Paris: Health Publication; 2009.

129. Hoebeke P, De Pooter J, De Caestecker K, et al. Solifenacin for therapy resistant overactive bladder. J Urol 2009;182(4 Suppl):2040–4.

130. Raes A, Hoebeke P, Segaert I, et al. Retrospective analysis of efficacy and tolerability of tolterodine in children with overactive bladder. Eur Urol 2004; 45(2):240–4.

131. Deshpande AV, Caldwell PHY, Sureshkumar P. Drugs for nocturnal enuresis in children (other than desmopressin and tricyclics). Cochrane Database Syst Rev 2012;(12):CD002238.

132. Yu J, Yan Z, Zhou S, et al. Desmopressin plus anticholinergic agent in the treatment of nocturnal enuresis: a meta-analysis. Exp Ther Med 2017; 14(4):2875–84.

Drugs Used in Circadian Sleep-Wake Rhythm Disturbances

Helen J. Burgess, PhD[a],*, Jonathan S. Emens, MD[b,c]

KEYWORDS

- Advance • Agonist • Circadian • Delay • Melatonin • Shift • Sleep

KEY POINTS

- Exogenous melatonin and other melatonin receptor agonists can be used to shift circadian timing and improve sleep in patients with sleep and circadian disturbances.
- Each medication varies in its circadian resetting and sleep-enhancing properties, and safety concerns.
- The latest exogenous melatonin treatment recommendations for circadian rhythm sleep-wake disorders are reviewed.

INTRODUCTION

The focus of this article is on the use of melatonin and other melatonin receptor agonists as chronobiotics; that is, drugs that shift central circadian timing (ie, reset the 24-hour biological clock) and that also have potential to improve sleep. The aim is to provide a relevant update from a recent review of melatonin and other melatonin receptor agonists[1] and highlight the practical use of these drugs. The authors recognize that other drugs have the potential to act as chronobiotics and that different medications, including hypnotics and alerting medications, may have potential for treating circadian rhythm sleep-wake disorders, but these are not addressed here because they remain to be tested in clinical trials examining circadian rhythm sleep-wake disorders.

This article provides a brief review of the circadian system and circadian rhythm sleep-wake disorders, followed by a summary of the relevant

agents available and the safety concerns surrounding their use. The circadian phase shifting and sleep-enhancing properties of these particular chronobiotics are reviewed, along with the latest American Academy of Sleep Medicine (AASM) clinical practice guidelines regarding the use of exogenous melatonin for treating intrinsic circadian rhythm disorders.[2] The article concludes with a discussion of the use of these medications in clinical practice.

THE CIRCADIAN SYSTEM AND CIRCADIAN RHYTHM SLEEP-WAKE DISORDERS

The circadian system orchestrates the near-24-hour endogenous rhythms seen in a wide variety of physiologic variables. The molecular "gears" of the clock exist in most organ systems and these disparate clocks are internally synchronized by a central pacemaker in the suprachiasmatic nuclei (SCN) of the hypothalamus, which is itself

This article originally appeared in June, 2018 issue of *Sleep Medicine Clinics* (Volume 13, Issue 2).

Disclosure: H.J. Burgess is a consultant for Natrol, LLC. J.S. Emens has nothing to disclose.

[a] Biological Rhythms Research Laboratory, Department of Behavioral Sciences, Rush University Medical Center, 1645 West Jackson Boulevard, Suite 425, Chicago, IL 60612, USA; [b] Department of Psychiatry, Oregon Health & Science University, VA Portland Health Care System, 3710 Southwest US Veterans Hospital, Road P3-PULM, Portland, OR 97239, USA; [c] Department of Medicine, Oregon Health & Science University, VA Portland Health Care System, 3710 Southwest US Veterans Hospital, Road P3-PULM, Portland, OR 97239, USA

* Corresponding author.

E-mail address: Helen_J_Burgess@rush.edu

synchronized (reset) by external time cues, primarily the light/dark cycle.[3] The timing of the clock (circadian phase) can be shifted to an earlier or later time (phase advances and phase delays, respectively) depending on when during the biological day or night a resetting stimulus is given. Circadian timing and sleep have a profound influence on mental and physical health (eg, see Refs.[4–7]), and circadian rhythm sleep-wake disorders result when wakefulness and sleep are scheduled in opposition to the timing of the biological clock (eg, attempting to sleep during the biological day). A key to understanding circadian rhythm sleep-wake disorders, and their treatment, is appreciating this difference between internal biological timing and external clock time.

The third edition of the International Classification of Sleep Disorders describes 6 circadian rhythm sleep-wake disorders that have been reviewed in depth previously.[2,8] These include the extrinsic circadian rhythm sleep-wake disorders (jet lag disorder and shift work disorder) and also the intrinsic circadian rhythm sleep-wake disorders (delayed sleep-wake phase disorder), advanced sleep-wake phase disorder, irregular sleep-wake rhythm disorder, and non-24-hour sleep-wake rhythm disorder (non-24). Their primary features and possible causes are summarized in **Table 1**.

MELATONIN AND OTHER MELATONIN RECEPTOR AGONISTS

The circadian resetting effects of melatonin are well documented[9–12] and both receptor subtypes have been shown to contribute to this effect.[13,14] Melatonin is available without a prescription in the United States both alone and in combination with other supplements, and in multiple formulations. It is estimated that 2% of US adults use exogenous melatonin, most commonly to improve sleep.[15,16] There are also melatonin formulations and other melatonin receptor agonists available via prescription in various countries, including Circadin, Tasimelteon, Ramelteon, and Agomelatine, which are summarized in **Table 2**.

TREATMENT SAFETY CONSIDERATIONS

Side effects are infrequent with exogenous melatonin, with the exception of sleepiness, but the side effects discussed in several meta-analyses are listed in **Table 2**. Because of the sleepiness side effect, patients should not drive or operate machinery after ingesting melatonin, and should test their individual response to particular doses and formulations in safe environments.

Bioavailability of melatonin can vary (eg, 1%–37%).[17] Meta-analyses have reported potential for melatonin to adversely affect people with epilepsy,[18] and for melatonin to interact with warfarin and potentially other oral anticoagulants.[18] There have also been concerns about potential effects of melatonin on development in children,[19] and so caution is advised in the administration of melatonin to prepubertal children unless the demonstrated benefits outweigh the potential risks (eg, in children with significant developmental delay or children with non-24-hour sleep-wake schedule disorder). It is also generally recommended that women who are pregnant, trying to get pregnant, or breastfeeding do not take exogenous melatonin.[20] Exogenous melatonin (5 mg) has been found to acutely impair glucose tolerance when administered with food[21] and further research on the effects of exogenous melatonin on glucose metabolism, and on which patients might be vulnerable to these effects,[22] is warranted. In general, large-scale randomized controlled trials are needed to evaluate the long-term safety of melatonin in children and adults.[20] Other prescription-based melatonin receptor agonists also carry their own potential side effect profiles, which are summarized in **Table 2**.

USING MELATONIN AND OTHER MELATONIN RECEPTOR AGONISTS TO SHIFT CIRCADIAN TIMING

As described in detail in our previous review,[1] both the dose and timing of exogenous melatonin administration need to be considered when attempting to reset the biological clock. The timing of melatonin administration simultaneously determines the direction and magnitude of the resulting circadian phase shift. Melatonin phase response curves (PRCs; eg, see Refs.[11,12]) are plots of average data that are similar to dose response curves, but instead of describing the effect of a drug at different doses, they describe the effect of a drug administered at different biological times. Biological timing can be determined by measuring a convenient marker of the biological clock, such as the onset of endogenous melatonin secretion assayed in plasma or saliva samples collected under dim light conditions (the dim light melatonin onset [DLMO]).[23–25] These PRCs indicate that exogenous melatonin typically causes phase advances when administered in the late biological afternoon and early evening (peaking about 5–7 hours before habitual bedtime), phase delays when administered late in the biological night and early morning (peaking around habitual wake time), and shifts from causing phase advances to

Table 1
International Classification of Sleep Disorders, Third Edition classification of circadian rhythm sleep-wake disorders

Disorder	Jet Lag Disorder	Shift Work Disorder	Delayed Sleep-Wake Phase Disorder	Advanced Sleep-Wake Phase Disorder	Irregular Sleep-Wake Rhythm Disorder	Non–24-h Sleep-Wake Rhythm Disorder
Primary Features	Insomnia and/or hypersomnolence with decreased total sleep time associated with transmeridian travel across ≥2 time zones	Insomnia and/or hypersomnolence with decreased total sleep time associated with work times during habitual sleep times	Sleep-wake timing is shifted ≥2 h later, sleep onset insomnia, morning somnolence, and an absence of difficulty when sleep timing is delayed	Sleep-wake timing is shifted ≥2 h earlier, evening somnolence, early morning insomnia, and an absence of difficulty when sleep timing is advanced	Irregular sleep/wake schedule with insomnia during scheduled sleep and somnolence during scheduled wake times	Sleep/wake timing that drifts progressively later (or earlier) across the 24-h day. In the blind: relapsing/remitting insomnia and somnolence while keeping a consistent sleep/wake schedule
Cause	Scheduling of sleep and wakefulness during the biological day and night, respectively, as a result of rapid transmeridian travel	Scheduling of work during the biological night with corresponding scheduling of sleep during the biological day	Altered circadian resetting (increased response to delaying evening light or decreased response to advancing morning light), altered exposure to resetting agents (eg, increased evening light exposure), and/or a long biological day (long circadian period)	Altered circadian resetting (increased response to advancing morning light or decreased response to delaying evening light), altered exposure to resetting agents (eg, increased morning light exposure), and/or a short biological day (short circadian period)	Seen in individuals with neurodegenerative or neurodevelopmental disorders	In the blind: a lack of light input to the circadian pacemaker In the sighted: possible self-selected light/dark schedule in conjunction with factors seen in delayed sleep-wake phase disorder

Data from American Academy of Sleep Medicine. Classification of Circadian Rhythm Sleep-Wake Disorders. In: International Classification of Sleep Disorders. 3rd ed. Darien, IL; 2014:191–224.

Table 2
A summary of the circadian, sleep, and possible side effects of melatonin and other melatonin receptor agonists

Drug	Approved for	Mechanism of Action	Circadian Phase Shifting Effects	Sleep Effects	Possible Side Effects
Melatonin	Available over the counter in the United States, via prescription in most other countries	MT1 and MT2 receptor agonist	Can phase advance and phase delay[11,12]	Decreases latency to sleep onset[32–34]; may increase total sleep time, sleep quality[33] Effects may be larger when endogenous melatonin levels are low[36]	Sleepiness, dizziness, headache, blood pressure changes, gastrointestinal upset[18,20,32]
Circadin	Insomnia in adults ≥55 y old	MT1 and MT2 receptor agonist	Not clear as a prolonged release melatonin formulation	Decreases latency to sleep onset, improves sleep quality[54]	Similar to exogenous melatonin[55]
Tasimelteon	Non–24-h sleep-wake rhythm disorder	MT1 and MT2 receptor agonist	Can phase advance[56,57]	Decreases latency to sleep onset; increases sleep efficiency when administered to enhance sleep 5 h before habitual bedtime[57]	Headache, increased liver enzyme levels, cardiac conduction changes, upper respiratory and urinary tract infections, nightmares[58]
Ramelteon	Insomnia in adults	MT1 and MT2 receptor agonist	Can phase advance[59]	Decreases latency to sleep onset; increases total sleep time, sleep efficiency, sleep quality[60]	Sleepiness, dizziness, headache, gastrointestinal upset, upper respiratory tract infections, dysmenorrhea[60]
Agomelatine	Depression	MT1 and MT2 receptor agonist, serotonin 5-HT2c receptor antagonist	Can phase advance[61,62]	Decreases latency to sleep onset in patients with major depressive disorder[63]	Liver injury[64,65]

Abbreviations: MT1, melatonin receptor 1; MT2, melatonin receptor 2.

phase delays in the biological evening (**Fig. 1**). It is therefore important to point out that exogenous melatonin causes the largest phase shifts when patients are likely to be awake (assuming they are maintaining a conventional sleep/wake schedule), and so low doses that will not result in somnolence are preferred, as discussed later.

The dose of melatonin can also affect the resulting phase shift. A wide range of doses have been examined for circadian resetting[11,12,26,27] and there is evidence that a therapeutic window exists for melatonin's chronobiotic effects: at lower doses of 0.02 to 0.30 mg, a dose response relationship has been shown,[27] whereas 0.5-mg and 3.0-mg doses cause similar resetting[12] and higher doses of 10 mg or more have smaller resetting effects.[26,28] This therapeutic window likely exists because increasing the dose of exogenous

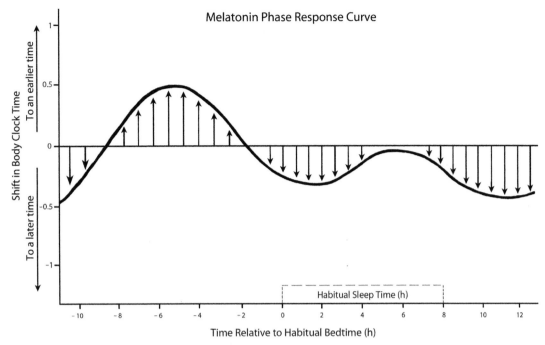

Fig. 1. A PRC rereferenced to habitual sleep timing. PRCs are usually referenced to a marker of circadian phase, but, for ease of use, the authors have rereferenced this PRC to habitual sleep timing. The melatonin phase response curve is adapted from a phase response curve generated to 3 days of a daily dose of 0.5 mg of exogenous melatonin.[12] Accordingly, we have reduced the amplitude of the melatonin phase response curve by a factor of 3, to better estimate the effects of a single dose. Any resulting phase shift will be a combined effect of exogenous melatonin plus concomitant light exposure.

melatonin also increases the duration of time that circulating levels of melatonin are increased. Within the lower part of this dose range, increasing doses simply result in increased resetting effects,[27] but with higher doses more and more of the melatonin PRC is stimulated until the opposite zone begins to be stimulated and less net circadian resetting occurs. This phenomenon of exogenous melatonin "spilling over"[28] onto the opposite zone of the melatonin PRC occurs, despite a half-life of 30 to 45 minutes,[17] because even doses of 0.5 to 1.0 mg of melatonin can produce supraphysiologic levels over several hours or more.[11,29] As reviewed later, melatonin also has soporific effects and therefore care should be taken to use the lowest dose possible when exogenous melatonin is taken during the habitual waking hours, as is often necessary for maximal circadian resetting effects.

The latest AASM clinical practice guidelines for the treatment of intrinsic circadian rhythm disorders with exogenous melatonin[2] are shown in **Table 3**. Details of the studies that formed the basis of the recommendations, including exogenous melatonin dose and timing of administration, are also summarized. Other reviews address how

exogenous melatonin can be used to reduce jet lag and improve adaptation to shift work.[30,31]

USING MELATONIN AND OTHER MELATONIN RECEPTOR AGONISTS TO IMPROVE SLEEP

Melatonin is well recognized to reduce the time taken to fall asleep (sleep onset latency).[32–34] The reports on whether melatonin can increase sleep duration and/or consolidation (eg, sleep efficiency) are mixed,[32–34] and it may not be soporific when administered during the biological night when endogenous melatonin levels are increased.[35] The soporific effects of exogenous melatonin can be larger in populations with lower levels of endogenous melatonin (eg, in hypertensive patients treated with β-blockers[36]). Nonetheless, the sleep-enhancing effects of exogenous melatonin are usually smaller than those associated with hypnotics, and sometimes are not considered clinically meaningful.[37] The sleep-enhancing effects of melatonin may in part be mediated via binding to melatonin receptors in the periphery, which can induce thermoregulatory changes that induce sleepiness and sleep.[38] Melatonin may also reduce circadian alerting signals by binding to melatonin receptors on the SCN.[39]

Table 3
Melatonin treatment recommendations from the 2015 clinical practice guideline for treatment of intrinsic circadian rhythm sleep-wake disorders

Disorder	Number of Studies That Formed Guideline	Effective Doses and Timing Tested	Treatment Guideline
Delayed sleep-wake phase disorder	3 Adult studies 3 Children studies	Adults: 0.3 mg or 3 mg fast release, 1.5–6.5 h before baseline DLMO, time pill taken advanced by 1 h after 2 wk[66] 5 mg fast release between 7 and 9 PM, treatment advanced by ~1 h after first week[67,68] Children: 0.15 mg/kg fast release 1.5–2.0 h before habitual bedtime[69] 3 or 5 mg fast release 6 or 7 PM[70,71]	Use strategically timed melatonin or other melatonin receptor agonists
Advanced sleep-wake phase disorder	No studies	NA	No recommendation
Irregular sleep-wake rhythm disorder (elderly with dementia)	1 Adult study	Null effects[72]	Do not use melatonin or other melatonin receptor agonists
Irregular sleep-wake rhythm disorder (children/adolescents with neurologic disorders)	1 Child study	2–10 mg fast release, ~30 min before planned bedtime[73]	Use strategically timed melatonin or other melatonin receptor agonists
Non–24-h sleep-wake rhythm disorder	3 Adult blind studies in patients whose circadian phase drifts later in time	10 mg 1 h before preferred bedtime[26] 0.5 mg[74] or 5 mg[75] at 9 PM	Use strategically timed melatonin or other melatonin receptor agonists

Note that a lack of recommendation does not indicate melatonin should not be used in those disorders but that the available evidence was insufficient to make a recommendation for or against treatment with melatonin and other melatonin receptor agonists.[76]
Abbreviation: NA, not available.
Data from refs[2,48,68–76].

PRACTICAL ASPECTS OF MELATONIN AND OTHER MELATONIN AGONIST TREATMENTS
Melatonin Preparations

The first practical consideration for clinicians is related to exogenous melatonin's classification as a dietary supplement by the US Food and Drug Administration (FDA): the purity and dose accuracy of different formulations is not necessarily assured.[40,41] In recent years, individual manufacturers have adopted improved testing procedures,[42] but ultimately clinicians may need to choose from among those formulations that have been subject to some type of outside review.[43,44] An important consideration for therapy with melatonin is the low cost (often <10 cents per pill[44]).

Melatonin Administration

As described earlier, the potential interactions between exogenous melatonin and prescription medications and/or other dietary supplements should be considered before recommending melatonin treatment. In addition, drugs metabolized by cytochrome P450 1A2 liver enzymes, including some antidepressants, caffeine, and oral contraceptives, can inadvertently increase levels of plasma melatonin after exogenous melatonin administration.[19,20] Clinicians should note that less than half of the general population are estimated to consult with their physicians about their use of supplements.[16]

Before beginning treatment, clinicians should first make sure the patient is maintaining a consistent light/dark schedule. This schedule is critical for ensuring that a correct biological time of administration is chosen and hence the desired circadian resetting effect is achieved. This schedule may also offer some benefit all on its own, because it minimizes the circadian misalignment associated with rapidly changing sleep/wake opportunities. Clinicians should be aware that exogenous melatonin, on its own, cannot overcome the resetting effect of a patient's self-selected light/dark cycle, and that it is important that the timing of melatonin and light act in concert to achieve the desired resetting effect. Evidence of this potential competition between melatonin and light can be seen in the larger resetting effects observed with exogenous melatonin administered in the laboratory (where light levels are controlled),[12] compared with administration at home.[11]

Once a patient is successfully maintaining a consistent light/dark schedule, the clinician should then administer melatonin about 5 to 6 hours before habitual bedtime to shift circadian timing to an earlier hour or at habitual wake time to shift circadian timing later. These administration times can be slowly moved an hour or less earlier or later, respectively, every few days,[45] if insomnia or somnolence symptoms have improved but sleep timing is still delayed or advanced. Just as consistent light/dark timing is critical to success, so is consistently timed administration of melatonin, and the use of alarms, such as on mobile phones, can help in this respect. In all cases, the aim is to achieve a normal and consistent relationship between the timing of sleep and the timing of the biological clock.

Non-24 in the blind is unique among the intrinsic circadian rhythm sleep-wake disorders, because the cause is clear but the treatment is more complex (for review of treatment see Ref.[46]). Non-24 arises in blind individuals because the biological clock is no longer reset by light. Most commonly, this results in circadian timing shifting ~20 minutes later every day.[47] Melatonin can arrest this drift,[26] but experiments have shown that the drift in circadian timing often does not immediately cease, nor does the eventual timing of the clock necessarily correspond with the timing of melatonin administration. As a result, clinicians should initially administer melatonin 6 hours before the desired bedtime and, as discussed earlier, slowly shift the administration time earlier or later if there are remaining symptoms that indicate a phase delay or phase advance, respectively. Less frequently, circadian timing shifts earlier each day[47] and melatonin should be administered at the desired wake time[48] (note that this is more likely to be the case in female patients[47,49]).

Melatonin and Light Combination Treatment

Apart from the case of blind patients, patients generally receive exogenous melatonin or other melatonin receptor agonists while exposed to a light-dark cycle, which is, as noted earlier, the strongest circadian resetting agent.[1] In general, light has opposite phase shifting effects to melatonin, such that evening light phase delays and morning light phase advances.[1] Consequently, when administering melatonin or other melatonin receptor agonists, phase shifting effects can be altered depending on whether the concomitant light exposure is facilitating or opposing the melatonin agonist phase shift.[50–52] Thus, in the case of sighted patients, concomitant light exposure and/or light avoidance should also be included in the treatment plan.

EVALUATION OF OUTCOME

A continued limitation in the diagnosis and treatment of circadian rhythm sleep-wake disorders is the lack of an FDA approved test of circadian timing. Although some progress has been made in this regard[53] since our last review,[1] clinicians should still use symptom improvement to gauge treatment response. This approach is similar to the treatment of most insomnias, in which the use of sleep diaries and rating scales can be useful. Wrist actigraphy offers a more objective measure, although, in clinical practice, the authors find it is more useful in determining the consistency of rest/activity and light/dark timing (discussed earlier).

SUMMARY

This article focuses on melatonin and other melatonin receptor agonists and summarizes their circadian phase shifting and sleep-enhancing properties, along with their associated possible safety concerns. The circadian system and circadian rhythm sleep-wake disorders are described, along with the latest AASM recommendations for the use of exogenous melatonin in treating them. In addition, the practical aspects of using exogenous melatonin obtainable over the counter in the United States, consideration of the effects of concomitant light exposure, and assessing treatment response are discussed.

ACKNOWLEDGMENTS

The authors thank Muneer Rizvydeen for his assistance in creating the figure. H.J. Burgess and J.S. Emens are supported by grants from the National Center for Complementary and Integrative Health (R34AT008347); National Heart, Lung, and Blood Institute (R01HL125893), (R01HL140577); National Institute of Nursing Research (R21NR014377); and National Institute on Alcohol Abuse and Alcoholism (R01AA023839). The content is solely the responsibility of the authors and does not necessarily represent the official views of the National Institutes of Health.

REFERENCES

1. Emens J, Burgess HJ. Effect of light and melatonin and other melatonin receptor agonists on human circadian physiology. Sleep Med Clin 2015;10: 435–53.
2. Auger RR, Burgess HJ, Emens JS, et al. Clinical practice guideline for the treatment of intrinsic circadian rhythm sleep-wake disorders: advanced sleep-wake phase disorder (ASWPD), delayed sleep-wake phase disorder (DSWPD), non-24-hour sleep-wake rhythm disorder (N24SWD), and irregular sleep-wake rhythm disorder (ISWRD). An update for 2015: an American Academy of Sleep Medicine clinical practice guideline. J Clin Sleep Med 2015; 11(10):1199–236.
3. Buhr ED, Takahashi JS. Molecular components of the mammalian circadian clock. Handb Exp Pharmacol 2013;217:3–27.
4. Wright KP, Hull JT, Hughes RJ, et al. Sleep and wakefulness out of phase with internal biological time impairs learning in humans. J Cogn Neurosci 2006;18(4):508–21.
5. Scheer FA, Hilton MF, Mantzoros CS, et al. Adverse metabolic and cardiovascular consequences of circadian misalignment. Proc Natl Acad Sci U S A 2009;106(11):4453–8.
6. Levandovski R, Dantas G, Fernandes LC, et al. Depression scores associate with chronotype and social jetlag in a rural population. Chronobiol Int 2011;28(9):771–8.
7. Watson NF, Badr MS, Belenky G, et al. Recommended amount of sleep for a healthy adult: a joint consensus statement of the American Academy of Sleep Medicine and Sleep Research Society. Sleep 2015;38(6):843–4.
8. Reid KJ, Burgess HJ. Circadian rhythm sleep disorders. Prim Care 2005;32:449–73.
9. Redman J, Armstrong S, Ng KT. Free-running activity rhythms in the rat: entrainment by melatonin. Science 1983;219(4588):1089–91.
10. Arendt J, Bojkowski C, Folkard S, et al. Some effects of melatonin and the control of its secretion in humans. In: Evered D, Clark S, editors. Photoperiodism, melatonin, and the pineal. London: Pitman; 1985. p. 266–83.
11. Lewy AJ, Bauer VK, Ahmed S, et al. The human phase response curve (PRC) to melatonin is about 12 hours out of phase with the PRC to light. Chronobiol Int 1998;15:71–83.
12. Burgess HJ, Revell VL, Molina TA, et al. Human phase response curves to three days of daily melatonin: 0.5 mg versus 3.0 mg. J Clin Endocrinol Metab 2010;95(7):3325–31.
13. Reppert SM, Weaver DR, Godson C. Melatonin receptors step into the light: cloning and classification of subtypes. Trends Pharmacol Sci 1996;17: 100–2.
14. Dubocovich ML. Melatonin receptors: role on sleep and circadian rhythm regulation. Sleep Med 2007; 8(Suppl 3):34–42.
15. National Sleep Foundation. 2005 Sleep in America Poll. Available at: https://sleepfoundation.org/sleep-polls-data/sleep-in-america-poll/2005-adult-sleep-habits-and-styles. Accessed Jan 2, 2018.
16. Bliwise DL, Ansari FP. Insomnia associated with valerian and melatonin usage in the 2002 National Health Interview Survey. Sleep 2007;30(7):881–4.
17. Fourtillan JB, Brisson AM, Gobin P, et al. Bioavailability of melatonin in humans after day-time administration of D(7) melatonin. Biopharm Drug Dispos 2000;21(1):15–22.
18. Herxheimer A, Petrie KJ. Melatonin for the prevention and treatment of jet lag. Cochrane Database Syst Rev 2002;2:CD001520.
19. Kennaway DJ. Potential safety issues in the use of the hormone melatonin in paediatrics. J Paediatr Child Health 2015;51(6):584–9.
20. Andersen LP, Gogenur I, Rosenberg J, et al. The safety of melatonin in humans. Clin Drug Investig 2016;36(3):169–75.
21. Rubio-Sastre P, Scheer FA, Gomez-Abellan P, et al. Acute melatonin administration in humans impairs glucose tolerance in both the morning and evening. Sleep 2014;37(10):1715–9.
22. Garaulet M, Gomez-Abellan P, Rubio-Sastre P, et al. Common type 2 diabetes risk variant in MTNR1B worsens the deleterious effect of melatonin on glucose tolerance in humans. Metabolism 2015; 64(12):1650–7.

23. Lewy AJ, Cutler NL, Sack RL. The endogenous melatonin profile as a marker of circadian phase position. J Biol Rhythms 1999;14(3):227–36.

24. Klerman EB, Gershengorn HB, Duffy JF, et al. Comparisons of the variability of three markers of the human circadian pacemaker. J Biol Rhythms 2002; 17(2):181–93.

25. Burgess HJ, Wyatt JK, Park M, et al. Home circadian phase assessments with measures of compliance yield accurate dim light melatonin onsets. Sleep 2015;38(6):889–97.

26. Sack RL, Brandes RW, Kendall AR, et al. Entrainment of free-running circadian rhythms by melatonin in blind people. N Engl J Med 2000;343(15):1070–7.

27. Lewy AJ, Emens JS, Lefler BJ, et al. Melatonin entrains free-running blind people according to a physiological dose-response curve. Chronobiol Int 2005;22(6):1093–106.

28. Lewy AJ, Emens JS, Sack RL, et al. Low, but not high, doses of melatonin entrained a free-running blind person with long circadian period. Chronobiol Int 2002;19(3):649–58.

29. Dollins AB, Zhdanova IV, Wurtman RJ, et al. Effect of inducing nocturnal serum melatonin concentrations in daytime on sleep, mood, body temperature, and performance. Proc Natl Acad Sci USA 1994;91(5): 1824–8.

30. Burgess HJ. Using bright light and melatonin to reduce jet lag. In: Perlis M, Aloia M, Kuhn B, editors. Behavioral treatments for sleep disorders: a comprehensive primer of behavioral sleep medicine treatment protocols. Burlington (New Jersey): Elsevier; 2011. p. 151–7.

31. Burgess HJ. Using bright light and melatonin to adjust to night work. In: Perlis M, Aloia M, Kuhn B, editors. Behavioral treatments for sleep disorders: a comprehensive primer of behavioral sleep medicine treatment protocols. Burlington (New Jersey): Elsevier; 2011. p. 159–65.

32. Buscemi N, Vandermeer B, Hooton N, et al. The efficacy and safety of exogenous melatonin for primary sleep disorders. A meta-analysis. J Gen Int Med 2005;20:1151–8.

33. Ferracioli-Oda E, Qawasmi A, Bloch MH. Meta-analysis: melatonin for the treatment of primary sleep disorders. PLoS One 2013;8(5):e63773.

34. Auld F, Maschauer EL, Morrison I, et al. Evidence for the efficacy of melatonin in the treatment of primary adult sleep disorders. Sleep Med Rev 2017;34: 10–22.

35. Wyatt JK, Dijk DJ, Ritz-de Cecco A, et al. Sleep-facilitating effect of exogenous melatonin in healthy young men and women is circadian-phase dependent. Sleep 2006;29(5):609–18.

36. Scheer FA, Morris CJ, Garcia JI, et al. Repeated melatonin supplementation improves sleep in hypertensive patients treated with beta-blockers: a randomized controlled trial. Sleep 2012;35(10): 1395–402.

37. Sateia MJ, Buysse DJ, Krystal AD, et al. Clinical practice guideline for the pharmacologic treatment of chronic insomnia in adults: an American Academy of Sleep Medicine clinical practice guideline. J Clin Sleep Med 2017;13(2):307–49.

38. Krauchi K, Cajochen C, Pache M, et al. Thermoregulatory effects of melatonin in relation to sleepiness. Chronobiol Int 2006;23:475–84.

39. Reppert SM, Weaver DR, Rivkees SA, et al. Putative melatonin receptors in a human biological clock. Science 1988;242:78–81.

40. Erland LA, Saxena PK. Melatonin natural health products and supplements: presence of serotonin and significant variability of melatonin content. J Clin Sleep Med 2017;13(2):275–81.

41. Hahm H, Kujawa J, Augsburger L. Comparison of melatonin products against USP's nutritional supplements standards and other criteria. J Am Pharm Assoc (Wash) 1999;39(1):27–31.

42. Available at: http://well.blogs.nytimes.com/2015/03/30/gnc-to-strengthen-supplement-quality-controls. Accessed Jan 2, 2018.

43. Available at: http://www.usp.org/verification-services/program-participants. Accessed Jan 2, 2018.

44. ConsumerLab.com. Product review: melatonin supplements. Available at: www.consumerlab.com/results/melatonin.asp. Accessed Jan 2, 2018.

45. Crowley SJ, Eastman CI. Melatonin in the afternoons of a gradually advancing sleep schedule enhances the circadian rhythm phase advance. Psychopharmacol (Berl) 2013;225(4):825–37.

46. Emens JS, Eastman CI. Diagnosis and treatment of non-24-h sleep-wake disorder in the blind. Drugs 2017;77:637–50.

47. Emens JS, Laurie AL, Songer JB, et al. Non-24-hour disorder in blind individuals revisited: variability and the influence of environmental time cues. Sleep 2013;36(07):1091–100.

48. Emens J, Lewy A, Yuhas K, et al. Melatonin entrains free-running blind individuals with circadian periods less than 24 hours. Sleep 2006;29(Suppl):A62.

49. Duffy JF, Cain SW, Chang AM, et al. Sex difference in the near-24-hour intrinsic period of the human circadian timing system. Proc Natl Acad Sci USA 2011; 108(Suppl 3):15602–8.

50. Revell VL, Burgess HJ, Gazda CJ, et al. Advancing human circadian rhythms with afternoon melatonin and morning intermittent bright light. J Clin Endocr Metab 2006;91:54–9.

51. Paul MA, Gray GW, Lieberman HR, et al. Phase advance with separate and combined melatonin and light treatment. Psychopharmacology (Berl) 2011;214(2):515–23.

52. Burke TM, Markwald RR, Chinoy ED, et al. Combination of light and melatonin time cues for phase

advancing the human circadian clock. Sleep 2013; 36(11):1617–24.

53. Burgess HJ, Park M, Wyatt JK, et al. Home dim light melatonin onsets with measures of compliance in delayed sleep phase disorder. J Sleep Res 2016; 25(3):314–7.

54. Wade A, Ford I, Crawford G, et al. Efficacy of prolonged release melatonin in insomnia patients aged 55-80 years: quality of sleep and next-day alertness outcomes. Curr Med Res Opin 2007; 23(10):2597–605.

55. Available at: http://www.ema.europa.eu/docs/en_GB/document_library/EPAR_-_Summary_for_the_public/human/000695/WC500026805.pdf. Accessed Jan 2, 2018.

56. Lockley SW, Dressman MA, Licamele L, et al. Tasimelteon for non-24-hour sleep-wake disorder in totally blind people (SET and RESET): two multicentre, randomised, double-masked, placebo-controlled phase 3 trials. Lancet 2015;386:1754–64.

57. Rajaratnam SM, Polymeropoulos MH, Fisher DM, et al. Melatonin agonist tasimelteon (VEC-162) for transient insomnia after sleep-time shift: two randomised controlled multicentre trials. Lancet 2009; 373(9662):482–91.

58. Available at: https://wayback.archive-it.org/7993/20170405224953/https://www.fda.gov/downloads/AdvisoryCommittees/CommitteesMeetingMaterials/Drugs/PeripheralandCentralNervousSystemDrugsAdvisoryCommittee/UCM374388.pdf. Accessed Jan 2, 2018.

59. Richardson GS, Zee PC, Wang-Weigand S, et al. Circadian phase-shifting effects of repeated ramelteon administration in healthy adults. J Clin Sleep Med 2008;4(5):456–61.

60. Kuriyama A, Honda M, Hayashino Y. Ramelteon for the treatment of insomnia in adults: a systematic review and meta-analysis. Sleep Med 2014;15(4): 385–92.

61. Krauchi K, Cajochen C, Mori D, et al. Early evening melatonin and S-20098 advance circadian phase and nocturnal regulation of core body temperature. Am J Physiol 1997;272:R1178–88.

62. Leproult R, Onderbergen AV, L'Hermite-Baleriaux M, et al. Phase-shifts of 24-h rhythms of hormonal release and body temperature following early evening administration of the melatonin agonist agomelatine in healthy older men. Clin Endocrinol 2005;63: 298–304.

63. Quera-Salva MA, Hajak G, Philip P, et al. Comparison of agomelatine and escitalopram on nighttime sleep and daytime condition and efficacy in major depressive disorder patients. Int Clin Psychopharmacol 2011;26(5):252–62.

64. Freiesleben SD, Furczyk K. A systematic review of agomelatine-induced liver injury. J Mol Psychiatry 2015;3(1):4.

65. Taylor D, Sparshatt A, Varma S, et al. Antidepressant efficacy of agomelatine: meta-analysis of published and unpublished studies. BMJ 2014;348:g1888.

66. Mundey K, Benloucif S, Harsanyi K, et al. Phase-dependent treatment of delayed sleep phase syndrome with melatonin. Sleep 2005;28:1271–8.

67. Kayumov L, Brown G, Jindal R, et al. A randomized, double-blind, placebo-controlled crossover study of the effect of exogenous melatonin on delayed sleep phase syndrome. Psychosom Med 2001;63:40–8.

68. Rahman SA, Kayumov L, Shapiro CM. Antidepressant action of melatonin in the treatment of delayed sleep phase syndrome. Sleep Med 2010;11(2): 131–6.

69. van Geijlswijk IM, van der Heijden KB, Egberts AC, et al. Dose finding of melatonin for chronic idiopathic childhood sleep onset insomnia: an RCT. Psychopharmacology (Berl) 2010;212(3):379–91.

70. Smits MG, Nagtegaal EE, van der Heijden J, et al. Melatonin for chronic sleep onset insomnia in children: a randomized placebo-controlled trial. J Child Neurol 2001;16(2):86–92.

71. Van der Heijden KB, Smits MG, Van Someren EJ, et al. Effect of melatonin on sleep, behavior, and cognition in ADHD and chronic sleep-onset insomnia. J Am Acad Child Adolesc Psychiatry 2007;46(2):233–41.

72. Serfaty M, Kennell-Webb S, Warner J, et al. Double blind randomised placebo controlled trial of low dose melatonin for sleep disorders in dementia. Int J Geriatr Psychiatry 2002;17(12):1120–7.

73. Wright B, Sims D, Smart S, et al. Melatonin versus placebo in children with autism spectrum conditions and severe sleep problems not amenable to behaviour management strategies: a randomised controlled crossover trial. J Autism Dev Disord 2011;41(2):175–84.

74. Hack LM, Lockley SW, Arendt J, et al. The effects of low-dose 0.5-mg melatonin on the free-running circadian rhythms of blind subjects. J Biol Rhythms 2003;18:420–9.

75. Lockley SW, Skene DJ, James K, et al. Melatonin administration can entrain the free-running circadian system of blind subjects. J Endocrinol 2000;164: R1–6.

76. Auger RR, Burgess HJ, Emens J, et al. Do evidence-based treatments for circadian rhythm sleep-wake disorders make the GRADE? Updated guidelines point to need for more clinical research. J Clin Sleep Med 2015;11(10):1079–80.

Sleep in the Aging Population

Brienne Miner, MD, MHS[a],*, Meir H. Kryger, MD, FRCP(C)[a,b]

KEYWORDS

- Aging • Insomnia • Sleep disorders • Multimorbidity • Polypharmacy • Geriatric syndromes

KEY POINTS

- Changes to sleep architecture with normal aging include decreases in total sleep time, sleep efficiency, slow wave sleep, and REM sleep, and an increase in wake after sleep onset.
- Although sleep disturbance is common with aging, it is not an inherent part of the aging process; medical, psychiatric, and psychosocial factors overshadow age as risk factors.
- Sleep disturbance in older adults is associated with increased morbidity and mortality.
- The evaluation and management of sleep disturbances in older adults is best approached as a multifactorial geriatric health condition, arising from impairments in multiple domains.

INTRODUCTION

Sleep is an important component for health and wellness across the lifespan. The number of people in the United States who are 65 years or older is steadily increasing, and is expected to double over the next 25 years to about 72 million. By 2030, roughly 1 in 5 people in this country will be over the age of 65.[1] Sleep complaints are common among older adults, and as this segment of the population grows, so too will the prevalence of sleep disturbances. However, sleep problems are not an inherent part of the aging process. There are changes to sleep architecture over the lifespan that are not, in themselves, pathologic, but can be viewed as making older adults more vulnerable to sleep disturbances.[2] It is the consequences of aging, in the form of medical and psychiatric comorbidity, medication and substance use, psychosocial factors, and primary sleep disorders that put older adults at risk for sleep disturbance. The increasing prevalence of multimorbidity (ie, having at least 2 concurrent diseases in the same individual)[3] among older adults means that sleep disorders might arise from multiple different domains. Thus, sleep disturbance in this age group should be considered a multifactorial geriatric health condition (previously referred to as a geriatric syndrome),[4] requiring consideration of multiple risk factors and a comprehensive treatment approach.

NORMAL AGE-RELATED CHANGES TO SLEEP–WAKE PHYSIOLOGY

Physicians addressing sleep complaints in older adults are commonly asked about how much sleep is enough. The National Sleep Foundation recommends 7 to 8 hours of sleep for adults aged 65 and older.[5] This recommendation is supported by evidence that older adults sleeping anywhere from 6 to 9 hours have better cognition, mental and physical health, and quality of life compared with older adults with shorter or longer sleep durations. Thus, the need for sleep is not reduced in older adults, but the ability to get the

This article originally appeared in March 2017 issue of *Sleep Medicine Clinics* (Volume 12, Issue 1).

Funding Sources: Dr B. Miner is supported by T32AG1934, the John A. Hartford Center of Excellence at Yale and the Yale Claude D. Pepper Older Americans Independence Center (P30AG021342).

Disclosure Statement: Drs B. Miner and M.H. Kryger have no commercial or financial conflicts of interest to disclose.

[a] Department of Internal Medicine, Yale School of Medicine, 333 Cedar Street, New Haven, CT 06520, USA;
[b] VA Connecticut Healthcare System, 950 Campbell Avenue, West Haven, CT 06516, USA
* Corresponding author.
E-mail address: brienne.miner@yale.edu

Sleep Med Clin 15 (2020) 311–318
https://doi.org/10.1016/j.jsmc.2020.02.016
1556-407X/20/© 2020 Elsevier Inc. All rights reserved.

required sleep may be decreased owing to normal changes in sleep architecture through the lifespan.[6]

Age-related changes in sleep physiology have been well-documented using polysomnography (**Table 1**). Most age-dependent changes in sleep parameters occur by age 60 years,[7] with the exception of sleep efficiency. Sleep efficiency (percentage of time spent asleep while in bed), in contrast, continues to show an age-dependent decrease beyond age 90 years. Older adults also have a decrease in total sleep time, with corresponding decreases in the percentage of time in slow wave sleep and REM sleep.[7] Slow wave sleep and REM sleep are thought to promote metabolic and cognitive recovery, and to enhance learning and memory, respectively.[2] Older adults also have an increase in time awake after sleep onset.[7] Although the number of arousals from sleep increases in healthy older adults, evidence suggests they do not have greater difficulty falling back to sleep.[8] There is an increase in sleep latency (the time it takes to fall asleep) up to age 60, with no clear age effect beyond that point.[7]

Circadian rhythms also change over the lifespan. These rhythms are 24-hour intrinsic physiologic cycles that are involved in control of sleep-wake and many other physiologic processes (eg, blood pressure, bone remodeling, release of certain hormones).[9] Aging is associated with a phase advance, resulting in an earlier onset of sleepiness in the evening and earlier morning awakening.[10] Daytime wakefulness is affected by phase advance, with older adults being more alert in the morning and more somnolent in the evening. Although napping is common in older adults, results with regard to the benefit or harm of this practice are mixed. Some studies show beneficial and potentially protective effects of napping in later life, whereas others show it to be a risk factor for morbidity and mortality.[11] There is some evidence to suggest that naps are protective for mortality if

nighttime sleep duration is short, but are associated with increased mortality risk if nighttime sleep duration is longer than 9 hours.[12]

SLEEP COMPLAINTS IN OLDER ADULTS
Epidemiology

Major sleep complaints include insomnia and drowsiness. Symptoms of insomnia consist of difficulties with initiating or maintaining sleep (including early morning awakening).[13] Drowsiness has to do with the propensity for sleep and is often established by napping behavior.[14] Many large studies documenting the epidemiology of sleep complaints in older adults have shown that insomnia symptoms and drowsiness are common in this age group. The Established Populations for Epidemiologic Studies of the Elderly included 9282 community-dwelling adults aged 65 and older, and found that 43% of participants reported difficulty with sleep onset or maintenance, and 25% reported napping.[15] The National Sleep Foundation's 2003 Sleep in America Poll confirmed the prevalence of these symptoms, stating that 46% of community-dwelling adults aged 65 to 74 reported insomnia symptoms, and 39% of people in this age group reported napping. These prevalence rates increased to 50% and 46%, respectively, in participants aged 75 to 84 years.[16] It is estimated that 40% to 70% of older adults have chronic sleep problems, and up to 50% of cases are undiagnosed.[6]

The major sleep complaint depends on the cause of the sleep disturbance. Symptoms of insomnia are common in people using activating medications or substances, in those with comorbid medical or psychiatric illness, or in those with restless leg syndrome (RLS). Daytime drowsiness can result from sedating medications, chronic medical illness, or obstructive sleep apnea (OSA). With respect to OSA, whereas drowsiness and snoring are the most common complaints, older adults may also complain of choking or gasping on awakening, observed apneas, morning headache, nocturia, wandering, or confusion.[17,18]

Consequences of Poor Sleep

Sleep complaints, whether related to insomnia symptoms or drowsiness, have important consequences in older adults. Beyond being distressing for the subject, these symptoms predict poor physical and mental health-related quality of life.[19] In longitudinal studies, insomnia complaints have been associated with many different detrimental outcomes, including poor self-reported health status, cognitive decline, depression, disability in basic activities of daily living, poorer

Table 1		
Age-related changes in sleep architecture		
	Decreased	**Increased**
Sleep parameter	• Total sleep time • Sleep efficiency • Slow wave sleep • Rapid eye movement sleep	• Time awake after sleep onset • Number of arousals from sleep • Sleep latency

quality of life, and a greater risk of institutionalization.[2,17] Insomnia is also associated with impaired physical function and an increased risk for falls.[11,17] Daytime drowsiness has also been associated with harmful outcomes in longitudinal studies, including cardiovascular disease, falls, and death.[2] Healthy older adults who have sleep latencies of greater than 30 minutes, sleep efficiencies of less than 80%, or REM sleep percentage of less than 16% or greater than 25% of total sleep are at increased mortality risk, even after controlling for age, gender, and baseline medical burden.[20]

PATHOLOGIC AND PSYCHOSOCIAL FACTORS AFFECTING SLEEP IN THE AGING POPULATION
Pathologic Factors

Although aging per se does not lead to sleep pathology, the aging process is associated commonly with multiple pathologic problems that can affect sleep. Older adults commonly suffer from pain syndromes, arthritis, digestive disease, heart disease, lung disease, renal and urologic diseases, and cancer, all of which can contribute to sleep disturbance through specific symptoms or because of complications or anxiety associated with these diseases.[21] Psychiatric illness is as important as medical comorbidity in its effect on sleep, and has long been recognized to significantly and independently increase the risk for insomnia in older adults.[21,22] Sleep disruption features prominently in many psychiatric conditions, including depression and anxiety, which are common in older adults.[21] Sleep disturbance and depression are intertwined, as insomnia may be a result of depression but also increases the risk of developing depression in older adults.[23]

More so than the impact that a single condition has on sleep problems, one of the major issues leading to a higher risk of sleep problems in older adults is the accumulation of comorbidities. More than 1 in 4 Americans is living with 2 or more chronic conditions, and the prevalence of multiple chronic conditions increases with age.[24] A recent report of fee-for-service Medicare beneficiaries found that the rate of 2 or more chronic conditions was 62% for those aged 65 to 74 years and increased to 82% for those aged 85 years and older.[25] In fact, this situation has become so common that there has been a shift from looking at comorbidity (which focuses on the effect of a single cooccurring disease with respect to an index disease) to multimorbidity. Multimorbidity refers to the coexistence of 2 or more chronic medical conditions in the same person.[25] However, a more nuanced definition takes into account the both number and the severity of conditions, and considers the link between multimorbidity and cognitive and physical dysfunction, as well as psychosocial factors.[3]

With an increasing number of health problems, the likelihood of sleep complaints increases. This was demonstrated in the 2003 National Sleep Foundation survey, which showed that, among people aged 65 years and older without comorbid illness, 36% reported a sleep problem. This percentage increased to 52% among people with 1 to 3 comorbid conditions, and to 69% among people with 4 or more comorbid conditions.[16] The cumulative effects of multiple chronic conditions on sleep complaints is not surprising, considering that single diseases are known to affect sleep quality in older adults; if one is bad, more than one is likely to be worse.

Medications and Substance Use

Medication use is another factor that may increase risk for sleep disturbances in older adults. The use of prescription medications, over-the-counter medications, and dietary supplements is increasing in this age group. A recent study of a nationally representative sample of community-dwelling adults aged 62 to 85 years found that 88% used at least 1 prescription medication, 38% used over-the-counter medications, and 64% used dietary supplements.[26]

Different classes of medications commonly used in older adults can impact sleep directly through multiple mechanisms. One such effect is increased daytime drowsiness, as can be seen with antihistamines, anticholinergic and anticonvulsant medications, and opiates. Medications can be activating or stimulating, as is the case with pseudoephedrine, beta agonists, corticosteroids, certain antidepressants, methylphenidate, or selegiline. Other medications can exacerbate primary sleep disorders or directly influence sleep architecture. For example, RLS and periodic limb movements of sleep (PLMS) can worsen with the use of certain antidepressants, and sleep disordered breathing can worsen with the use of opiates or benzodiazepines.[21] With respect to sleep architecture, certain beta-blockers have been shown to suppress melatonin secretion and increase sleep fragmentation. Others can worsen parasomnias, induce REM sleep behavior disorder (RBD), or change the amount of time spent in REM sleep.[21] A final factor to consider is whether a medication might be interfering with sleep by worsening other conditions or causing sleep-disruptive symptoms. Several examples of such effects include medications that worsen heart failure, have diuretic effects, create bothersome coughing, or cause nocturnal hypoglycemia.

Polypharmacy may also contribute to heightened risk for sleep disturbance in older adults. Although it is generally defined as the use of multiple medications, there is no consensus definition about the number of medications that constitutes polypharmacy.[27] In epidemiologic studies, polypharmacy is frequently defined as taking 5 or more medications. A 2003 survey of Medicare beneficiaries found that 46% of those surveyed met this definition for polypharmacy.[28] This condition is increasingly common as age-related comorbidities increase, putting older adults at risk for drug–drug and drug–disease interactions.[26,29] Polypharmacy may be compounded by the cascade effect, which refers to the use of medications to treat side effects caused by other medications.[21]

Substance use merits consideration in the older adult with sleep disruption, especially with respect to alcohol, caffeine, and tobacco consumption. Although acute consumption of alcohol may decrease sleep latency, it can increase arousal, leading to sleep that is of poorer quality and shorter duration. Alcohol can also exacerbate sleep-disordered breathing by decreasing pharyngeal muscle tone.[21] The stimulating effects of caffeine can increase sleep latency and number of arousals, leading to a shorter sleep duration.[21] Tobacco consumption has been associated with insomnia in several studies. Nicotine is a potential mediator of this effect, because it may promote wakefulness via an effect on acetylcholine transmission in the central nervous system.[21] However, a causal relationship has not been established.[30]

Psychosocial Factors

Psychosocial factors can impact sleep in older adults in multiple ways. Particularly relevant are the effects of caregiving, social isolation, loss of physical function, and bereavement.

Caregiving is common to the process of aging. Recent evidence from the National Alliance for Caregiving indicates that 43.5 million adults in the United States provided unpaid care to an adult or child in the prior year, and that approximately 1 in 5 of these caregivers was 65 years of age or older.[31] Providing intensive assistance can result in psychological stress, physical strain, and erratic schedules, all of which may contribute to diminished sleep quality and disruptions in normal sleep patterns. In addition, caregiving is associated with depressed mood as well as erosion of physical health in the caregiver, further increasing the risk for sleep disturbance.[31,32] This can be a vicious cycle, because poor sleep can further erode physical health. Poor overnight sleep in caregivers has also been associated with reduced quality of life and increased inflammatory markers,[32] and is one of the strongest factors leading to institutionalization of a care recipient with dementia.[33]

Rates of social isolation increase after retirement and because 28.3% of adults aged 65 and older live alone.[34] Isolation can impact sleep through its effect on sleep hygiene and zeitgebers (see below). Sleep hygiene refers to a set of behavioral and environmental recommendations that are intended to promote sleep. These recommendations include avoiding caffeine or alcohol, getting regular exercise, and maintaining a regular sleep schedule while avoiding daytime naps.[35] However, the loss of a regular schedule and decreased social contact can lead to loneliness, inactivity, and boredom, potentially promoting behaviors like napping and irregular bedtimes that are counter to the promotion of healthy sleep. Zeitgebers are cues from the environment that entrain circadian rhythms to a 24-hour cycle length, promoting normal sleep–wake habits. Zeitgebers may be light based, but also include exercise, scheduled meals, and other social cues.[36] For socially isolated older adults, there may be inadequate exposure to zeitgebers, leading to irregular sleep–wake patterns. Previous evidence has shown that reports of insomnia and drowsiness were greater in older adults who felt socially isolated,[16] whereas activity and satisfaction with social life protected those aged 65 and older against insomnia symptoms.[37]

Loss of physical function is common among older adults. In 2009, 30% of Medicare enrollees aged 65 and older reported needing assistance with basic activities of daily living.[38] Although this loss has many implications for the health of older adults, it also affects their level of activity and exposure to zeitgebers. Thus, its effects on sleep are similar to those described for social isolation. In a National Sleep Foundation survey, older adults with decreased physical function (defined as difficulty walking one-half mile without help and/or difficulty walking a flight of stairs without help) were more likely to report insomnia symptoms (66% vs 44%) and daytime sleepiness (28% vs 12%).[16] Loss of physical function has also been associated significantly with the development of insomnia symptoms.[15]

Bereavement, the experience of losing a loved one to death,[39] is another factor that may contribute to sleep disturbance in older adults. A recent study found that more than 70% of older adults experienced bereavement over a 2.5-year period.[40] Bereavement is experienced more often in older adults because the loss of a spouse, siblings, or friends is common in this age group.[40,41] The grief experienced from such a loss has been associated with worsening health and functional impairment in older adults,[41] as well as an increased risk for the development of mood and anxiety disorders and substance abuse.[39] Importantly, bereavement in older adults has also been associated with increased loneliness and social isolation.[41] Thus, as with the other psychosocial factors mentioned, worsening health, psychiatric illness, and social isolation play a role in increasing the risk for sleep disturbance in bereavement. Multiple studies have shown an association between bereavement and sleep disturbance.[15,42,43] Older adults are at higher risk for complicated grief after bereavement, a condition in which grief symptoms are more severe and prolonged. The physical and mental health consequences of complicated grief are more severe than those associated with acute grief, and sleep impairment may be worse in these individuals.[41]

SLEEP DISORDERS IN OLDER ADULTS
Insomnia

A diagnosis of insomnia disorder is made clinically via a complaint of dissatisfaction with sleep quality and/or quantity, difficulty initiating or maintaining sleep, waking up too early, and/or nonrestorative or poor sleep, with a negative impact on daytime functioning and occurring at least 3 nights a week for more than 3 months.[44] The majority of insomnia diagnoses in older adults result from "comorbid insomnia."[45] This designation emphasizes the coexistence of insomnia with other medical and psychiatric comorbidities, and acknowledges that it may not be possible to determine whether insomnia is a cause or consequence of coexisting illnesses. As described, multimorbidity, polypharmacy and substance use, and psychosocial factors are common with the aging process and put older adults at risk for a diagnosis of insomnia.

The epidemiology of insomnia in older adults has been the subject of many studies, but summarizing the results is difficult because insomnia is defined differently in these studies. Some look only at insomnia symptoms (eg, difficulty initiating or maintaining sleep, complaints of nonrestorative sleep) with or without inclusion of criteria on frequency or severity of symptoms, whereas others look at insomnia diagnosis but use different diagnostic criteria. It is widely accepted that insomnia symptoms increase with advancing age, with prevalence rates approaching 50% in adults aged 65 and older.[13] The annual incidence rates

for insomnia symptoms have been estimated to be 3% to 5%,[15,22] and remission rates may be as high as 50% over 3 years.[15] With respect to an insomnia diagnosis, the prevalence has been estimated to be around 5%.[46] It is thought that prevalence of insomnia diagnosis increases after 45 years of age, but may remain the same in individuals after 65 years of age.[13] There are different theories about why the discrepancy between insomnia symptoms and diagnosis exists. Some authors have postulated that insomnia symptoms may be better tolerated or the daily demands less for older adults.[47] Others point to a "paradox of well-being" bias in questionnaires, in which older adults are less likely to report dissatisfaction or distress because their actual state of health exceeds the expected level.[11,48]

Obstructive Sleep Apnea

OSA increases with advancing age, with prevalence estimates differing depending on the definition used. Using a definition of 10 or more apneas and/or hypopneas per hour of sleep, OSA prevalence estimates in older adults may be as high as 70% in men and 56% in women. This is in contrast with prevalence estimates in the general adult population of 15% in men and 5% in women.[17] Although it is more common, this condition frequently goes undiagnosed because the phenotype of OSA can look very different in older adults. After the age of 60, the prevalence of OSA is equivalent in males and females, obesity is no longer a significant risk factor, and witnessed apneas and snoring are not reported as frequently.[49] Older adults are also more likely to present with more sleep-related complaints, including daytime sleepiness and nocturia.[50]

Older adults are at risk for OSA for several reasons. With aging, there is loss of tissue elasticity as well as sarcopenic muscle wasting.[11,49] There are also structural changes to the upper airway, including lengthening of soft palate and upper airway fat pad deposition.[11] These age-related changes increase the tendency for oropharyngeal collapse. In addition, ventilatory control instability may predispose older adults to apneic events.[11]

The negative consequences of OSA in older adults include excessive daytime sleepiness, decreased quality of life, neurocognitive impairment, nocturia, and worsening of cardiovascular disease, particularly hypertension, heart failure, and stroke. Diabetes mellitus and depression have also been found to be more common in older adults with OSA. The impact of untreated OSA in older adults on mortality is not clear.[17] However, older adults have similar adherence rates to treatment,[17,49] so there is no clear reason not to treat older adults with OSA.

Restless Leg Syndrome and Periodic Limb Movements of Sleep

RLS and PLMS increase in prevalence and severity with advancing age and have the potential to cause sleep complaints. RLS is a sensorimotor disorder characterized by unpleasant sensations in the limbs that cause an urge to move, especially in the evening. PLMS is a disorder characterized by repetitive episodes of stereotypic limb movements caused by muscle contractions during sleep.[17] In epidemiologic studies, the prevalence of RLS in older adults ranges from 9% to 20%, and PLMS is estimated to be present in 4% to 11% of older adults.[51] Of persons with RLS, 80% will have PLMS. However, PLMS occurs in the absence of RLS approximately 70% of the time.[2] These disorders can contribute to insomnia complaints through disruption of sleep onset or maintenance, as well as contributing to daytime drowsiness.

REM Sleep Behavior Disorder

RBD is a disorder resulting from a lack of the normal atonia seen in REM sleep. As a result, subjects with RBD are able to act out dreams in a way that can be violent and injurious. The majority of cases occur in older adults in the sixth or seventh decades of life, and the disorder is more common in men.[17] Although it may be idiopathic, RBD is associated with a neurodegenerative disorder in 48% to 73% of cases. Subjects with RBD may complain of sleep disruption or vivid dreams.[52]

TREATMENT OF SLEEP DISTURBANCES IN OLDER ADULTS

As we have seen in this article, sleep disturbance is highly pervasive among older adults owing to multiple factors common to the aging process. These include medical and psychiatric comorbidity, polypharmacy and substance use, psychosocial factors (such as caregiving, social isolation, and loss of physical function), and sleep disorders. With rates of multimorbidity increasing in older adults, it is likely that multiple processes in different domains are contributing to their sleep disturbance. Thus, sleep disturbance in this age group should be approached as a multifactorial geriatric health condition.[2,4] The implication of this designation is that evaluation of sleep disturbance requires consideration of multiple risk factors and a multifaceted treatment approach. Similar approaches have been used in other

multifactorial geriatric health conditions, including falls and delirium, and have successfully decreased occurrence of these events.[53,54]

SUMMARY

There are normal changes to sleep architecture throughout the lifespan. There is not, however, a decreased need for sleep and sleep disturbance is not an inherent part of the aging process. Sleep disturbance is common in older adults because aging is associated with an increasing prevalence of multimorbidity, polypharmacy, psychosocial factors affecting sleep, and certain primary sleep disorders. It is also associated with morbidity and mortality, making evaluation and management of sleep disturbance in older adults an important focus. Because many older adults will have several factors from different domains affecting their sleep, these complaints are best approached as a multifactorial geriatric health condition, necessitating a multifaceted treatment approach.

REFERENCES

1. Centers for Disease Control and Prevention. The state of aging and health in America 2013. Atlanta (GA): Centers for Disease Control and Prevention; 2013.
2. Vaz Fragoso CA, Gill TM. Sleep complaints in community-living older persons: a multifactorial geriatric syndrome. J Am Geriatr Soc 2007;55(11): 1853–66.
3. Marengoni A, Angleman S, Melis R, et al. Aging with multimorbidity: a systematic review of the literature. Ageing Res Rev 2011;10(4):430–9.
4. Inouye SK, Studenski S, Tinetti ME, et al. Geriatric syndromes: clinical, research, and policy implications of a core geriatric concept. J Am Geriatr Soc 2007;55(5):780–91.
5. Hirshkowitz M, Whiton K, Albert SM, et al. National Sleep Foundation's sleep time duration recommendations: methodology and results summary. Sleep Health 2015;1(1):40–3.
6. Avidan AY. Normal sleep in humans. In: Kryger MH, Avidan AY, Berry RB, editors. Atlas of clinical sleep medicine. 2nd edition. Philadelphia: Saunders; 2014. p. 65–97.
7. Ohayon MM, Carskadon MA, Guilleminault C, et al. Meta-analysis of quantitative sleep parameters from childhood to old age in healthy individuals: developing normative sleep values across the human lifespan. Sleep 2004;27(7):1255–73.
8. Klerman EB, Davis JB, Duffy JF, et al. Older people awaken more frequently but fall back asleep at the same rate as younger people. Sleep 2004;27(4): 793–8.

9. Tranah G, Stone K, Ancoli-Israel S. Circadian rhythms in older adults. In: Kryger MH, Roth T, Dement WC, editors. Principles and practice of sleep medicine. 6th edition. Philadelphia: Elsevier; 2016. p. 1510–5.

10. Monk TH. Aging human circadian rhythms: conventional wisdom may not always be right. J Biol Rhythms 2005;20(4):366–74.

11. Bliwise DL. Normal aging. In: Kryger MH, Roth T, Dement WC, editors. Principles and practice of sleep medicine. 6th edition. Philadelphia: Elsevier; 2016. p. 25–38.

12. Cohen-Mansfield J, Perach R. Sleep duration, nap habits, and mortality in older persons. Sleep 2012; 35(7):1003–9.

13. Ohayon MM. Epidemiology of insomnia: what we know and what we still need to learn. Sleep Med Rev 2002;6(2):97–111.

14. Johns MW. Sleepiness in different situations measured by the Epworth Sleepiness Scale. Sleep 1994;17(8):703–10.

15. Foley DJ, Monjan A, Simonsick EM, et al. Incidence and remission of insomnia among elderly adults: an epidemiologic study of 6,800 persons over three years. Sleep 1999;22(Suppl 2):S366–72.

16. National Sleep Foundation. Sleep in America Poll. 2003. Available at: https://sleepfoundation.org/sites/ default/files/2003SleepPollExecSumm.pdf. Accessed July 13, 2016.

17. Bloom HG, Ahmed I, Alessi CA, et al. Evidence-based recommendations for the assessment and management of sleep disorders in older persons. J Am Geriatr Soc 2009;57(5):761–89.

18. Ancoli-Israel S, Kripke DF, Klauber MR, et al. Sleep-disordered breathing in community-dwelling elderly. Sleep 1991;14(6):486–95.

19. Reid KJ, Martinovich Z, Finkel S, et al. Sleep: a marker of physical and mental health in the elderly. Am J Geriatr Psychiatry 2006;14(10):860–6.

20. Dew MA, Hoch CC, Buysse DJ, et al. Healthy older adults' sleep predicts all-cause mortality at 4 to 19 years of follow-up. Psychosom Med 2003;65(1): 63–73.

21. Barczi SR, Teodorescu MC. Psychiatric and medical comorbidities and effects of medications in older adults. In: Kryger MH, Roth T, Dement WC, editors. Principles and practices of sleep medicine. 6th edition. Philadelphia: Elsevier; 2016. p. 1484–95.

22. Morgan K, Clarke D. Risk factors for late-life insomnia in a representative general practice sample. Br J Gen Pract 1997;47(416):166–9.

23. Livingston G, Blizard B, Mann A. Does sleep disturbance predict depression in elderly people? A study in inner London. Br J Gen Pract 1993;43(376):445–8.

24. U.S. Department of Health and Human Services. Multiple chronic conditions - a strategic framework: optimum health and quality of life for individuals with multiple chronic conditions. Washington, DC: 2010. Available at: http://www.hhs.gov/sites/default/files/ ash/initiatives/mcc/mcc_framework.pdf. Accessed November 14, 2016.

25. Salive ME. Multimorbidity in older adults. Epidemiol Rev 2013;35:75–83.

26. Qato DM, Wilder J, Schumm L, et al. Changes in prescription and over-the-counter medication and dietary supplement use among older adults in the United States, 2005 vs 2011. JAMA Intern Med 2016;176(4):473–82.

27. Fried TR, O'Leary J, Towle V, et al. Health outcomes associated with polypharmacy in community-dwelling older adults: a systematic review. J Am Geriatr Soc 2014;62(12):2261–72.

28. Safran DG, Neuman P, Schoen C, et al. Prescription drug coverage and seniors: findings from a 2003 national survey. Health Aff (Millwood) 2005;Suppl Web Exclusives:W5-152. W5-166.

29. Hines LE, Murphy JE. Potentially harmful drug–drug interactions in the elderly: a review. Am J Geriatr Pharmacother 2011;9(6):364–77.

30. Wetter DW, Young TB. The relation between cigarette smoking and sleep disturbance. Prev Med 1994;23(3):328–34.

31. AARP, National Alliance for Caregiving. Caregiving in the US. 2015. Available at: http://www.aarp.org/ content/dam/aarp/ppi/2015/caregiving-in-the-united-states-2015-report-revised.pdf. Accessed July 13, 2016.

32. Peng HL, Chang YP. Sleep disturbance in family caregivers of individuals with dementia: a review of the literature. Perspect Psychiatr Care 2013;49(2):135–46.

33. Hope T, Keene J, Gedling K, et al. Predictors of institutionalization for people with dementia living at home with a carer. Int J Geriatr Psychiatry 1998; 13(10):682–90.

34. West LA, Cole S, Goodkind D, et al. 65+ in the United States: 2010. Washington, DC: United States Census Bureau; 2014.

35. Irish LA, Kline CE, Gunn HE, et al. The role of sleep hygiene in promoting public health: a review of empirical evidence. Sleep Med Rev 2015;22:23–36.

36. Gabehart RJ, Van Dongen, Hans PA. Circadian rhythms in sleepiness, alertness, and performance. In: Kryger MH, Roth T, Dement WC, editors. Principles and practice of sleep medicine. 6th edition. Philadelphia: Elsevier; 2016. p. 388–95.

37. Ohayon MM, Zulley J, Guilleminault C, et al. How age and daytime activities are related to insomnia in the general population: consequences for older people. J Am Geriatr Soc 2001;49(4):360–6.

38. Federal Interagency Forum on Aging Statistics. Older Americans 2012: key indicators of well-being. Available at: http://www.agingstats.gov/main_site/data/2012_ documents/docs/entirechartbook.pdf. Accessed June 26, 2016.

39. Shear MK. Clinical practice. Complicated grief. N Engl J Med 2015;372(2):153–60.
40. Williams BR, Sawyer Baker P, Allman RM, et al. Bereavement among African American and white older adults. J Aging Health 2007;19(2):313–33.
41. Shear MK, Ghesquiere A, Glickman K. Bereavement and complicated grief. Curr Psychiatry Rep 2013; 15(11):406.
42. Boelen PA, Lancee J. Sleep difficulties are correlated with emotional problems following loss and residual symptoms of effective prolonged grief disorder treatment. Depress Res Treat 2013;2013: 739804.
43. Byrne GJ, Raphael B. The psychological symptoms of conjugal bereavement in elderly men over the first 13 months. Int J Geriatr Psychiatry 1997;12(2): 241–51.
44. American Psychiatric Association. Diagnostic and statistical manual of mental disorders. 5th edition. Arlington (VA): American Psychiatric Publishing; 2013.
45. National Institutes of Health. National Institutes of Health State of the Science Conference statement on Manifestations and management of chronic insomnia in adults, June 13-15, 2005. Sleep 2005; 28(9):1049–57.
46. Gooneratne NS, Vitiello MV. Sleep in older adults: normative changes, sleep disorders, and treatment options. Clin Geriatr Med 2014;30(3):591–627.
47. Roth T, Coulouvrat C, Hajak G, et al. Prevalence and perceived health associated with insomnia based on DSM-IV-TR; International Statistical Classification of diseases and related health problems, Tenth Revision; and Research Diagnostic Criteria/International Classification of Sleep Disorders, Second Edition criteria: results from the America Insomnia Survey. Biol Psychiatry 2011;69(6):592–600.
48. Levy BR. Mind matters: cognitive and physical effects of aging self-stereotypes. J Gerontol B Psychol Sci Soc Sci 2003;58(4):P203–11.
49. Phillips B. Obstructive sleep apnea in the elderly. In: Kryger MH, Roth T, Dement WC, editors. Principles and practices of sleep medicine. 6th edition. Philadelphia: Elsevier; 2016. p. 1496–502.
50. Endeshaw Y. Clinical characteristics of obstructive sleep apnea in community-dwelling older adults. J Am Geriatr Soc 2006;54(11):1740–4.
51. Hornyak M, Trenkwalder C. Restless legs syndrome and periodic limb movement disorder in the elderly. J Psychosom Res 2004;56(5):543–8.
52. Schenck CH, Mahowald MW. REM sleep behavior disorder: clinical, developmental, and neuroscience perspectives 16 years after its formal identification in SLEEP. Sleep 2002;25(2):120–38.
53. Inouye SK, Bogardus ST Jr, Charpentier PA, et al. A multicomponent intervention to prevent delirium in hospitalized older patients. N Engl J Med 1999; 340(9):669–76.
54. Tinetti ME, Baker DI, McAvay G, et al. A multifactorial intervention to reduce the risk of falling among elderly people living in the community. N Engl J Med 1994;331(13):821–7.

Sleep, Health, and Society

Michael A. Grandner, PhD, MTR, CBSM

KEYWORDS

- Sleep • Sleep disorders • Epidemiology • Social factors • Health • Disparities • Society

KEY POINTS

- Insufficient sleep and sleep disorders are highly prevalent in the population and are associated with significant morbidity and mortality.
- Adverse outcomes of insufficient sleep and/or sleep disorders are weight gain and obesity, cardiovascular disease, diabetes, accidents and injuries, stress, pain, neurocognitive dysfunction, psychiatric symptoms, and mortality.
- Exposure to sleep difficulties varies by age, sex, race/ethnicity, and socioeconomic status; significant sleep health disparities exist in the population.
- Societal influences, such as globalization, technology, and public policy, affect sleep at a population level.

CONCEPTUALIZING SLEEP IN A SOCIAL CONTEXT

Sleep represents an emergent set of many physiologic processes under primarily neurobiological regulation that impact many physiologic systems. As such, many advances have been made over the past several decades that have shed light on these neurobiologic mechanisms of sleep-wake,[1–4] with especially exciting work in the area of functional genetics/genomics[5,6] and molecular mechanisms of sleep-related regulation.[7–9] Still, the phenomenon of sleep exists outside the nucleus and the cell membrane—sleep is experienced phenomenologically. Sleep is a biological requirement for human life, alongside food, water, and air. Like consumption of food and unlike breathing air, achieving this biological need requires the individual to engage in volitional behaviors. Although many of these behaviors are genetically and intrapersonally driven (eg, it is not a coincidence that most people prefer to sleep at night, and that most humans sleep in a stereotypical posturally recumbent manner), there is still much variability in sleep behaviors and practices. Because of this, sleep is also socially driven, dictated by the environment, and subject to interpersonal and societal factors.

Sleep in most humans occupies between 20% and 40% of the day. Even prehistoric evidence suggests the importance of sleep in human life[10]; this is consistent with archaeological and historical accounts of sleep having a prominent and important role in even early human society. Sleep was a universal phenomenon that was inescapable and thus was incorporated in social structures. In this way, sleep became not just a set of physiologic processes, but one represented in sociocultural structures. Thus, the timing, environment, and constraints surrounding sleep across human societies began to differ between rich and poor, powerful and powerless, rural and urban, and so forth. As sociologist, Simon Williams, writes, "Where we sleep, when we sleep, and with whom we sleep are all important markers or indicators of social status, privilege, and prevailing power relations."[11]

Conceptualizing Downstream Consequences

The downstream consequences of insufficient sleep duration and/or inadequate sleep quality

This article originally appeared in March 2017 issue of *Sleep Medicine Clinics* (Volume 12, Issue 1).
Dr M.A. Grandner is supported by National Heart, Lung, and Blood Institute (K23HL110216).
Department of Psychiatry, College of Medicine, University of Arizona, 1501 North Campbell Avenue, PO Box 245002, BUMC Suite 7326, Tucson, AZ 85724-5002, USA
E-mail address: grandner@email.arizona.edu

Sleep Med Clin 15 (2020) 319–340
https://doi.org/10.1016/j.jsmc.2020.02.017

(including sleep disorders and circadian misalignment of sleep) are varied and impact many physiologic systems. Conceptualizing these is therefore difficult. One way to do so is to acknowledge domains of outcomes and recognize the overlaps and relationships among those domains. The recent position statement from the American Academy of Sleep Medicine and Sleep Research Society[12–15] broadly categorizes effects of insufficient sleep as pertaining to the following categories: general health, cardiovascular health, metabolic health, mental health, immunologic health, human performance, cancer, pain, and mortality.

Conceptualizing Upstream Influences: Social Ecological Models

Upstream social and environmental influences on sleep are also complex and overlapping and implicate many potential pathways. With this in mind, a social-ecological framework may be best suited to describe this relationship. The social-ecological model was originally developed to describe the complex ways that an individual's behavior related to their health is a product of influences at the individual level, but that the individual operates in the context of social structures that they are a member of, but these structures exist outside of the individual.[16] For example, an individual has genetic, psychological, and other reasons for consuming a healthy diet, but social structures that they are a part of but exist outside of that individual (like their neighborhood, which may have healthy food; their job, which may or may not have a cafeteria; their family, which may have other food

restrictions, and so forth) play a role in that individual's behavior.

This model may also be appropriate for understanding sleep. At the individual level, factors that influence a person's sleep include that person's genetics, knowledge, beliefs, and attitudes about sleep, their overall health, and so forth. The individual level is embedded, though, within a social level, which includes the home (family, bedroom, and so forth), neighborhood, work/school, socioeconomics, religion, culture, race/ethnicity, and other factors. All of these factors influence sleep through the individual. Still, this social level is embedded within a societal level, which includes social forces that exist outside of things like work, family, and neighborhood, including globalization, geography, technology, public policy. These factors, at this high of a level, filter through the social structures that eventually come to bear on the individual. For example, as society embraced the Internet, it caused changes in jobs and families, which led to individual changes that play a role in sleep (such as social networking in bed or browsing the Internet late at night). **Fig. 1** displays a social-ecological model of sleep, illustrating of sleep duration and quality are influenced by factors at the individual level, which is embedded within a social level, which itself is embedded within a societal level. **Fig. 2** brings these models together, with sleep as the fulcrum (shown in **Fig. 1**) at the interface of upstream social-environmental influences (shown in more detail in **Fig. 3**) and downstream health and functional outcomes (shown in more detail in **Fig. 2**). This model brings all of these concepts together to describe how sleep is influenced by

Fig. 1. Social ecological model of sleep.

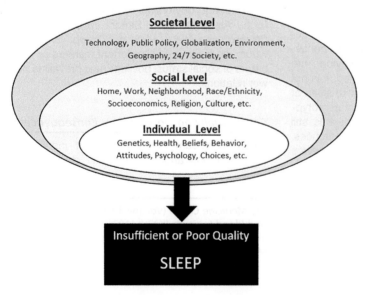

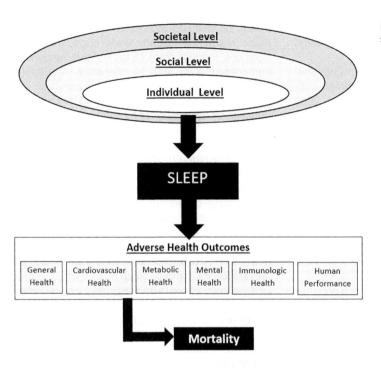

Fig. 2. Social ecological model of sleep and health.

these societal factors and how those influences, through sleep, may play a role in health. The first version of this model was published in 2010,[17] and it has appeared in several other publications since then.[14,18–20] It may serve as a useful framework for conceptualizing the physiologic processes of sleep in a social context.

POPULATION PREVALENCE OF SLEEP DURATION AND SLEEP DISTURBANCES
Sleep Duration

Population estimates of habitual sleep duration are variable, because few studies used identical methods to derive estimates. The best population-level estimates come from 1 of 3 sources: (1) self-reported time use data, (2) self-reported typical weeknight/work-night sleep, and (3) self-reported average sleep within 24 hours. For US-based data, the primary sources of these estimates come from the American Time Use Survey (ATUS) for time use data, the National Health Interview Survey or National Health and Nutrition Examination Survey (NHANES) for weeknight sleep, and the Behavioral Risk Factor Surveillance System (BRFSS) for 24-hour sleep.

Longitudinal analysis of time-use diaries by Knutson and colleagues[21] found that the proportion of Americans reporting short (<6 hours) sleep was 7.6% in 1975 and 9.3% in 2006. Bin and colleagues[22] examined similar time use data from several countries and showed that, in the United States, sleep duration has generally declined since the 1960s, if only by a small amount. The most comprehensive analysis of time use data related to sleep was recently undertaken by Basner and colleagues.[23] They report that the age group that receives the most sleep is young adults (8.86 hours on weeknights and 10.02 hours on weekends) and that those aged 25 to 64 report about 0.70 to 0.99

Fig. 3. Health belief model.

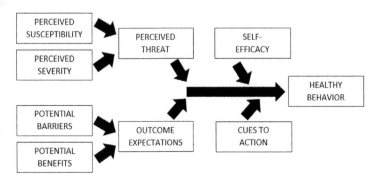

fewer hours on weeknights and 0.62 to 1.16 fewer hours on weekends. Prevalence of sleep duration by hour is not reported, though.

Regarding weekday sleep duration, Grandner and colleagues[24] reported census-weighted estimates of sleep duration using the 2007 to 2008 wave of the NHANES. They report that 6.2% of the population reports less than 5 hours of sleep, 33.78% reports 5 to 6 hours of sleep, 52.68% report 7 to 8 hours of sleep, and 7.38% report at least 9 hours of sleep per typical weeknight. These values from NHANES is similar to values reported from Krueger and Friedman,[25] who assessed similar data from the NHIS using data from 2004 to 2007. They report prevalence of 5 hours or less being 7.8%, 6 hours being 20.5%, 7 hours being 30.8%, 8 hours being 32.5%, and 9 or more hours being 8.5%.

Regarding typical 24-hour sleep, which presumably includes napping, recent data from the Centers for Disease Control and Prevention (CDC) released data from the 2014 BRFSS, which included data from 444,306 American adults. Based on the recently published guidelines,[12,15] the CDC calculated the prevalence of less than 7 hours of sleep duration across all 50 states.[26] The median prevalence of less than 7 hours of sleep was 35.1%, with a range of 28.4% (South Dakota) to 43.9% (Hawaii). This report also documents that the prevalence of 5 hours or less was 11.8%, with prevalence of 6, 7, 8, 9, and 10 or more hours being 23.0%, 29.5%, 27.7%, 4.4%, and 3.6%, respectively.

Taken together, the time diaries generally show more sleep than other retrospective reports, perhaps because they may better capture time in bed but not actual sleep. Indeed, most retrospective sleep reports have this issue,[27] although perhaps it is particularly problematic for time diaries. In general, though, at least one-third of the population seems to be reporting habitual sleep of 6 hours or less. The proportion of those with 6 hours or less is salient, given the risk factors associated with sleep duration described in more detail in later discussion.

Sleep Disturbances

Sleep disturbances are difficult to measure at the population level. Often, population-level assessments of general sleep disturbances subsume insufficient sleep duration and/or sleep disorders that may not expressly fit into this category. The 2006 BRFSS asked the following question to more than 150,000 residents of 36 US states/territories: "Over the last 2 weeks, how many days have you had trouble falling asleep or staying asleep or sleeping too much?" In an analysis of these responses, values were coded in whole numbers ranging from 0 to 14, but responses aggregated at 0 and 14; therefore, responses were dichotomized as either endorsing or not endorsing "sleep disturbance."[28,29] For men, the prevalence of sleep disturbance ranged from 13.7% (ages 70–74) to 18.1% (ages 18–24), and for women, the prevalence ranged from 17.7% (ages 80 or older) to 25.1% (ages 18–24).[29] Interestingly, reports of sleep disturbance generally declined with age. This finding was recently replicated using data from the 2009 BRFSS, which showed a similar pattern of declining self-report of insufficient sleep with age.[30]

Regarding sleep symptoms, data from the 2007 to 2008 NHANES were examined with regards to prevalence of various sleep symptoms.[31] Long sleep latency (more than 30 minutes) was reported by 18.8% of Americans. Self-reported difficulty falling asleep was reported at a rate of 11.71% for mild symptoms (1–3 times per week) and 7.7% for moderate-severe symptoms (at least half of nights). Similarly, sleep maintenance difficulties were reported by 13.21% endorsing mild and 7.7% endorsing moderate-severe symptoms, and early morning awakenings were reported at a rate of 10.7% for mild and 5.8% for moderate-severe symptoms. Daytime sleepiness and nonrestorative sleep were reported at a rate of 13.0% and 17.8% for mild symptoms, respectively, and 5.8% and 10.9% for moderate-severe symptoms, respectively. Frequent snoring was reported by 31.5% of adults and snorting/gasping during sleep was reported by 6.6% "occasionally" and 5.8% "frequently."

SLEEP EFFECTS ON HEALTH AND LONGEVITY

Because sleep is involved with many physiologic systems, insufficient sleep duration and poor sleep quality have been associated with several adverse health outcomes. Separate literature texts have emerged describing some of the negative effects of insufficient sleep duration, sleep apnea, and insomnia.

Mortality

The first report documenting the relationship between sleep duration and mortality risk was published more than 50 years ago.[32] This first study, an analysis of data from the American Cancer Society's first Cancer Prevention Study of more than one million US adults, found that increased mortality risk was associated with both short (6 hours or less) and long (9 hours or more) sleep duration. Since that time, many other studies have been published, from both large and small cohorts, covering both short and long follow-up periods, from 6 continents. Taken together, this overall pattern of findings, that both short and long sleep are associated with mortality risk, has generally remained consistent across studies, although not all studies found this pattern.[17] Two meta-analyses have been published, using slightly different methods and controls.[33,34] Still, their findings were highly consistent, indicating a 10% to 12% increased risk for short sleep and a 30% to 38% increased risk associated with long sleep duration. Much controversy remains, though, regarding this issue. For example, the precision of measurement of sleep in these studies is often poor.[17,27,35] Self-reported sleep time may better approximate time in bed, and although an actigraphic study found a similar pattern,[36] the cutoffs for short and long sleep indicated an overestimate among self-reports. Also, there is still a lack of clarity on the biological plausibility of the long sleep relationship, although some ideas have been proposed.[37,38] For this reason, most of the attention has been focused on risks associated with short sleep duration, which may be far more prevalent.

Weight Gain and Obesity

Many studies have found associations between sleep duration and adiposity and obesity.[39–41] Although most of these studies are cross-sectional, precluding causality, several other studies have longitudinally examined this relationship, demonstrating that short sleep duration is associated with increased weight gain over time.[42–46] These studies include individuals with otherwise low obesity risk, diverse community samples, and samples where effectiveness of weight loss interventions was mitigated by sleep and circadian factors. Several important caveats seem to be present in this relationship. First, this relationship is dependent on age, with the strongest relationships among younger adults and U-shaped relationships more common in middle-aged adults.[47] Also, this relationship may be moderated by race/ethnicity, with stronger relationships between sleep and obesity among non-Hispanic white and black/African American adults.[24]

Diabetes and Metabolism

Several studies have documented a cross-sectional relationship between insufficient sleep and diabetes risk.[40,48–51] A recent meta-analysis showed that insufficient sleep is associated with a 33% increased risk of incident diabetes.[52] These studies are supported by laboratory findings that show that physiologic sleep loss is associated with diabetes risk factors, including insulin resistance,[53–56] and other diabetes risk factors, such as increased consumption of unhealthy foods.[57–59] Physiologic studies also show that sleep loss can influence metabolism through changes in metabolic hormones,[60,61] adipocyte function,[62] and beta-cell function.[63]

Inflammation

Laboratory studies have shown that physiologic sleep restriction is associated with a proinflammatory state, including elevations in inflammatory cytokines, such as interleukin 1B (IL-1B),[64,65] IL-6,[64,66–68] IL-17,[64,69] tumor necrosis factor-α,[64,68,70–72] and C-reactive protein.[64,69,73–76] Findings at the population level have been more difficult to assess,[64] but similar relationships were found. A recent meta-analysis found no consistent relationship between sleep duration and inflammation,[77] but this may be because it did not include some studies that were more generalizable and with larger samples (eg, Ref.[76]). Also, it is plausible that population-level samples did not optimally measure these markers, because relationships with sleep vary across 24 hours and single time-point blood draws may miss the window of difference.[68]

Cardiovascular Disease

In addition to increased likelihood of obesity, diabetes, and inflammation, insufficient sleep is associated with increased risk of cardiovascular disease. Many studies have found that short sleep duration is associated with hypertension.[24,78–80] Although directionality is difficult to ascertain, several of these studies were longitudinal in nature. A meta-analysis of these longitudinal studies indicated that habitual short-sleep duration is associated with a 20% increased likelihood of hypertension, relative to normal sleep duration.[81] Other studies have supported this association, showing increased 24-hour blood pressure in short sleepers.[82] Other studies have also shown short sleep to be associated with hypercholesterolemia[24,79] and atherosclerosis risk.[83] Regarding cardiovascular endpoints, there is some evidence that habitual short sleep increases likelihood of cardiovascular events,[84] although meta-analyses do not generally show short sleep to be associated with increased cardiovascular mortality.[33,34,85]

Neurocognitive Functioning

Many studies have examined the relationship between laboratory-induced sleep loss and neurocognitive function. The domain that is most often studied is vigilant attention,[86,87] most often operationalized with the psychomotor vigilance task.[87,88] These studies show that as sleep time declines, attentional lapses increase in a somewhat dose-dependent manner.[86,89] Furthermore, these impairments often become cumulative over time[90] and do not seem to level off even after weeks in a laboratory. Other domains of neurocognitive function have also been assessed. For example, reduced sleep duration has been shown to cause impairments in working memory,[91] executive function,[92] processing speed,[93–95] and cognitive throughput.[96] Although some of these effects may be rescued with stimulants such as caffeine, the effects on executive function particularly do not seem to be rescued.[92] Although studies of this phenomenon in the general population are scarce, some studies show that reduced sleep time is associated with drowsy driving[97] and occupational accidents.[98–100]

Mental Health

Many studies have shown that short sleep duration is associated with poor mental health. Sleep disruptions are a common diagnostic feature of many mental health disorders.[101] Patients with mood disorders and anxiety disorders frequently experience short sleep duration. Sleep duration has also been identified as a suicide risk factor.[102] In the general population, overall mental health has been identified as the leading predictor of self-reported insufficient sleep.[30]

BELIEFS AND ATTITUDES ABOUT SLEEP

Real-world sleep may be driven by many of the same factors that drive other health-related behaviors, such as diet and exercise. With this in mind, previous literature from health behavior researchers has identified several models that explain healthy behavior, identifying the roles of beliefs and attitudes.

The Health Belief Model and Application to Sleep

The Health Belief Model was originally developed in the 1960s,[103,104] but has since been used in the study of many health-related behaviors. See **Fig. 3** for a schematic of this model. This model can be applied to sleep behaviors. For example, a person will engage in healthy sleep behaviors (eg, making time for sufficient sleep or adhering to treatment) if they (1) believe that they are susceptible to the adverse effects of insufficient/poor sleep, (2) believe that the adverse effects

are severe enough to warrant action, (3) believe that the action will mitigate the adverse effects, (4) believe that barriers to performing the action are sufficiently reduced, (5) are reminded to engage in the action, and (6) believe that performing the action is under their control. According to the health belief model, all of these are required for action. Therefore, just educating patients about the severity of outcomes of inaction, for example, is not sufficient to motivate behavior.

The Integrated Behavioral Model and Application to Sleep

The Integrated Behavioral Model arose from the Theory of Planned Behavior and Theory of Reasoned Action[105] to describe why people engage in behaviors. A schematic for this model is presented in **Fig. 4**. According to this model, attitudes, norms, and agency need to be addressed. Regarding attitudes, this would involve leading individuals to not only endorse helpful beliefs and attitudes about healthy sleep but also associate healthy sleep with positive feelings. Regarding norms, more research is needed to understand how the sleep of a person's (perceived) peers and those to which that individual wishes to conform influences individual sleep behaviors.

Beliefs and Attitudes About Sleep

Across segments of society, sleep practices and beliefs can vary to a great extent. For example, bed-sharing with infants and other family members differentially exists across cultures.[106–111] The cultural impact of dreaming also varies widely across cultures.[112] As globalization and technology penetrate society, sleep-related beliefs and practices can change, including the provision of longer working hours,[113–120] shift work,[121–124] and discouraging otherwise culturally appropriate naps.[125–127] There have been a few studies that examined beliefs and attitudes about sleep. In a sample from Brooklyn, New York, blacks/African Americans who were at high risk of obstructive sleep apnea had higher scores on the Dysfunctional Beliefs and Attitudes about Sleep scale, compared with those who were not at high risk.[128] In a study in the Philadelphia area among older black and white women,[129] participants were administered a questionnaire to evaluate sleep-related beliefs and practices. Black women were more likely to endorse incorrect and unhelpful statements. Sell and colleagues[130] examined sleep knowledge among Mexican Americans in San Diego. Non-Hispanic whites were more likely than Mexican Americans to know what sleep apnea was, but when describing the symptoms,

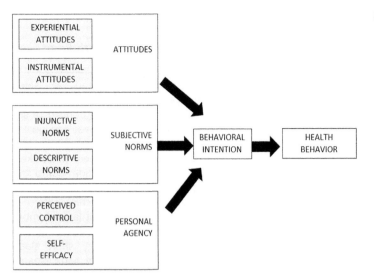

Fig. 4. Integrated behavior model.

both groups had similar knowledge that such a problem existed. Taken together, the role of sleep and health in society is driven by healthy behavior choices. These behavioral decisions, as described in the models above, are largely influenced by beliefs and attitudes about sleep. These beliefs and attitudes, though, are differentially endorsed by racial/ethnic groups, which may underlie sleep difficulties in those populations.

GENDER AND AGE IMPACTS SLEEP IN THE POPULATION

Sleep Changes with Normal Aging in the Population

Physiologic changes in sleep have been well-documented. In a landmark meta-analysis by Ohayon and colleagues,[131] polysomnographic sleep characteristics across the lifespan were examined across 65 studies spanning more than 40 years. This analysis found that with age, polysomnographic total sleep time, sleep efficiency, slow-wave sleep, rapid eye movement (REM) sleep, and REM latency decline, whereas sleep latency, wake after sleep onset, stage 1 sleep, and stage 2 sleep increase. This finding suggests a phenomenon of more disturbed and lighter sleep. In addition to these changes, melatonin secretion declines with age, which may also impact sleep consolidation in older adults.[132] Risk for many sleep disorders also increases with age.[133–135] In particular, sleep disorders, such as insomnia,[136] restless legs syndrome,[137,138] sleep apnea,[139] and REM behavior disorder,[140] include older age as a risk factor. However, a paradox exists, which was highlighted in a large, international cohort

study by Soldatos and colleagues.[141] In this study, older adults were more likely to report difficulties initiating and maintaining sleep. However, they did not endorse a greater level of dissatisfaction with their sleep. A lack of dissatisfaction is similar to results reported in Italy by Zilli and colleagues,[142] who found that younger adults were more likely to report dissatisfaction with sleep than older adults. In the US population, general dissatisfaction with sleep associated with age was examined using the 2006 BRFSS. In a study of more than 150,000 US adults, general sleep disturbance (general difficulties with sleep) was most frequently reported in young adults, and rates generally declined with age.[29] In controlled analyses, no age groups were statistically less likely to report sleep disturbances than the oldest adults, aged 80 or older, although many of the younger groups reported higher levels. These results were replicated using the 2009 BRFSS, which examined self-reported perceived insufficient sleep among greater than 350,000 US adults and found a decline in general sleep insufficiency associated with age.[30] Thus, it appears that sleep objectively worsens with age, but that subjective dissatisfaction with sleep is not associated with normal aging. In fact, this may be a sign of illness or depression.[143]

Population-Level Differences in Sleep Between Men and Women

Differences in sleep between men and women have been widely reported in the literature for decades.[144–149] Overall, in the general population, women report shorter sleep duration,[150] more sleep symptoms,[31] greater rates of insomnia,[151] and lower rates of sleep apnea.[152] In an analysis of sleep disturbances reported in the 2006 BRFSS, it was found that women reported more nighttime sleep disturbances and daytime tiredness than men. Across all age groups, sleep disturbance was reported by between 13.7% and 18.1% of men, depending on age group, and between 17.7% and 25.1% of women.[29] Similarly, for daytime tiredness, rates were 16.4% to 22.9% of men and 20.5% to 29.9% of women, depending on age. In all age groups, women reported nominally more disturbances than men. Statistically, after adjusting for demographics, socioeconomics, health variables, and depression, rates of sleep disturbances were more prevalent among women for all age groups between 25 and 69 years old and rates of daytime tiredness were more common in women for all age groups from 18 to 59 and 75 to 79.

Other issues regarding sleep differences exist between men and women. For example, sleep disturbances are common in pregnancy,[153–155] especially the first and third trimesters. These sleep disturbances can include insomnia, short sleep duration, sleep fragmentation, and gestational sleep apnea. Sleep disturbance in pregnant women can result in adverse outcomes for both the mother and the fetus.[156,157] Sleep in new parents (especially mothers) is also frequently disturbed,[158,159] especially in the first few months after birth. Sleep disturbances among parents of infants are associated with increased postpartum depression,[160–162] increased sleep disturbances among infants, and other adverse outcomes. Women also experience sleep disturbances around menopause. Sleep during the menopausal transition is often characterized by insomnia symptoms and increased sleep fragmentation.[163] Hot flashes are also a common source of sleep disturbance around the menopausal transition.[164]

Some sleep disturbances are disproportionately experienced by men. For example, men are more likely to have obstructive sleep apnea,[139] are more likely to have difficulty adhering to sleep apnea treatment,[165,166] and are more likely to die as a result of complications or consequences of sleep apnea.[167] In addition, men are more likely to be diagnosed with REM Behavior Disorder, which is typically diagnosed among older adults and likely predates neurodegenerative disorders.[168] During the aging process, men are also more likely to demonstrate a steeper decline in slow-wave sleep generation,[131] with lower amounts of slow-wave sleep among older man versus older women.

RACE, ETHNICITY, AND CULTURE ASSOCIATED WITH SLEEP
Insufficient Sleep Associated with Race/Ethnicity

Many studies have documented a "sleep disparity" in the population,[19,39] such that racial/ethnic minorities, especially in the context of socioeconomic disadvantage, achieve less quality sleep. Most studies in this area have shown that, overall, blacks/African Americans are more likely to experience short sleep duration compared with non-Hispanic whites.[19,39] One nationally representative study found that this pattern is robust even after adjustment for a large number of other demographic and socioeconomic covariates, such that the rate of very short sleep ($\leq$4 hours) was 2.5 times those of non-Hispanic whites and the rate of short (5–6 hours) sleep was about twice as high.[150] A similar pattern was seen for Asians/others, who reported very short sleep at a rate of 4 times that seen in non-Hispanic whites and a short sleep about twice as frequently. Among Hispanics/Latinos, there is less clear evidence of habitual short sleep, especially among Mexican Americans. In addition to epidemiologic studies, some laboratory studies have also examined this issue. For example, blacks/African Americans have been shown to sleep less in the laboratory.[169–171] Also, this group has been shown to demonstrate less slow-wave sleep, compensated by increased stage 2 sleep. Other studies have shown similar patterns for sleep duration in other samples that included minority groups,[172,173] and this topic was the subject of multiple recent reviews.[19,174,175]

Sleep Disturbances Associated with Race/Ethnicity in the Population

Less work has been done to characterize rates of sleep disturbances in racial/ethnic minorities. One previous study showed that racial/ethnic minorities demonstrated a lower sleep efficiency based on actigraphy.[176] A study in the Philadelphia area found that race differences in poor sleep quality largely depended on socioeconomic status.[177] A nationally representative study found that black/African Americans were 60% more likely than non-Hispanic whites to report sleep latency more than 30 minutes, although they (along with Hispanics/Latinos) were less likely to report "difficulty falling asleep."[31] This discrepancy between self-reported "problems" and computed long sleep latency suggests that symptom reports may vary based on the question asked. Overall, minority groups were less likely to report insomnia symptoms, nonrestorative sleep, and daytime sleepiness, although non-Mexican Hispanics/Latinos were more likely to endorse sleep apnea symptoms such as snoring.

Several studies have examined the role of racial discrimination as a unique stressor that impacts sleep. A study of residents in Michigan and Wisconsin found that exposure to racial discrimination was associated with sleep disturbances, above the effects of race, sociodemographics, and even depressed mood.[178] This finding, that sleep disturbance is associated with exposure to racism was consistent with other findings that showed that exposure to discrimination was associated with shorter sleep and more sleep difficulties[179] and that these findings are also seen in objective sleep assessments.[169,170] Interestingly, polysomnographic differences in slow-wave sleep between black/African American and non-Hispanic white individuals (ie, reduced slow-wave sleep) were mediated by exposure to discrimination.

Sleep, Acculturation, and Immigration

Few studies have examined sleep related to acculturation. Sell and colleagues[130] found that Mexican Americans who were more acculturated to American lifestyle were more familiar with information about sleep disorders. Also, in a nationally representative sample, speaking only Spanish at home was associated with a decreased likelihood of sleep duration in the short (5–6 hours) and very short (≤4 hours) categories compared with 7 to 8 hours. In this same sample, being born in Mexico (but not any other country) was associated with decreased likelihood of both short and very short sleep duration, but these effects were not significant after adjusting for other demographic and socioeconomic factors, which likely explain this finding.[129]

EMPLOYMENT, NEIGHBORHOOD, AND SOCIOECONOMICS

Although sleep is an important factor in overall health, society has incentivized insufficient sleep. Many of these incentives involve finances and employment. Because of this, there is evidence that one of the strongest societal determinants of sleep is work. The relationship between work and sleep is especially important for safety-sensitive occupations that not only incentivize insufficient sleep but also for which the associated fatigue also jeopardizes the public safety.

Trading Sleep for Work Hours

Replicating and extending prior work in this area, Basner and colleagues[23] examined data from greater than 100,000 Americans over a 9-year period who participated in the ATUS, which is performed annually by the US Bureau of Labor Statistics and uses time diaries to determine work and other activities across 24 hours.[180] In a recent report, Basner and colleagues[23] show that work time, including actual work and other related activities (such as commuting), was the primary determinant of sleep duration. In addition, later start times of school and work were associated with longer sleep, such that each hour of delayed work or training start time was associated with 20 more minutes of sleep. Also, those holding multiple jobs were at greater risk for short sleep duration compared with those only working one job at a time. Although work is a strong determinant of sleep duration, other studies show that employed individuals report the lowest rates of self-reported sleep disturbance.[28] Unemployment, on the other hand, is associated with more sleep problems.[28,30]

Sleep Deprivation and Sleep Disorders in Occupational Settings

Recognition of the role of sleep disorders and sleep deprivation in occupational settings is gaining increased attention. Rosekind and colleagues[181] showed that the typical well-rested worker costs an employer about $1300 per year in lost sleep-related productivity, and this number increases to about $3000 for those with insomnia or insufficient sleep. Furthermore, the loss to productivity permeates many areas of functioning, including time management, mental and interpersonal demands, output demands, and physical job demands. Hui and Grandner[182] show that not only is self-reported poor sleep quality associated with decreased work performance but also worsening sleep longitudinally predicts worsening performance over time. In addition, difficulty sleeping is associated with increased health care costs. Those with difficulty sleeping "often" or "always" were associated with additional health care costs of $3600 to $5200 per person per year more than those who "never" have sleep problems, and these costs increased over time if sleep became worse. Additional analyses from this dataset also showed that poor sleep may motivate employees to make healthy changes as part of a workplace wellness program, but it may also limit those employees' ability to maintain healthy change.[183]

Regarding safety-sensitive occupations such as medicine, law enforcement, and transportation, sleep plays a critical role in safety. For example, sleep apnea occurs at high rates among commercial drivers[184–186] and impairs their ability to drive safely. Accordingly, workplace programs to increase screening and treatment of sleep apnea may have financial benefits for companies.[184] Similar efforts may show effectiveness in rail workers as well.[187,188] Airline pilots face similar challenges, in addition to challenges presented by crossing many time zones. To address these concerns, sleep disorders screening in addition to circadian approaches and scheduled napping have shown effectiveness in improving safety.[189–197] Among law enforcement and first responders, several studies have shown that sleep disturbances are common among police officers[198–203] and firefighters.[204,205] In particular, issues such as sleep apnea, insomnia, and shift work are the most common problems.[206] In a landmark study by Rajaratnam and colleagues,[198] police officers who were at greatest risk of sleep disorders were also more likely to be at risk for job-related problems, such as falling asleep at meetings and using unnecessary violence against citizens. Studies have shown that sleep disturbances in police officers and firefighters are associated with reduced ability to maintain job performance and safety.[198,203,207]

Several studies have been conducted among medical residents and nurses. For nurses, shift work and long work hours have been shown to be related to adverse health outcomes and indicators of reduced functioning.[208–217] Among medical residents, long work hours and shift work have been shown to lead to insufficient sleep duration.[218–221] Furthermore, longer work hours in medical residents have been associated with markers of reduced work performance, although impacts on actual work performance are more inconsistent.[115,222] In a landmark study that compared 2 groups of residency programs, those that gave more time off for sleep did not show measurable changes in work performance.[223] Paradoxically, residents given more time to sleep were more worried about decreases in their quality of work as a result of working less, yet they were more satisfied with the quality of their life and social functioning.

Sleep, Poverty, and Neighborhood Factors

Several studies have shown that poverty is associated with both shorter sleep duration and worse sleep quality.[30] However, once the benefits of income are accounted for (by statistically covarying education, access to health care, and so forth), associations with income are often nonexistent and may go in the opposite direction. For example, in an analysis of data from greater than 350,000 US adults, insufficient sleep was associated with poverty before adjusting for covariates, but after adjustment, the opposite relationship was seen.[30] A positive relationship between income and insufficient sleep after adjusting for covariates suggests that money may not buy sleep, but many of the benefits of income may contribute to healthy sleep. One aspect of this relationship is neighborhood quality. Several studies have investigated the role of the neighborhood in an individual's sleep quality, showing that neighborhoods that are crime-ridden, not socially cohesive, and dirty, are associated with worse sleep quality.[224–227] Furthermore, sleep quality may partially mediate the relationship between neighborhood quality and both mental[227] and physical[225] health. One way that a neighborhood may directly influence sleep would be via the physical environment. There is substantial literature showing that environmental noise[228,229] and light[230–233] can adversely impact sleep and that neighborhoods that are active at night may directly impact sleep through these.

INFLUENCES OF HOME, FAMILY, AND SCHOOL ENVIRONMENT

The home, family, and school environments also likely play important roles in an individual's sleep. For example, household size is negatively associated with sleep, such that more crowded homes are more likely to foster insufficient sleep.[30] Also, as mentioned above, the physical sleep environment can also play a role. Bedrooms that have levels of light, noise, and temperature that are not conducive to sleep may contribute to insufficient sleep.[234–236] Although data on beds and other sleeping surfaces are relatively scarce, an uncomfortable sleeping environment may also reduce sleep ability.[237–239]

Another key issue of the home and family environment on sleep regards the marital relationship. Although most sleep research is performed on individuals sleeping alone in a laboratory, most adults do not sleep alone most nights.[240,241] With this in mind, several studies have explored the important role of marital and relationship quality in sleep quality and how this relates to health. For example, relationship quality has been shown to be an important predictor of sleep health, especially among women, and relationship quality may be an important moderator between sleep quality and health.[241–244]

TECHNOLOGY IN AND OUT OF THE BEDROOM

In 2011, the National Sleep Foundation polled Americans regarding their use of technology in the bedroom. In a report of the findings of this survey, Gradisar and colleagues[245] note that 90% of Americans use some sort of electronic device in the hour before bed. Also, more than two-thirds of adolescents and young adults used a Smartphone in the hour before bed, compared with approximately one-third of middle-aged adults and about one-fifth of older adults. Furthermore, the more engaging the technology application, the more the electronic device use was associated with difficulties falling asleep and nonrestorative sleep. This finding is supported by other work that shows that not only is electronic media use near bedtime prevalent[246] but also the light emitted by the devices[247] as well as the mental engagement[248] can interfere with sleep. Growing awareness of the influence of mobile electronic device use on sleep is a key example of a societal-level change (use of technology) impacting an individual's sleep.

GLOBALIZATION AND 24/7 SOCIETY

Another societal-level factor that impacts sleep is the advent of globalization and a 24/7 society. In the past, social interactions, commercial activities, and work responsibilities were dictated by more local factors. Now, though, the advent of globalization and 24/7 operations often impinge on sleep. Regarding globalization, individuals and organizations are connected across the globe. In combination with a society that institutes shift work and 24-hour operations, entire segments of the population are awake across all hours of the 24-hour day, and access to individuals across time zones is easier than ever. Because of this, social interactions (such as interactions with friends, family, and even online groups), commercial activities (such as eCommerce and availability of entertainment around the clock on demand), and work responsibilities (such as e-mails outside of business hours and business conducted across the globe) can impinge on sleep. The influence of globalization and 24/7 society on sleep behaviors is particularly relevant, because shift work has been repeatedly shown in both laboratory and field studies to be related to adverse health outcomes.

PUBLIC SAFETY AND PUBLIC POLICY

As mentioned above, many safety-sensitive occupations, such as those in transportation, law enforcement, and medicine, require healthy sleep for optimal performance. The problem is that these professions often institute policies that make healthy sleep difficult. As a result, the sleep of an individual in one of those occupations may have

ramifications for others in the public. For example, when a large commercial truck crashes, it causes more damage and a greater likelihood of fatal injury.[249,250] For this reason, several policy approaches to sleep and public safety have been proposed. The Accreditation Council for Graduate Medical Education has already instituted duty hour restrictions on medical residents, based on results from a report by the Institute of Medicine.[218] These restrictions, although controversial,[115,251–253] are likely resulting in increased sleep among medical residents.[222] In the transportation industry, recommendations by the National Highway Transportation and Safety Administration address the need for sleep disorders screening and fatigue mitigation among commercial drivers,[250] although formal regulations have not yet been passed. The Federal Aviation Administration also recently issued guidelines to address sleep issues in pilots.[254] More work is needed in this area, and although regulations to ensure public safety have been proposed, they still have not yet been passed.

Another domain of public safety is drowsy driving. Even among non–commercial drivers, drowsy driving is an important public safety issue. Drowsy driving is prevalent, reported among about 5% of the US population over a 6-month period.[255] Population-level data suggest that short sleep duration is an independent risk factor for drowsy driving, even if respondents believe that they are completely well rested.[97]

Another area of public policy related to sleep involves school start times. Existing evidence suggests that most US schools, especially high schools, start too early for most adolescents.[256–259] Earlier start times not only promote shorter sleep duration among adolescents (who need more sleep than adults) but also do not take into account natural circadian delays that occur in adolescence.[260] It has been proposed that delaying school start times can improve academic performance, improve mental health, and improve overall health in students.[261–266]

Other public policy initiatives have addressed the issue of environmental light and noise in neighborhoods. There are several policies in place, and more being proposed, that limit the brightness of street lights in neighborhoods, increase "quiet time" regulations at night, direct airplanes to avoid some residential areas at night, reduce traffic and train noise at night, and so forth. These approaches are usually regional, and many efforts are ongoing.

One more public policy implication relevant to sleep would be health policy legislation. For example, improving mental health parity laws will do much to intervene on perhaps the most important determinant of sleep health at the population level[30] and will facilitate treatment of insomnia with the most well supported therapy.[267] In addition, health equity legislation may help to address some of the disparities seen in sleep in the population.[20] These and other future approaches may better promote healthy sleep from a policy standpoint.

IMPORTANT LIMITATIONS OF THE EXISTING LITERATURE

There are several important limitations to the existing literature, which constrain interpretations and generalizations of the data. The most important limitation is that there is a lack of consistency in sleep assessment methods across studies, and this is a problem for several reasons. First, retrospective self-report (eg, survey), prospective self-report (eg, diary), laboratory-based objective (eg, polysomnography), and field-based objective (eg, actigraphy) estimates of sleep tend to disagree with each other, because they capture different elements of sleep well. It is likely that physiologic sleep is substantially less than that which is self-reported.[27] Even among survey methods, there seems to be systematic variation.[35] Second, because there is still no nationally representative dataset that includes any well-validated estimate of sleep duration or quality, generalizability from one dataset to the next is limited. Third, cutoffs and categories used to describe sleep are often inconsistent across studies; for example, the cutoff for the shortest sleep duration category can be as low as 4 hours or less or as high as 7 hours.

Another important limitation is a general lack of physiologic sleep measures at the societal level. Because these measures are typically more expensive and require more infrastructure to implement, they are often infeasible for large studies that require assessment of thousands of people. Until sleep assessment becomes more of a priority, otherwise rich datasets will continue to have just a few nonvalidated survey items measuring sleep. Suboptimal measurement of sleep will make data interpretation difficult, because it is unclear the degree to which associations are referring to physiologic sleep or other factors that become subsumed in self-reported sleep experience.

A third important limitation regards the complexity of social environments. As shown in the Social-Ecological Model, the influences that may play a role in sleep are many, varied, and exist at several levels. Still, most studies do not address the complex nature of social-environmental influences on health. Also, future studies that will examine epigenetic effects will need to better account for gene-environment interactions, and this will require a better operationalization of environmental variables in many cases. An example of one study that brought these methodologies together is cited by Watson and colleagues,[268] who combined geospatial neighborhood analyses with sleep genetic information to characterize a social-environmental influence on sleep duration.

A fourth important limitation to the existing literature is a lack of interventional studies. If, for example, sleep represents a modifiable factor in health disparities, it is plausible that improvements in sleep at the community level could reduce effects of health disparities. However, there is a lack of interventional studies that can demonstrate this; rather, the best examples of investigations in this area use mediational analysis to show that changes in sleep account for changes in health outcomes across groups, such as blood pressure.[269] More sleep interventions at the community level are going to be needed in order to understand the causal role of sleep in these outcomes. Also, there is a general lack of empirically supported interventions for sleep health. Although many interventions exist to promote healthy diet, physical activity, and substance cessation, a lack of standardized sleep health interventions limits knowledge in this area.

FUTURE RESEARCH DIRECTIONS

Several potential future research directions may help advance knowledge in this area. First, expanded epigenetic studies are needed to explore gene-environment interactions. As the science of human sleep genetics develops, more research into how genetic vulnerabilities interact with environmental influences is needed. For example, although it is unlikely that genetics explains racial disparities in sleep, it is plausible that some genetic adaptations to one geographic region may confer risk in another region (eg, less sunlight, different food availability). Also, it may be possible that certain genetic vulnerabilities (eg, airway collapse) may differentially affect groups because body mass indexes increase in the presence of increasing obesity rates due to westernized diets.

Another important direction in research will be to clarify the sleep phenotypes and endophenotypes. Currently, typing of sleep at the community and population level is frequently based on broad sleep duration groups (eg, "short sleepers") or sleep symptoms ("difficulty falling asleep"), although these groups can be highly heterogeneous. Genetic studies are limited by this limited clarity in sleep phenotypes. Short sleepers, for example, may comprise individuals who are "true" short sleepers and need less sleep, those who need more sleep but are able to tolerate less sleep for an extended period of time ("resilient"), and those who are insufficient sleepers. Still, insufficient sleepers may belong to groups that demonstrate neurocognitive and metabolic impairments at variable rates (eg, some individuals may demonstrate more metabolic impairments and some more cognitive). Perhaps more clarity regarding phenotypes will help move forward an agenda of better human sleep genetics.

More intervention studies are also needed at the laboratory, clinical, and community levels that address real-world sleep concerns. As mentioned above, there is a lack of healthy sleep interventions, relative to healthy diet or physical activity recommendations. Without these data, it is difficult to make recommendations in addition to just stating a problem. Also, interventions need to address issues that have generally been ignored yet carry real-world significance For example, despite many adults sleeping between 6 and 7 hours per night, this sleep duration is almost never included in the literature, either because epidemiologic studies categorize at the hour (including them in either 6- or 7-hour groups) or because laboratory studies try to maximize difference between groups (usually comparing 8–6, 5, or 4 hours but not between 6 and 7).[14] These and other real-world issues need to be better captured in intervention studies.

Finally, intervention studies are needed that identify real-world approaches to increasing sleep time among chronically sleep-deprived individuals. Unlike traditional intervention study designs, where changing sleep is the intervention and some health marker is the outcome (which would address the question of whether changing sleep impacts health), study designs are needed whereby changing sleep itself is the outcome. For example, it is known that smoking cessation can positively impact health. However, how does one quit smoking? Just recommending that someone quit is not enough, and literature has emerged that proposes novel ways to achieve this difficult behavioral change. Likewise, changing sleep duration in a real-world setting (with home, work, and other societal pressures) may be difficult, and useful strategies besides simply making recommendations need to be explored.

REFERENCES

1. Cajochen C, Chellappa S, Schmidt C. What keeps us awake?–the role of clocks and hourglasses, light, and melatonin. Int Rev Neurobiol 2010;93: 57–90.

2. Fuller PM, Lu J. Neurobiology of sleep. In: Amlaner CJ, Fuller PM, editors. Basics of sleep guide. 2nd edition. Westchester (IL): Sleep Research Society; 2009. p. 53–62.

3. Mackiewicz M, Naidoo N, Zimmerman JE, et al. Molecular mechanisms of sleep and wakefulness. Ann N Y Acad Sci 2008;1129:335–49.

4. Schwartz JR, Roth T. Neurophysiology of sleep and wakefulness: basic science and clinical implications. Curr Neuropharmacol 2008;6(4):367–78.

5. Franken P. A role for clock genes in sleep homeostasis. Curr Opin Neurobiol 2013;23(5):864–72.

6. Feng D, Lazar MA. Clocks, metabolism, and the epigenome. Mol Cell 2012;47(2):158–67.

7. Gerstner JR, Lenz O, Vanderheyden WM, et al. Amyloid-beta induces sleep fragmentation that is rescued by fatty acid binding proteins in Drosophila. J Neurosci Res 2016. [Epub ahead of print].

8. Xu M, Chung S, Zhang S, et al. Basal forebrain circuit for sleep-wake control. Nat Neurosci 2015; 18(11):1641–7.

9. Cox J, Pinto L, Dan Y. Calcium imaging of sleep-wake related neuronal activity in the dorsal pons. Nat Commun 2016;7:10763.

10. Park DA. The fire within the eye: a historical essay on the nature and meaning of light. Princeton (NJ): Princeton University Press; 1997.

11. Williams S. Sleep and society: sociological ventures into the (Un)known. London: Taylor & Francis; 2005.

12. Watson NF, Badr MS, Belenky G, et al. Recommended amount of sleep for a healthy adult: a joint consensus statement of the American Academy of Sleep Medicine and Sleep Research Society. Sleep 2015;38(6):843–4.

13. Consensus Conference Panel, Watson NF, Badr MS, et al. Joint consensus statement of the American Academy of Sleep Medicine and Sleep Research Society on the recommended amount of sleep for a healthy adult: methodology and discussion. J Clin Sleep Med 2015;11(8): 931–52.

14. Consensus Conference Panel, Watson NF, Badr MS, et al. Joint consensus statement of the American Academy of Sleep Medicine and Sleep Research Society on the recommended amount of sleep for a healthy adult: methodology and discussion. Sleep 2015;38(8):1161–83.

15. Consensus Conference Panel, Watson NF, Badr MS, et al. Recommended amount of sleep for a healthy adult: a joint consensus statement of the American Academy of Sleep Medicine and Sleep Research Society. J Clin Sleep Med 2015; 11(6):591–2.

16. Bronfenbrenner U. Toward an experimental ecology of human development. Am Psychol 1977;32: 513–31.

17. Grandner MA, Patel NP, Hale L, et al. Mortality associated with sleep duration: the evidence, the possible mechanisms, and the future. Sleep Med Rev 2010;14:191–203.

18. Grandner MA. Addressing sleep disturbances: an opportunity to prevent cardiometabolic disease? Int Rev Psychiatry 2014;26(2):155–76.

19. Grandner MA, Williams NJ, Knutson KL, et al. Sleep disparity, race/ethnicity, and socioeconomic position. Sleep Med 2016;18:7–18.

20. Grandner MA. Sleep disparities in the American population: prevalence, potential causes, relationships to cardiometabolic health disparities, and future drections for research and policy. In: Kelly R, editor. Health disparities in America. Washington, DC: US Congress; 2015. p. 126–32.

21. Knutson KL, Van Cauter E, Rathouz PJ, et al. Trends in the prevalence of short sleepers in the USA: 1975-2006. Sleep 2010;33(1):37–45.

22. Bin YS, Marshall NS, Glozier N. Secular trends in adult sleep duration: a systematic review. Sleep Med Rev 2012;16(3):223–30.

23. Basner M, Spaeth AM, Dinges DF. Sociodemographic characteristics and waking activities and their role in the timing and duration of sleep. Sleep 2014;37(12):1889–906.

24. Grandner MA, Chakravorty S, Perlis ML, et al. Habitual sleep duration associated with self-reported and objectively determined cardiometabolic risk factors. Sleep Med 2014;15(1):42–50.

25. Krueger PM, Friedman EM. Sleep duration in the United States: a cross-sectional population-based study. Am J Epidemiol 2009;169(9):1052–63.

26. Liu Y, Wheaton AG, Chapman DP, et al. Prevalence of healthy sleep duration among adults –United States, 2014. MMWR Morb Mortal Wkly Rep 2016;65(6):137–41.

27. Kurina LM, McClintock MK, Chen JH, et al. Sleep duration and all-cause mortality: a critical review of measurement and associations. Ann Epidemiol 2013;23(6):361–70.

28. Grandner MA, Patel NP, Gehrman PR, et al. Who gets the best sleep? Ethnic and socioeconomic factors related to sleep disturbance. Sleep Med 2010;11:470–9.

29. Grandner MA, Martin JL, Patel NP, et al. Age and sleep disturbances among American men and women: data from the U.S. Behavioral Risk Factor Surveillance System. Sleep 2012;35(3):395–406.

30. Grandner MA, Jackson NJ, Izci-Balserak B, et al. Social and behavioral determinants of perceived insufficient sleep. Front Neurol 2015;6:112.

31. Grandner MA, Petrov MER, Rattanaumpawan P, et al. Sleep symptoms, race/ethnicity, and socioeconomic position. J Clin Sleep Med 2013; 9(9):897–905, 905A–D.

32. Hammond EC. Some preliminary findings on physical complaints from a prospective study of 1,064,004 men and women. Am J Public Health Nations Health 1964;54:11–23.

33. Gallicchio L, Kalesan B. Sleep duration and mortality: a systematic review and meta-analysis. J Sleep Res 2009;18(2):148–58.

34. Cappuccio FP, D'Elia L, Strazzullo P, et al. Sleep duration and all-cause mortality: a systematic review and meta-analysis of prospective studies. Sleep 2010;33(5):585–92.

35. Grandner MA, Patel NP, Gehrman PR, et al. Problems associated with short sleep: bridging the gap between laboratory and epidemiological studies. Sleep Med Rev 2010;14:239–47.

36. Kripke DF, Langer RD, Elliott JA, et al. Mortality related to actigraphic long and short sleep. Sleep Med 2011;12(1):28–33.

37. Youngstedt SD, Kripke DF. Long sleep and mortality: rationale for sleep restriction. Sleep Med Rev 2004;8(3):159–74.

38. Grandner MA, Drummond SP. Who are the long sleepers? Towards an understanding of the mortality relationship. Sleep Med Rev 2007;11(5): 341–60.

39. Adenekan B, Pandey A, McKenzie S, et al. Sleep in America: role of racial/ethnic differences. Sleep Med Rev 2013;17(4):255–62.

40. Morselli LL, Guyon A, Spiegel K. Sleep and metabolic function. Pflugers Arch 2012;463(1):139–60.

41. Knutson KL. Does inadequate sleep play a role in vulnerability to obesity? Am J Hum Biol 2012; 24(3):361–71.

42. Watanabe M, Kikuchi H, Tanaka K, et al. Association of short sleep duration with weight gain and obesity at 1-year follow-up: a large-scale prospective study. Sleep 2010;33(2):161–7.

43. Chaput JP, Bouchard C, Tremblay A. Change in sleep duration and visceral fat accumulation over 6 years in adults. Obesity (Silver Spring) 2014; 22(5):E9–12.

44. Chaput JP, Despres JP, Bouchard C, et al. The association between sleep duration and weight gain in adults: a 6-year prospective study from the Quebec Family Study. Sleep 2008;31(4):517–23.

45. Baron KG, Reid KJ, Kern AS, et al. Role of sleep timing in caloric intake and BMI. Obesity (Silver Spring) 2011;19(7):1374–81.

46. Shechter A, Grandner MA, St-Onge MP. The role of sleep in the control of food intake. Am J Lifestyle Med 2014;8(6):371–4.

47. Grandner MA, Schopfer EA, Sands-Lincoln M, et al. Relationship between sleep duration and body mass index depends on age. Obesity (Silver Spring) 2015;23(12):2491–8.

48. Barone MT, Menna-Barreto L. Diabetes and sleep: a complex cause-and-effect relationship. Diabetes Res Clin Pract 2011;91(2):129–37.

49. Aldabal L, Bahammam AS. Metabolic, endocrine, and immune consequences of sleep deprivation. Open Respir Med J 2011;5:31–43.

50. Bopparaju S, Surani S. Sleep and diabetes. Int J Endocrinol 2010;2010:759509.

51. Zizi F, Jean-Louis G, Brown CD, et al. Sleep duration and the risk of diabetes mellitus: epidemiologic evidence and pathophysiologic insights. Curr Diab Rep 2010;10(1):43–7.

52. Shan Z, Ma H, Xie M, et al. Sleep duration and risk of type 2 diabetes: a meta-analysis of prospective studies. Diabetes Care 2015;38(3):529–37.

53. Buxton OM, Pavlova M, Reid EW, et al. Sleep restriction for 1 week reduces insulin sensitivity in healthy men. Diabetes 2010;59(9):2126–33.

54. Morselli L, Leproult R, Balbo M, et al. Role of sleep duration in the regulation of glucose metabolism and appetite. Best Pract Res Clin Endocrinol Metab 2010;24(5):687–702.

55. Tasali E, Leproult R, Spiegel K. Reduced sleep duration or quality: relationships with insulin resistance and type 2 diabetes. Prog Cardiovasc Dis 2009;51(5):381–91.

56. Spiegel K, Knutson K, Leproult R, et al. Sleep loss: a novel risk factor for insulin resistance and Type 2 diabetes. J Appl Physiol 2005;99(5):2008–19.

57. Spaeth AM, Dinges DF, Goel N. Sex and race differences in caloric intake during sleep restriction in healthy adults. Am J Clin Nutr 2014;100(2):559–66.

58. Kim S, Deroo LA, Sandler DP. Eating patterns and nutritional characteristics associated with sleep duration. Public Health Nutr 2011;14(5):889–95.

59. Nedeltcheva AV, Kilkus JM, Imperial J, et al. Sleep curtailment is accompanied by increased intake of calories from snacks. Am J Clin Nutr 2009;89(1):126–33.

60. Van Cauter E, Spiegel K, Tasali E, et al. Metabolic consequences of sleep and sleep loss. Sleep Med 2008;9(Suppl 1):S23–8.

61. Spiegel K, Tasali E, Penev P, et al. Brief communication: sleep curtailment in healthy young men is associated with decreased leptin levels, elevated ghrelin levels, and increased hunger and appetite. Ann Intern Med 2004;141(11):846–50.

62. Hayes AL, Xu F, Babineau D, et al. Sleep duration and circulating adipokine levels. Sleep 2011;34(2):147–52.

63. Perelis M, Ramsey KM, Marcheva B, et al. Circadian transcription from beta cell function to diabetes pathophysiology. J Biol Rhythms 2016;31(4):323–36.

64. Grandner MA, Sands-Lincoln MR, Pak VM, et al. Sleep duration, cardiovascular disease, and proinflammatory biomarkers. Nat Sci Sleep 2013;5:93–107.

65. Frey DJ, Fleshner M, Wright KP Jr. The effects of 40 hours of total sleep deprivation on inflammatory markers in healthy young adults. Brain Behav Immun 2007;21(8):1050–7.

66. Ferrie JE, Kivimaki M, Akbaraly TN, et al. Associations between change in sleep duration and inflammation: findings on C-reactive protein and interleukin 6 in the Whitehall II Study. Am J Epidemiol 2013;178(6):956–61.

67. Rohleder N, Aringer M, Boentert M. Role of interleukin-6 in stress, sleep, and fatigue. Ann N Y Acad Sci 2012;1261:88–96.

68. Vgontzas AN, Zoumakis E, Bixler EO, et al. Adverse effects of modest sleep restriction on sleepiness, performance, and inflammatory cytokines. J Clin Endocrinol Metab 2004;89(5):2119–26.

69. van Leeuwen WM, Lehto M, Karisola P, et al. Sleep restriction increases the risk of developing cardiovascular diseases by augmenting proinflammatory responses through IL-17 and CRP. PLoS One 2009;4(2):e4589.

70. Chennaoui M, Sauvet F, Drogou C, et al. Effect of one night of sleep loss on changes in tumor necrosis factor alpha (TNF-alpha) levels in healthy men. Cytokine 2011;56(2):318–24.

71. Shearer WT, Reuben JM, Mullington JM, et al. Soluble TNF-alpha receptor 1 and IL-6 plasma levels in humans subjected to the sleep deprivation model of spaceflight. J Allergy Clin Immunol 2001;107(1):165–70.

72. Patel SR, Zhu X, Storfer-Isser A, et al. Sleep duration and biomarkers of inflammation. Sleep 2009;32(2):200–4.

73. Meier-Ewert HK, Ridker PM, Rifai N, et al. Effect of sleep loss on C-reactive protein, an inflammatory marker of cardiovascular risk. J Am Coll Cardiol 2004;43(4):678–83.

74. Miller MA, Kandala NB, Kivimaki M, et al. Gender differences in the cross-sectional relationships between sleep duration and markers of inflammation: Whitehall II study. Sleep 2009;32(7):857–64.

75. Matthews KA, Zheng H, Kravitz HM, et al. Are inflammatory and coagulation biomarkers related to sleep characteristics in mid-life women?: Study of Women's Health across the Nation sleep study. Sleep 2010;33(12):1649–55.

76. Grandner MA, Buxton OM, Jackson N, et al. Extreme sleep durations and increased C-reactive protein: effects of sex and ethnoracial group. Sleep 2013;36(5):769–779E.

77. Irwin MR, Olmstead R, Carroll JE. Sleep disturbance, sleep duration, and inflammation: a systematic review and meta-analysis of cohort studies and

experimental sleep deprivation. Biol Psychiatry 2016;80(1):40–52.

78. von Ruesten A, Weikert C, Fietze I, et al. Association of sleep duration with chronic diseases in the European Prospective Investigation into Cancer and Nutrition (EPIC)-Potsdam study. PLoS One 2012;7(1):e30972.

79. Altman NG, Izci-Balserak B, Schopfer E, et al. Sleep duration versus sleep insufficiency as predictors of cardiometabolic health outcomes. Sleep Med 2012;13(10):1261–70.

80. Wang Q, Xi B, Liu M, et al. Short sleep duration is associated with hypertension risk among adults: a systematic review and meta-analysis. Hypertens Res 2012;35(10):1012–8.

81. Meng L, Zheng Y, Hui R. The relationship of sleep duration and insomnia to risk of hypertension incidence: a meta-analysis of prospective cohort studies. Hypertens Res 2013;36(11):985–95.

82. Mezick EJ, Hall M, Matthews KA. Sleep duration and ambulatory blood pressure in black and white adolescents. Hypertension 2012;59(3):747–52.

83. King CR, Knutson KL, Rathouz PJ, et al. Short sleep duration and incident coronary artery calcification. JAMA 2008;300(24):2859–66.

84. Amagai Y, Ishikawa S, Gotoh T, et al. Sleep duration and incidence of cardiovascular events in a Japanese population: the Jichi Medical School cohort study. J Epidemiol 2010;20(2):106–10.

85. Cappuccio FP, Cooper D, D'Elia L, et al. Sleep duration predicts cardiovascular outcomes: a systematic review and meta-analysis of prospective studies. Eur Heart J 2011;32(12):1484–92.

86. Goel N, Rao H, Durmer JS, et al. Neurocognitive consequences of sleep deprivation. Semin Neurol 2009;29(4):320–39.

87. Lim J, Dinges DF. Sleep deprivation and vigilant attention. Ann N Y Acad Sci 2008;1129:305–22.

88. Dinges DF, Powell JW. Microcomputer analyses of performance on a portable, simple visual RT task during sustained operations. Beh Res Meth Instr Comp 1985;17:652–5.

89. Banks S, Dinges DF. Behavioral and physiological consequences of sleep restriction. J Clin Sleep Med 2007;3(5):519–28.

90. Van Dongen HP, Baynard MD, Maislin G, et al. Systematic interindividual differences in neurobehavioral impairment from sleep loss: evidence of trait-like differential vulnerability. Sleep 2004;27(3):423–33.

91. Verweij IM, Romeijn N, Smit DJ, et al. Sleep deprivation leads to a loss of functional connectivity in frontal brain regions. BMC Neurosci 2014;15:88.

92. Killgore WD, Grugle NL, Balkin TJ. Gambling when sleep deprived: don't bet on stimulants. Chronobiol Int 2012;29(1):43–54.

93. Jackson ML, Croft RJ, Kennedy GA, et al. Cognitive components of simulated driving performance: sleep loss effects and predictors. Accid Anal Prev 2013;50:438–44.

94. Saint Martin M, Sforza E, Barthelemy JC, et al. Does subjective sleep affect cognitive function in healthy elderly subjects? The Proof cohort. Sleep Med 2012;13(9):1146–52.

95. Rupp TL, Wesensten NJ, Balkin TJ. Trait-like vulnerability to total and partial sleep loss. Sleep 2012;35(8):1163–72.

96. Banks S, Van Dongen HP, Maislin G, et al. Neurobehavioral dynamics following chronic sleep restriction: dose-response effects of one night for recovery. Sleep 2010;33(8):1013–26.

97. Maia Q, Grandner MA, Findley J, et al. Short and long sleep duration and risk of drowsy driving and the role of subjective sleep insufficiency. Accid Anal Prev 2013;59:618–22.

98. Chiu HY, Tsai PS. The impact of various work schedules on sleep complaints and minor accidents during work or leisure time: evidence from a national survey. J Occup Environ Med 2013;55(3):325–30.

99. Lilley R, Day L, Koehncke N, et al. The relationship between fatigue-related factors and work-related injuries in the Saskatchewan Farm Injury Cohort Study. Am J Ind Med 2012;55(4):367–75.

100. Kucharczyk ER, Morgan K, Hall AP. The occupational impact of sleep quality and insomnia symptoms. Sleep Med Rev 2012;16(6):547–59.

101. American Psychiatric Association. Diagnostic and statistical manual of mental disorders. 5th edition. Washington, DC: American Psychiatric Association; 2003. DSM-5.

102. Chakravorty S, Siu HY, Lalley-Chareczko L, et al. Sleep duration and insomnia symptoms as risk factors for suicidal ideation in a nationally representative sample. Prim Care Companion CNS Disord 2015;17(6).

103. Rosenstock IM. Why people use health services. Milbank Mem Fund Q 1966;44(3 Suppl):94–127.

104. Champion VL, Skinner CS. The health belief model. In: Glanz K, Rimer BK, Viswanath K, editors. Health behavior and health education: theory, research, and practice. San Francisco (CA): Jossey-Bass; 2008. p. 45–65.

105. Montano DE, Kasprzyk D. Theory of reasoned action, theory of planned behavior, and the integrated behavioral model. In: Glanz K, Rimer BK, Viswanath K, editors. Health behavior and health education: theory, research, and practice. San Francisco (CA): Jossey-Bass; 2008. p. 68–96.

106. Hooker E, Ball HL, Kelly PJ. Sleeping like a baby: attitudes and experiences of bedsharing in northeast England. Med Anthropol 2001;19(3):203–22.

107. Thoman EB. Co-sleeping, an ancient practice: is-sues of the past and present, and possibilities for the future. Sleep Med Rev 2006;10(6):407–17.

108. Mindell JA, Sadeh A, Wiegand B, et al. Cross-cul-tural differences in infant and toddler sleep. Sleep Med 2010;11(3):274–80.

109. Norton PJ, Grellner KW. A retrospective study on infant bed-sharing in a clinical practice population. Matern Child Health J 2011;15(4):507–13.

110. Gettler LT, McKenna JJ. Evolutionary perspectives on mother-infant sleep proximity and breastfeeding in a laboratory setting. Am J Phys Anthropol 2011; 144(3):454–62.

111. Jain S, Romack R, Jain R. Bed sharing in school-age children–clinical and social implications. J Child Adolesc Psychiatr Nurs 2011;24(3):185–9.

112. Shulman D, Strousma GG. Dream cultures: explo-rations in the comparative history of dreaming. Ox-ford (United Kingdom): Oxford University Press; 1999.

113. Spurgeon A, Harrington JM, Cooper CL. Health and safety problems associated with long working hours: a review of the current position. Occup Envi-ron Med 1997;54(6):367–75.

114. Goto A, Yasumura S, Nishise Y, et al. Association of health behavior and social role with total mortality among Japanese elders in Okinawa, Japan. Aging Clin Exp Res 2003;15(6):443–50.

115. Lockley SW, Landrigan CP, Barger LK, et al. When policy meets physiology: the challenge of reducing resident work hours. Clin Orthop Relat Res 2006; 449:116–27.

116. Ko GT, Chan JC, Chan AW, et al. Association be-tween sleeping hours, working hours and obesity in Hong Kong Chinese: the 'better health for better Hong Kong' health promotion campaign. Int J Obes (Lond) 2007;31(2):254–60.

117. Basner M, Dinges DF. Dubious bargain: trading sleep for Leno and Letterman. Sleep 2009;32(6): 747–52.

118. Gangwisch JE. All work and no play makes Jack lose sleep. Commentary on Virtanen et al. Long working hours and sleep disturbances: the White-hall II prospective cohort study. Sleep 2009;32: 737–45. Sleep 2009;32(6):717–8.

119. Virtanen M, Ferrie JE, Gimeno D, et al. Long work-ing hours and sleep disturbances: the Whitehall II prospective cohort study. Sleep 2009;32(6): 737–45.

120. Nakata A. Effects of long work hours and poor sleep characteristics on workplace injury among full-time male employees of small- and medium-scale businesses. J Sleep Res 2011;20(4):576–84.

121. Mahan RP, Carvalhais AB, Queen SE. Sleep reduc-tion in night-shift workers: is it sleep deprivation or a sleep disturbance disorder? Percept Mot Skills 1990;70(3 Pt 1):723–30.

122. Rajaratnam SM, Arendt J. Health in a 24-h society. Lancet 2001;358(9286):999–1005.

123. Nag PK, Nag A. Shiftwork in the hot environment. J Hum Ergol (Tokyo) 2001;30(1–2):161–6.

124. Costa G. Shift work and health: current problems and preventive actions. Saf Health Work 2010; 1(2):112–23.

125. Owens J. Sleep in children: cross-cultural perspec-tives. Sleep Biol Rhythms 2004;2:165–73.

126. Milner CE, Cote KA. Benefits of napping in healthy adults: impact of nap length, time of day, age, and experience with napping. J Sleep Res 2009;18(2): 272–81.

127. Worthman CM, Brown RA. Sleep budgets in a glob-alizing world: biocultural interactions influence sleep sufficiency among Egyptian families. Soc Sci Med 2013;79:31–9.

128. Pandey A, Gekhman D, Gousse Y, et al. Short sleep and dysfunctional beliefs and attitudes to-ward sleep among black men. Sleep 2011; 34(Abstract Suppl):261–2.

129. Grandner MA, Patel NP, Jean-Louis G, et al. Sleep-related behaviors and beliefs associated with race/ ethnicity in women. J Natl Med Assoc 2013;105(1): 4–15.

130. Sell RE, Bardwell W, Palinkas L, et al. Ethnic differ-ences in sleep-health knowledge. Sleep 2009; 32(Abstract Supplement):A392.

131. Ohayon MM, Carskadon MA, Guilleminault C, et al. Meta-analysis of quantitative sleep parameters from childhood to old age in healthy individuals: developing normative sleep values across the hu-man lifespan. Sleep 2004;27(7):1255–73.

132. Hardeland R. Melatonin in aging and disease -mul-tiple consequences of reduced secretion, options and limits of treatment. Aging Dis 2012;3(2): 194–225.

133. Neikrug AB, Ancoli-Israel S. Sleep disorders in the older adult - a mini-review. Gerontology 2010;56(2): 181–9.

134. Roepke SK, Ancoli-Israel S. Sleep disorders in the elderly. Indian J Med Res 2010;131:302–10.

135. Martin J, Shochat T, Gehrman PR, et al. Sleep in the elderly. Respir Care Clin N Am 1999;5(3):461–72, ix.

136. Ruiter ME, VanderWal GS, Lichstein KL. Insomnia in the elderly. In: Pandi-Perumal SR, Monti JR, Monjan AA, editors. Principles and practice of geri-atric sleep medicine. Cambridge (United Kingdom): Cambridge; 2010. p. 271–9.

137. Yeh P, Walters AS, Tsuang JW. Restless legs syn-drome: a comprehensive overview on its epidemi-ology, risk factors, and treatment. Sleep Breath 2012;16(4):987–1007.

138. Spiegelhalder K, Hornyak M. Movement disorders in the elderly. In: Pandi-Perumal SR, Monti JR, Monjan AA, editors. Principles and practice of

geriatric sleep medicine. Cambridge (United Kingdom): Cambridge; 2010. p. 233–40.

139. Peppard PE, Young T, Barnet JH, et al. Increased prevalence of sleep-disordered breathing in adults. Am J Epidemiol 2013;177(9):1006–14.

140. Ferini Strambi L. REM sleep behavior disorder in the elderly. In: Pandi-Perumal SR, Monti JR, Monjan AA, editors. Principles and practice of geriatric sleep medicine. Cambridge (United Kingdom): Cambridge; 2010. p. 241–7.

141. Soldatos CR, Allaert FA, Ohta T, et al. How do individuals sleep around the world? Results from a single-day survey in ten countries. Sleep Med 2005;6(1):5–13.

142. Zilli I, Ficca G, Salzarulo P. Factors involved in sleep satisfaction in the elderly. Sleep Med 2009; 10(2):233–9.

143. Grandner MA, Patel NP, Gooneratne NS. Difficulties sleeping: a natural part of growing older? Aging Health 2012;8(3):219–21.

144. Roehrs T, Kapke A, Roth T, et al. Sex differences in the polysomnographic sleep of young adults: a community-based study. Sleep Med 2006;7(1): 49–53.

145. Kimura M. Minireview: gender-specific sleep regulation. Sleep Biol Rhythms 2005;3:75–9.

146. Vitiello MV, Larsen LH, Moe KE. Age-related sleep change: gender and estrogen effects on the subjective-objective sleep quality relationships of healthy, noncomplaining older men and women. J Psychosom Res 2004;56(5):503–10.

147. Voderholzer U, Al-Shajlawi A, Weske G, et al. Are there gender differences in objective and subjective sleep measures? A study of insomniacs and healthy controls. Depress Anxiety 2003;17(3): 162–72.

148. Mohsenin V. Gender differences in the expression of sleep-disordered breathing: role of upper airway dimensions. Chest 2001;120(5):1442–7.

149. Armitage R, Hudson A, Trivedi M, et al. Sex differences in the distribution of EEG frequencies during sleep: unipolar depressed outpatients. J Affect Disord 1995;34(2):121–9.

150. Whinnery J, Jackson N, Rattanaumpawan P, et al. Short and long sleep duration associated with race/ethnicity, sociodemographics, and socioeconomic position. Sleep 2014;37(3):601–11.

151. Green MJ, Espie CA, Hunt K, et al. The longitudinal course of insomnia symptoms: inequalities by sex and occupational class among two different age cohorts followed for 20 years in the west of Scotland. Sleep 2012;35(6):815–23.

152. Ye L, Pien GW, Weaver TE. Gender differences in the clinical manifestation of obstructive sleep apnea. Sleep Med 2009;10(10):1075–84.

153. Del Campo F, Zamarron C. Sleep apnea and pregnancy. An association worthy of study. Sleep Breath 2013;17(2):463–4.

154. Ibrahim S, Foldvary-Schaefer N. Sleep disorders in pregnancy: implications, evaluation, and treatment. Neurol Clin 2012;30(3):925–36.

155. Facco FL, Kramer J, Ho KH, et al. Sleep disturbances in pregnancy. Obstet Gynecol 2010; 115(1):77–83.

156. Chen YH, Kang JH, Lin CC, et al. Obstructive sleep apnea and the risk of adverse pregnancy outcomes. Am J Obstet Gynecol 2012;206(2):136. e1–5.

157. Okun ML, Luther JF, Wisniewski SR, et al. Disturbed sleep, a novel risk factor for preterm birth? J Womens Health (Larchmt) 2012;21(1): 54–60.

158. Moore M, Meltzer LJ, Mindell JA. Bedtime problems and night wakings in children. Sleep Med Clin 2007;2:377–85.

159. Mindell JA, Kuhn B, Lewin DS, et al. Behavioral treatment of bedtime problems and night wakings in infants and young children. Sleep 2006;29(10): 1263–76.

160. Okun ML, Luther J, Prather AA, et al. Changes in sleep quality, but not hormones predict time to postpartum depression recurrence. J Affect Disord 2011;130(3):378–84.

161. Chang JJ, Pien GW, Duntley SP, et al. Sleep deprivation during pregnancy and maternal and fetal outcomes: is there a relationship? Sleep Med Rev 2010;14(2):107–14.

162. Pires GN, Andersen ML, Giovenardi M, et al. Sleep impairment during pregnancy: possible implications on mother-infant relationship. Med Hypotheses 2010;75(6):578–82.

163. Ameratunga D, Goldin J, Hickey M. Sleep disturbance in menopause. Intern Med J 2012;42(7): 742–7.

164. Regestein QR. Do hot flashes disturb sleep? Menopause 2012;19(7):715–8.

165. Baron KG, Smith TW, Berg CA, et al. Spousal involvement in CPAP adherence among patients with obstructive sleep apnea. Sleep Breath 2011; 15(3):525–34.

166. McDowell A. Spousal involvement and CPAP adherence: a two-way street? Sleep Breath 2011; 15(3):269–70.

167. Punjabi NM, Caffo BS, Goodwin JL, et al. Sleep-disordered breathing and mortality: a prospective cohort study. PLoS Med 2009;6(8):e1000132.

168. Mahowald MW, Schenck CH. REM sleep behaviour disorder: a marker of synucleinopathy. Lancet Neurol 2013;12(5):417–9.

169. Tomfohr L, Pung MA, Edwards KM, et al. Racial differences in sleep architecture: the role of ethnic discrimination. Biol Psychol 2012;89(1):34–8.

170. Thomas KS, Bardwell WA, Ancoli-Israel S, et al. The toll of ethnic discrimination on sleep architecture and fatigue. Health Psychol 2006;25(5):635–42.

171. Profant J, Ancoli-Israel S, Dimsdale JE. Are there ethnic differences in sleep architecture? Am J Hum Biol 2002;14(3):321–6.

172. Ruiter ME, Decoster J, Jacobs L, et al. Normal sleep in African-Americans and Caucasian-Americans: a meta-analysis. Sleep Med 2011; 12(3):209–14.

173. Ruiter ME, DeCoster J, Jacobs L, et al. Sleep disorders in African Americans and Caucasian Americans: a meta-analysis. Behav Sleep Med 2010; 8(4):246–59.

174. Grandner MA, Knutson KL, Troxel W, et al. Implications of sleep and energy drink use for health disparities. Nutr Rev 2014;72(Suppl 1):14–22.

175. Knutson KL. Sociodemographic and cultural determinants of sleep deficiency: implications for cardiometabolic disease risk. Soc Sci Med 2013;79: 7–15.

176. Mezick EJ, Matthews KA, Hall M, et al. Influence of race and socioeconomic status on sleep: Pittsburgh SleepSCORE project. Psychosom Med 2008;70(4):410–6.

177. Patel NP, Grandner MA, Xie D, et al. "Sleep disparity" in the population: poor sleep quality is strongly associated with poverty and ethnicity. BMC Public Health 2010;10(1):475.

178. Grandner MA, Hale L, Jackson N, et al. Perceived racial discrimination as an independent predictor of sleep disturbance and daytime fatigue. Behav Sleep Med 2012;10(4):235–49.

179. Slopen N, Williams DR. Discrimination, other psychosocial stressors, and self-reported sleep duration and difficulties. Sleep 2014;37(1):147–56.

180. Bureau of Labor Statistics. American time use survey fact sheet. Washington, DC: Bureau of Labor Statistics; 2013.

181. Rosekind MR, Gregory KB, Mallis MM, et al. The cost of poor sleep: workplace productivity loss and associated costs. J Occup Environ Med 2010;52(1):91–8.

182. Hui SK, Grandner MA. Trouble sleeping associated with lower work performance and greater health care costs: longitudinal data from Kansas State Employee Wellness Program. J Occup Environ Med 2015;57(10):1031–8.

183. Hui SK, Grandner MA. Associations between poor sleep quality and stages of change of multiple health behaviors among participants of Employee Wellness Program. Prev Med Rep 2015;2:292–9.

184. Gurubhagavatula I, Nkwuo JE, Maislin G, et al. Estimated cost of crashes in commercial drivers supports screening and treatment of obstructive sleep apnea. Accid Anal Prev 2008;40(1):104–15.

185. Pack AI, Maislin G, Staley B, et al. Impaired performance in commercial drivers: role of sleep apnea and short sleep duration. Am J Respir Crit Care Med 2006;174(4):446–54.

186. Xie W, Chakrabarty S, Levine R, et al. Factors associated with obstructive sleep apnea among commercial motor vehicle drivers. J Occup Environ Med 2011;53(2):169–73.

187. Moore-Ede M, Heitmann A, Guttkuhn R, et al. Circadian alertness simulator for fatigue risk assessment in transportation: application to reduce frequency and severity of truck accidents. Aviat Space Environ Med 2004;75(3 Suppl):A107–18.

188. Paterson JL, Dorrian J, Clarkson L, et al. Beyond working time: factors affecting sleep behaviour in rail safety workers. Accid Anal Prev 2012; 45(Suppl):32–5.

189. Darwent D, Dawson D, Roach GD. Prediction of probabilistic sleep distributions following travel across multiple time zones. Sleep 2010;33(2): 185–95.

190. Dorrian J, Darwent D, Dawson D, et al. Predicting pilot's sleep during layovers using their own behaviour or data from colleagues: implications for biomathematical models. Accid Anal Prev 2012; 45(Suppl):17–21.

191. Drury DA, Ferguson SA, Thomas MJ. Restricted sleep and negative affective states in commercial pilots during short haul operations. Accid Anal Prev 2012;45(Suppl):80–4.

192. Gander PH, Signal TL, van den Berg MJ, et al. In-flight sleep, pilot fatigue and Psychomotor Vigilance Task performance on ultra-long range versus long range flights. J Sleep Res 2013;22(6): 697–706.

193. Holmes A, Al-Bayat S, Hilditch C, et al. Sleep and sleepiness during an ultra long-range flight operation between the Middle East and United States. Accid Anal Prev 2012;45(Suppl):27–31.

194. Powell DM, Spencer MB, Petrie KJ. Fatigue in airline pilots after an additional day's layover period. Aviat Space Environ Med 2010;81(11): 1013–7.

195. Roach GD, Darwent D, Dawson D. How well do pilots sleep during long-haul flights? Ergonomics 2010;53(9):1072–5.

196. Roach GD, Petrilli RM, Dawson D, et al. Impact of layover length on sleep, subjective fatigue levels, and sustained attention of long-haul airline pilots. Chronobiol Int 2012;29(5):580–6.

197. Roach GD, Sargent C, Darwent D, et al. Duty periods with early start times restrict the amount of sleep obtained by short-haul airline pilots. Accid Anal Prev 2012;45(Suppl):22–6.

198. Rajaratnam SM, Barger LK, Lockley SW, et al. Sleep disorders, health, and safety in police officers. JAMA 2011;306(23):2567–78.

199. Charles LE, Gu JK, Andrew ME, et al. Sleep duration and biomarkers of metabolic function among police officers. J Occup Environ Med 2011;53(8):831–7.

200. Fekedulegn D, Burchfiel CM, Hartley TA, et al. Shift-work and sickness absence among police officers: the BCOPS study. Chronobiol Int 2013;30(7):930–41.

201. Gu JK, Charles LE, Burchfiel CM, et al. Long work hours and adiposity among police officers in a US northeast city. J Occup Environ Med 2012;54(11):1374–81.

202. McCanlies EC, Slaven JE, Smith LM, et al. Metabolic syndrome and sleep duration in police officers. Work 2012;43(2):133–9.

203. Neylan TC, Metzler TJ, Henn-Haase C, et al. Prior night sleep duration is associated with psychomotor vigilance in a healthy sample of police academy recruits. Chronobiol Int 2010;27(7):1493–508.

204. Aisbett B, Wolkow A, Sprajcer M, et al. "Awake, smoky, and hot": providing an evidence-base for managing the risks associated with occupational stressors encountered by wildland firefighters. Appl Ergon 2012;43(5):916–25.

205. Vargas de Barros V, Martins LF, Saitz R, et al. Mental health conditions, individual and job characteristics and sleep disturbances among firefighters. J Health Psychol 2013;18(3):350–8.

206. Grandner MA, Pack AI. Sleep disorders, public health, and public safety. JAMA 2011;306(23):2616–7.

207. Sharwood LN, Elkington J, Meuleners L, et al. Use of caffeinated substances and risk of crashes in long distance drivers of commercial vehicles: case-control study. BMJ 2013;346:f1140.

208. Grundy A, Sanchez M, Richardson H, et al. Light intensity exposure, sleep duration, physical activity, and biomarkers of melatonin among rotating shift nurses. Chronobiol Int 2009;26(7):1443–61.

209. Ruggiero JS, Redeker NS, Fiedler N, et al. Sleep and psychomotor vigilance in female shiftworkers. Biol Res Nurs 2012;14(3):225–35.

210. Chang YS, Wu YH, Hsu CY, et al. Impairment of perceptual and motor abilities at the end of a night shift is greater in nurses working fast rotating shifts. Sleep Med 2011;12(9):866–9.

211. Chung MH, Kuo TB, Hsu N, et al. Recovery after three-shift work: relation to sleep-related cardiac neuronal regulation in nurses. Ind Health 2012;50(1):24–30.

212. Demir Zencirci A, Arslan S. Morning-evening type and burnout level as factors influencing sleep quality of shift nurses: a questionnaire study. Croat Med J 2011;52(4):527–37.

213. Dorrian J, Paterson J, Dawson D, et al. Sleep, stress and compensatory behaviors in Australian nurses and midwives. Rev Saude Publica 2011;45(5):922–30.

214. Eldevik MF, Flo E, Moen BE, et al. Insomnia, excessive sleepiness, excessive fatigue, anxiety, depression and shift work disorder in nurses having less than 11 hours in-between shifts. PLoS One 2013;8(8):e70882.

215. Geiger-Brown J, Rogers VE, Han K, et al. Occupational screening for sleep disorders in 12-h shift nurses using the Berlin Questionnaire. Sleep Breath 2013;17(1):381–8.

216. Geiger-Brown J, Rogers VE, Trinkoff AM, et al. Sleep, sleepiness, fatigue, and performance of 12-hour-shift nurses. Chronobiol Int 2012;29(2):211–9.

217. Geiger-Brown J, Trinkoff A, Rogers VE. The impact of work schedules, home, and work demands on self-reported sleep in registered nurses. J Occup Environ Med 2011;53(3):303–7.

218. Ulmer C, Wolman DM, Johns MME. Institute of Medicine committee on optimizing graduate medical trainee (resident) hours and work schedules to improve patient safety. Resident duty hours: enhancing sleep, supervision, and safety. Washington, DC: National Academies Press; 2009.

219. Amin MM, Graber M, Ahmad K, et al. The effects of a mid-day nap on the neurocognitive performance of first-year medical residents: a controlled interventional pilot study. Acad Med 2012;87(10):1428–33.

220. Arora VM, Georgitis E, Woodruff JN, et al. Improving sleep hygiene of medical interns: can the sleep, alertness, and fatigue education in residency program help? Arch Intern Med 2007;167(16):1738–44.

221. Kim HJ, Kim JH, Park K-D, et al. A survey of sleep deprivation patterns and their effects on cognitive functions of residents and interns in Korea. Sleep Med 2011;12(4):390–6.

222. Reed DA, Fletcher KE, Arora VM. Systematic review: association of shift length, protected sleep time, and night float with patient care, residents' health, and education. Ann Intern Med 2010;153(12):829–42.

223. Bilimoria KY, Chung JW, Hedges LV, et al. National cluster-randomized trial of duty-hour flexibility in surgical training. N Engl J Med 2016;374(8):713–27.

224. Hale L. Do DP. Racial differences in self-reports of sleep duration in a population-based study. Sleep 2007;30(9):1096–103.

225. Hale L, Hill TD, Burdette AM. Does sleep quality mediate the association between neighborhood disorder and self-rated physical health? Prev Med 2010;51(3–4):275–8.

226. Hale L, Hill TD, Friedman E, et al. Perceived neighborhood quality, sleep quality, and health status:

evidence from the Survey of the Health of Wisconsin. Soc Sci Med 2013;79:16–22.

227. Hill TD, Burdette AM, Hale L. Neighborhood disorder, sleep quality, and psychological distress: testing a model of structural amplification. Health Place 2009;15(4):1006–13.

228. Pirrera S, De Valck E, Cluydts R. Nocturnal road traffic noise: a review on its assessment and consequences on sleep and health. Environ Int 2010; 36(5):492–8.

229. Kawada T. Noise and health: sleep disturbance in adults. J Occup Health 2011;53(6):413–6.

230. Fonken LK, Kitsmiller E, Smale L, et al. Dim nighttime light impairs cognition and provokes depressive-like responses in a diurnal rodent. J Biol Rhythms 2012;27(4):319–27.

231. Hu RF, Jiang XY, Zeng YM, et al. Effects of earplugs and eye masks on nocturnal sleep, melatonin and cortisol in a simulated intensive care unit environment. Crit Care 2010;14(2):R66.

232. Wood B, Rea MS, Plitnick B, et al. Light level and duration of exposure determine the impact of self-luminous tablets on melatonin suppression. Appl Ergon 2013;44(2):237–40.

233. Herljevic M, Middleton B, Thapan K, et al. Light-induced melatonin suppression: age-related reduction in response to short wavelength light. Exp Gerontol 2005;40(3):237–42.

234. Pigeon WR, Grandner MA. Creating an optimal sleep environment. In: Kushida CA, editor. Encyclopedia of sleep. Oxford (United Kingdom): Elsevier; 2013. p. 72–6.

235. Buxton OM, Ellenbogen JM, Wang W, et al. Sleep disruption due to hospital noises: a prospective evaluation. Ann Intern Med 2012;157(3):170–9.

236. Parmeggiani PL. Sleep behaviour and temperature. In: Parmeggiani PL, Velluti RA, editors. The physiologic nature of sleep. London: Imperial College Press; 2005. p. 387–405.

237. McCall WV, Boggs N, Letton A. Changes in sleep and wake in response to different sleeping surfaces: a pilot study. Appl Ergon 2012;43(2):386–91.

238. Shanmugan B, Roux F, Stonestreet C, et al. Lower back pain and sleep: mattresses, sleep quality and daytime symptoms. Sleep Diagn Ther 2007; 2(5):36–40.

239. Verhaert V, Haex B, De Wilde T, et al. Ergonomics in bed design: the effect of spinal alignment on sleep parameters. Ergonomics 2011;54(2):169–78.

240. Troxel WM. It's more than sex: exploring the dyadic nature of sleep and implications for health. Psychosom Med 2010;72(6):578–86.

241. Troxel WM, Robles TF, Hall M, et al. Marital quality and the marital bed: examining the covariation between relationship quality and sleep. Sleep Med Rev 2007;11(5):389–404.

242. Troxel WM, Buysse DJ, Hall M, et al. Marital happiness and sleep disturbances in a multi-ethnic sample of middle-aged women. Behav Sleep Med 2009;7(1):2–19.

243. Troxel WM, Buysse DJ, Monk TH, et al. Does social support differentially affect sleep in older adults with versus without insomnia? J Psychosom Res 2010;69(5):459–66.

244. Troxel WM, Cyranowski JM, Hall M, et al. Attachment anxiety, relationship context, and sleep in women with recurrent major depression. Psychosom Med 2007;69(7):692–9.

245. Gradisar M, Wolfson AR, Harvey AG, et al. The sleep and technology use of Americans: findings from the National Sleep Foundation's 2011 Sleep in America poll. J Clin Sleep Med 2013;9(12): 1291–9.

246. Orzech K, Grandner MA, Roane BM, et al. Electronic media use within 2 hours of bedtime predicts sleep variables in college students. Sleep 2012; 35(Abstract Suppl):A73.

247. Chang AM, Aeschbach D, Duffy JF, et al. Evening use of light-emitting eReaders negatively affects sleep, circadian timing, and next-morning alertness. Proc Natl Acad Sci U S A 2015;112(4): 1232–7.

248. Weaver E, Gradisar M, Dohnt H, et al. The effect of presleep video-game playing on adolescent sleep. J Clin Sleep Med 2010;6(2):184–9.

249. NHTSA. Drowsy driving. Wahinton, DC: US Department of Transportation; 2011.

250. Strohl KP, Blatt J, Council F, et al. Drowsy driving and automobile crashes: NCSDR/NHTSA expert panel on driver fatigue and sleepiness. Washington, DC: National Highway Traffic Safety Administration; 1998.

251. Borman KR, Biester TW, Jones AT, et al. Sleep, supervision, education, and service: views of junior and senior residents. J Surg Educ 2011;68(6): 495–501.

252. Borman KR, Fuhrman GM. "Resident duty hours: enhancing sleep, supervision, and safety": response of the Association of Program Directors in Surgery to the December 2008 report of the Institute of Medicine. Surgery 2009;146(3):420–7.

253. Sataloff RT. Resident duty hours: concerns and consequences. Ear Nose Throat J 2009;88(3): 812–6.

254. Federal Aviation Administration. Fact sheet–sleep apnea in aviation. Washington, DC: FAA; 2015.

255. McKnight-Eily LR, Liu Y, Wheaton AG, et al. Unhealthy sleep-related behaviors—12 States, 2009. MMWR Morb Mortal Wkly Rep 2011;60(8):233–8.

256. Lufi D, Tzischinsky O, Hadar S. Delaying school starting time by one hour: some effects on attention levels in adolescents. J Clin Sleep Med 2011;7(2):137–43.

257. Moore M, Meltzer LJ. The sleepy adolescent: causes and consequences of sleepiness in teens. Paediatr Respir Rev 2008;9(2):114–20 [quiz: 120–1].

258. Wahlstrom K. School start time and sleepy teens. Arch Pediatr Adolesc Med 2010;164(7):676–7.

259. Wolfson AR, Spaulding NL, Dandrow C, et al. Middle school start times: the importance of a good night's sleep for young adolescents. Behav Sleep Med 2007;5(3):194–209.

260. Roenneberg T, Kuehnle T, Pramstaller PP, et al. A marker for the end of adolescence. Curr Biol 2004;14(24):R1038–9.

261. Barnes M, Davis K, Mancini M, et al. Setting adolescents up for success: promoting a policy to delay high school start times. J Sch Health 2016;86(7):552–7.

262. Meltzer LJ, Shaheed K, Ambler D. Start later, sleep later: school start times and adolescent sleep in homeschool versus public/private school students. Behav Sleep Med 2016;14(2):140–54.

263. Millman RP, Boergers J, Owens J. Healthy school start times: can we do a better job in reaching our goals? Sleep 2016;39(2):267–8.

264. Minges KE, Redeker NS. Delayed school start times and adolescent sleep: a systematic review of the experimental evidence. Sleep Med Rev 2016;28:86–95.

265. Thacher PV, Onyper SV. Longitudinal outcomes of start time delay on sleep, behavior, and achievement in high school. Sleep 2016;39(2):271–81.

266. Wheaton AG, Chapman DP, Croft JB. School start times, sleep, behavioral, health, and academic outcomes: a review of the Literature. J Sch Health 2016;86(5):363–81.

267. Siebern AT, Manber R. Insomnia and its effective non-pharmacologic treatment. Med Clin North Am 2010;94(3):581–91.

268. Watson NF, Horn E, Duncan GE, et al. Sleep duration and area-level deprivation in twins. Sleep 2016;39(1):67–77.

269. Knutson KL, Van Cauter E, Rathouz PJ, et al. Association between sleep and blood pressure in midlife: the CARDIA sleep study. Arch Intern Med 2009;169(11):1055–61.

Printed and bound by CPI Group (UK) Ltd, Croydon, CR0 4YY

03/10/2024

01040371-0004